CONTROVERSIES IN NEURO-ONCOLOGY

Volume 1: Avastin and Malignant Gliomas

EDITOR

Thomas C. Chen

eBooks End User License Agreement

CONTENT

CHAPTERS

I.   BASIC SCIENCE AND RATIONALE

II.   BEVACIZUMAB TREATMENT FOR RECURRENT MALIGNANT GLIOMAS

III.   BEVACIZUMAB TREATMENT FOR NEWLY DIAGNOSED MALIGNANT GLIOMAS

IV.   BEVACIZUMAB TOXCICITY

V.   BEVACIZUMAB-OPTIMAL DOSING

XI. CONCLUSION

FOREWORD

Controversies in Neuro-Oncology: Avastin and Malignant Gliomas, edited by Thomas Chen and Marc Chamberlain, is a timely book for the clinician treating patients with high-grade gliomas. The book will find a ready audience among today's physicians practising neuro-oncology, medical oncology, and radiation oncology. Bevacizumab (avastin) was recently approved by the FDA for use in patients with glioblastoma. The book that follows is a collation of 25 chapters from North America and Europe that discuss current knowledge that forms the basis for bevacizumab action, experience using bevacizumab in the treatment of high-grade gliomas, its impact on neuroimaging studies, its use with radiation therapy, and its use to ameliorate radiation damage to the CNS. In addition and for comparison, there are 5 chapters that discuss other drugs that have, as one site of action, inhibition of VEGF receptor(s). The editor and authors should be congratulated for compiling an informative book that helps us to understand how best to use bevacizumab in neuro-oncology practice.

Victor A. Levin, *M.D.*
The University of Texas,
M. D. Anderson Cancer Center

PREFACE

This is the first issue of our new series entitled Controversies **in Neuro-oncology**. The goal of this series is to stimulate timely discussion in different areas of neuro-oncology where is still considerable debate on a specific topic, hopefully leading to new studies that will result in a better understanding of the problem.

Our first issue "Avastin and Maligant Gliomas" certainly illustrates this point. Avastin is now approved by the FDA as standalone therapy for patients with recurrent glioblastoma multiforme (GBM). It is the third FDA approved therapy for GBM, besides Gliadel (BCNU wafers) and temozolomide. However, the role, usage, and treatment endpoint of Avastin , still remains undefined in many instances. This issue highlights this point.

Hofman and Chen review the basic science and rationale for the use of Avastin as an anti-angiogenesis agent. The use of Avastin and CPT-11 (irinotecan) in the setting of recurrent GBM is highlighted in the Duke experience presented by Desjardins and Vredenburgh. Subsequently, the use of Avastin alone was demonstrated by Kreisl *et al.* to be similar to Avastin and CPT-11 in a National Cancer Institute (NCI) trial, leading to FDA approval of Avastin alone in the treatment of recurrent GBM, vs Avastin and CPT-11. Iwamoto and Gutin demonstrate that the addition of radiosurgery to previously radiatied patients does not increase radiation necrosis in the setting of Avastin. Norden presents the clinical and radiographic progression of recurrent glioma patients that have become resistant to Avastin, leading to rapid clinical progression and death.

The role of Avastin in upfront therapy is still to be defined. Reardon *et al.* present an update on the role of Avastin for newly diagnosed glioblastoma. Patel *et al.* discuss the effects of radiation therapy when combined with Avastin in the upfront setting. Wu and Gilbert discuss the upcoming Radiation Therapy Oncology Group (RTOG 0825) in which newly diagnosed patients are randomized to standard of care (radiation and temozolomide, followed by temozolomide alone) vs standard of care plus Avastin.

Kamsheh *et al.* discuss the various protocols to define the optimal dose and schedule for Avastin administration to minimize systemic toxicity. Avastin toxicity is discussed by Agregawi and Schiff. Rogers discusses her experience with anticoagulation for thromboembolism in patients receiving Avastin.

Defining the response to chemotherapy is currently based on the MacDonald criteria of changes in tumor size using contrast enhanced T1 MRI scans. However, Avastin actually decreases the "leakiness" of the blood tumor barrier, leading to decreased gadolinium enhancement of the GBM. As a result, standard methods of evaluation of tumor responses need to be clarified. Neuroradiographic evaluation of response to Avastin therapy is presented in a comprehensive chapter by Pope based on the UCLA experience with Avastin administration. Butowski and Chang present the problem with Avastin effects on the tumor vasculature, leading to mistaken interpretations on tumor response. Thind *et al* and Henson *et al.* present further insights into the imaging responses to Avastin, and response to therapy.

From the neurosurgical standpoint, Avastin therapy presents challenges from the standpoint of wound breakdown, and increased medical complications of thromboembolism, proteinuria, and hypertension. These considerations are well presented in chapters by Aghi and Berger, and by Rahmathulla and Vogelbaum.

Other potential novel applications of Avastin therapy are presented by Chamberlain in the use of Avastin for other cancers, including metastatic carcinoma and meningiomas. Wu and Levin present a unique chapter on the use of Avastin for radiation necrosis. Chamberlain reviews the use of Avastin for recurrent anaplastic gliomas.

Although the use of Avastin has been well received in the United States, its reception in Europe is much more guarded. European perspectives are presented by Stupp, van den Bent, Weller, and Wick *et al.* who advocate the use of further randomized trials for Avastin application in malignant gliomas.

Lastly, the use of other angiogenesis inhibitors that are currently in development is presented. Bart details the use of the tyrosine kinase inhibitor sunitinib for gliomas, and Nabors presents the use of the integrin inhibitor cilengitide for malignant gliomas. Grossman and Blakeley detail the development of another tyrosine kinase inhibitor sorafenib for treatment of malignant gliomas, and Drappatz *et al.* describe the use of the VEGF-trap Aflibercept in high grade gliomas. Lastly, Gerstner *et al.* outline the use of the VEGF receptor inhibitor cerdiranib for treatment of glioblastomas.

Finally, to put everything into perspective, Gu and Chen present a comparative study of how the use of Avastin is similar and different from Avastin therapy for other malignant cancers.

It is our hope that this ebook will highlight the nuances and complexities involved in Avastin therapy for malignant gliomas. Although Avastin therapy is still controversial in many ways, it has also become another pinnacle of hope for malignant glioma patients who otherwise would have no other therapy once they have progressed on temozolomide.

Thomas Chen
University of Southern California
USA

CONTRIBUTORS

Aghi, Manish K.

Department of Neurological Surgery, 505 Parnassus Avenue, Rm M779 San Francisco, CA 94143-0112

Aregawi, Dawit

University of Michigan Hematology/Oncology, C369 Med Inn Building, 1500 E Medical Center SPC 5848, Ann Arbor, MI 48109-5848

Bart, Neyns

UZ Brussel, Laarbeeklaan 101, 1090 Brussel, Belgium

Batchelor, Tracy

Stephen E. and Catherine Pappas Center for Neuro-Oncology, Yawkey 9E, Massachusetts General Hospital Cancer Center, 55 Fruit Street Boston, MA 02114, USA

Berger, Mitchel S.

Department of Neurological Surgery, 505 Parnassus Avenue, Rm M779 San Francisco, CA 94143-0112

Blakeley, Jaishri

Department of Neurology, The Johns Hopkins Oncology Center, 600 North Wolfe Street Baltimore, MD, 21287, USA

Butowski, Nicholas

Department of Neuro-Oncology, Brain Tumor Research Center, University of California, San Francisco 400 Parnassus Avenue, A808, San Francisco, California 94143-0350

Chakravarti, Arnab

Ohio State University, Columbus Ohio, USA

Chamberlain, Marc C.

Fred Hutchinson Cancer Center, Seattle Cancer Care Alliance, 825 Eastlake Ave E, POB 10923, MS: G4-940, Seattle, WA 98109-1023

Chang, Susan

Department of Neuro-Oncology , Brain Tumor Research Center, University of California, San Francisco 400 Parnassus Avenue, A808, San Francisco, California 94143-0350

Chen, Thomas C.

Departments of Neurosurgery, Keck School of Medicine, University of Southern California, Los Angeles, CA 90033, USA

Desjardins, Annick

Duke University Medical Center DUMC, Box 3624, Durham, NC 27710

Dietrich, Jörg H.

Stephen E. and Catherine Pappas Center for Neuro-Oncology, Yawkey 9E, Massachusetts General Hospital Cancer Center, 55 Fruit Street Boston, MA 02114, USA

Drappatz, Jan

Center for Neuro-Oncology, Dana Farber Cancer Institute, 44 Binney Street, SW-430D, Boston, MA 02115, USA

Gerstner, Elizabeth R.

Stephen E. and Catherine Pappas Center for Neuro-Oncology, Yawkey 9E, Massachusetts General Hospital Cancer Center, 55 Fruit Street Boston, MA 02114, USA

Gilbert, Mark R.

M. D. Anderson Cancer Center 1515 Holcombe Blvd., Unit 431 Houston, Texas 77030

Grossman, Rachel

Department of Neurosurgery, The Johns Hopkins Oncology Center, 600 North Wolfe Street, Baltimore, MD, 21287, USA

Gu, Helen

Norris Cancer Center, 1441 Eastlake Ave., Los Angeles CA 90033, USA

Gutin, Philip H.

Department of Neurological Surgery, Weill Medical College of Cornell University, New York, USA

Henson, John W.

Neurology, Swedish Neuroscience Institute, 550 17th Avenue, Suite 500 Seattle, WA 98122

Hofman, Florence M.

Departments of Pathology, Keck School of Medicine, University of Southern California, USA

Iwamoto, Fabio M.

Neuro-Oncology Branch, National Cancer Institute, National Institute of Neurological Disorders and Stroke, National Institutes of Health, Bethesda, Maryland

Kamsheh, L.

Northwestern University, Feinberg School of Medicine, Robert H. Lurie Comprehensive Cancer Center, 710 N. Lake Shore Drive, Abbott Hall, Room 1123, Chicago, IL 60611

Keogh, Bart

Neuroradiology, Swedish Neuroscience Institute , 550 17th Avenue, Suite 500, Seattle, WA 98122

Kreisl, Teri N.

Neuro-Oncology Branch – NCI 9030, Old Georgetown Road, Bldg. 82, Rm. 243 Bethesda, MD 20892, USA

Levin, Victor A.

Department of Neuro-Oncology, The University of Texas, M. D. Anderson Cancer Center, Houston, TX 77030

Mehta, Minesh

University of Wisconsin, Madison WI, USA

Mikkelsen, T.

Hermelin Brain Tumor Center, Depts. Neurology & Neurosurgery, E&R3096 Henry Ford Hospital 2799 West Grand Blvd., Detroit, MI 48202

Mohan, Y.S.

Hermelin Brain Tumor Center, Depts. Neurology & Neurosurgery, E&R3096 Henry Ford Hospital 2799 West Grand Blvd., Detroit, MI 48202

Nabors, L. Burt

Neuro oncology Program, University of Alabama at Birmingham 510 20th Street South, FOT 1020, Birmingham, AL 35294 USA

Norden, Andrew D.

Brigham and Women's Hospital , Dana-Farber/Brigham and Women's Cancer Center, Harvard Medical School, Boston MA 02115, USA

Patel, Disha

Ohio State University, Columbus Ohio, USA

Platten, Michael

Department of Neurooncology, University Hospital of Heidelberg, Im Neuenheimer Feld 400, D-69120 Heidelberg, Germany

Pope, Whitney B.

David Geffen School of Medicine, Department of Radiology, University of California Los Angeles

Rahmathulla, Gazanfar

Brain Tumor and NeuroOncology Center, Cleveland Clinic, 9500 Euclid Ave., Cleveland, OH 44195

Raizer, Jeffrey

Northwestern University, Feinberg School of Medicine, Robert H. Lurie Comprehensive Cancer Center, 710 N. Lake Shore Drive, Abbott Hall, Room 1123, Chicago, IL 60611

Reardon, David A.

Preston Robert Tisch Brain Tumor Center at Duke, Duke University Medical Center, Box 3624, Durham, NC 27710, USA

Rogers, Lisa R.

University Hospitals, Case Western Reserve Medical Center, 11100 Euclid Avenue, Hanna House 517, Cleveland, Ohio 44106

Sathornsumetee, Sith

Neuro-Oncology Program, Department of Medicine, Faculty of Medicine, Siriraj Hospital, Mahidol University, Bangkok, Thailand

Schiff, David

University of Virginia, Health System, Box 800432, Charlottesville VA 22908-0432

Stupp, Roger

Department of Neurosurgery, University Hospital (CHUV), Rue du Bugnon 46 CH-1011 Lausanne, Switzerland `

Thind, R.

Hermelin Brain Tumor Center, Depts. Neurology & Neurosurgery, E&R3096 Henry Ford Hospital 2799 West Grand Blvd., Detroit, MI 48202

Van den Bent, M.J.

Dept Neuro-Oncology, Daniel den Hoed Cancer Center, Erasmus University Hospital, Rotterdam, The Netherlands

Vogelbaum, Michael A.

Brain Tumor and Neuro-Oncology Center, Center for Translational Therapeutics, Department of Neurological Surgery, Cleveland Clinic / Neurological Institute, 9500 Euclid Ave., Cleveland, OH 44195

Vredenburgh, James V.

Department of Medicine, The Preston Robert Tisch Brain Tumor Center, Duke University Medical Center, Durham, NC 27710

Wang, Daphne

Stephen E. and Catherine Pappas Center for Neuro-Oncology, Yawkey 9E, Massachusetts General Hospital Cancer Center, 55 Fruit Street Boston, MA 02114, USA

Weller, Michael

University Hospital Zurich, Switzerland

Wen, Patrick Y.

Center for Neuro-Oncology, Dana Farber Cancer Institute, 44 Binney Street, SW-430D, Boston, MA 02115, USA

Wick, Antje

Department of Neurooncology, University Hospital of Heidelberg, Im Neuenheimer Feld 400, D-69120 Heidelberg, Germany

Wick, Wolfgang

Department of Neurooncology, University Hospital of Heidelberg, Im Neuenheimer Feld 400, D-69120 Heidelberg, Germany

Wu, Jing

Dept of Neuro-Oncology, M. D. Anderson Cancer Center, 1515 Holcombe Blvd., Unit 431, Houston, Texas 77030

CHAPTER 1

The Basic Science of Avastin (Bevacizumab) Therapy

Florence M. Hofman[1,2] and Thomas C. Chen[1,2,*]

[1]Departments of Pathology and [2]Neurosurgery, Keck School of Medicine, University of Southern California

Abstract: Malignant gliomas are characterized by an extensive vasculature. The most potent pro-angiogenic factor, vascular endothelial growth factor (VEGF), is therefore a therapeutic target for anti-angiogenic therapy. This chapter focuses on different functional characteristics of VEGF and its receptors in the angiogenesis process. Furthermore, the effects of decreasing or blocking VEGF using the humanized monoclonal antibody to VEGF, bevacizumab (Avastin), are discussed. The possible mechanisms of activity of this agent, as well as potential problems with this drug are also discussed.

INTRODUCTION

Malignant gliomas are devastating tumors that are associated with a poor prognosis. The mean survival time from initial diagnosis is approximately 15 months [1]. There are currently limited therapies available for treatment these patients. One outstanding characteristic of the glioblastoma (GBM) tumors is the high degree of vascularity. Many studies have shown that tumor growth is dependent on the proliferation and expansion of the vasculature [2]. The tumor-associated blood vessels provide the essential elements to sustain tumor growth. Therefore therapies which target the tumor vasculature play an important role in the treatment of these tumors. Understanding the elements that regulate blood vessel growth is critical to identifying the appropriate drugs for treatment.

ANGIOGENESIS

The vasculature provides tissues with nutrients, oxygen, and waste removal, and serves as a mechanism for the distribution of hormones and other growth factors [3]. The critical cellular component of blood vessels are the inner, or luminal, layer of cells, the endothelial cells, which are a very stable and static population. Endothelial cells have been shown to divide once in several years [4]. In normal individuals, new blood vessel growth is limited to wound healing and the female reproductive system. However angiogenesis, the formation of new blood vessels from pre-existing blood vessels, is a very dynamic process.

Angiogenesis involves a sequence of events, initiated by the activation of endothelial cells. Blocking or interfering with any of these events will inhibit or decrease the formation of new vessels. Endothelial cells can be activated by a number of stimulatory signals including hypoxia, decreased nutrients, changes in flow rate, and inflammation [4]. Once this activation process occurs, endothelial cells release an array of enzymes which break down the extracellular matrix (ECM) surrounding the endothelial cells, the basement membrane. This enables endothelial cells to migrate out of the existing blood vessel causing sprouting. The enzymes responsible for sprouting include matrix metalloproteases (MMP)2, MMP9, and urokinase plasminogen activator (uPA). In addition to disrupting the physical barrier around the vessels to allow vessel growth, the destruction of the ECM releases proangiogenic factors which further stimulate the endothelial cells. These proangiogenic factors include vascular endothelial growth factor (VEGF), interleukin-8 (IL-8), platelet-derived growth factor (PDGF), placental growth factor (PLGF), and endothelin-1 (Et-1) [5]. These factors comprise the proangiogenic environment which continues to stimulate blood vessel growth. Proangiogenic factors can function to induce endothelial cells to sprout, migrate, and proliferate, thereby culminating in the formation of new vessels. Inhibition of endothelial cell activity during any of these processes will block new vessel formation.

The principal pro-angiogenic growth factor is Vascular Endothelial Growth Factor (VEGF). VEGF is produced by the tissues surrounding the blood vessels, and induced by glucose deprivation, hypoxia, and chemical inducers of endoplasmic reticulum (ER) stress. Inflammatory cytokines also stimulate VEGF secretion [6,7].

*Address correspondence to the Dr. Thomas C. Chen:** Department of Neurosurgery, Keck School of Medicine, University of Southern California, Los Angeles, CA 90033, Tel: 323-442-3918, E-mail: tchen@usc.edu

In sharp contrast to normal blood vessels, the tumor vasculature is morphologically and functionally different; especially in brain tumors. Morphologically, the glioma vessels exhibit increased numbers of caveolae, abnormal pericyte distribution, and discontinuous basement membranes [9]. The vasculature in gliomas is considerably denser as compared to normal brain tissue. The vessels are also irregular in distribution, thicker walled with blind outpouchings, and shunts from arterioles to venuoles, without the typical capillary structures [3,9]. These abnormalities cause decreased blood flow and blood pooling. Tumor vessels are also more permeable, resulting in a loss of interstitial pressure. On the cellular level, endothelial cells isolated from brain tumors function very differently from normal brain endothelial cells. These tumor-associated brain endothelial cells constutively produce a variety of proangiogenic cytokines and growth factors, migrate more rapidly, but proliferate more slowly than control endothelial cells [10]. What is particularly critical for cancer therapy is that these tumor-associated endothelial cells are generally resistant to chemotherapeutic agents [11]. The mechanism of this chemoresistance is under investigation.

Tumor growth depends on the expansion of the tumor vasculature. Tumor cells can only survive within a 1-2 mm^3 distance from the blood vessels, without succumbing to hypoxic death [12]. Without a parallel expansion of the blood supply, tumors will not grow, but remain dormant for years or die [2]. The mechanism responsible for this extensive angiogenesis in tumors is a result of the production of pro-angiogenic growth factors, particularly VEGF. Studies have shown that VEGF is produced by tumor cells and present in the tumor microenvironment. Thus targeting VEGF has been a primary goal for an anti-angiogenic therapy for cancer.

VASCULAR ENDOTHELIAL GROWTH FACTOR (VEGF)

To date, the most effective pro-angiogenic growth factor is Vascular Endothelial Growth Factor (VEGF), also known as Vascular Permeability Factor (VPF) [13,14]. This growth factor is a key regulator for angiogenesis, responsible for endothelial cell proliferation, migration, and survival. VEGF also induces the recruitment of endothelial cell progenitor cells, from the bone marrow into the circulation [15]. VEGF induces several pro-survival proteins such as Bcl-2 and survivin, through the PI3K/Akt signaling pathway [13]. VEGF also enhances vascular permeability [14]. VEGF stimulates actin polymerization and rapid formation of focal adhesion leading to cytosketon reorganization and cellular migration [16]. The signaling pathway for migration can also be mediated by the p38 MAPK pathway [17]. VEGF upregulates ICAM-1 expression, enhancing migration and leukocyte adhesion to the vessel wall [18]. Under normal circumstances, there is little new blood vessels formation, so there are minimal amounts of VEGF in the tissue environment. However, during wound healing and other non-neoplastic pathologic events, VEGF is produced by macrophages, pericytes and stromal cells [19]. In cancer, the tumor cells, as well as infiltrating macrophages, secrete this angiogenic factor [15, 20]. Hypoxia stimulates VEGF by inducing HIF-1a, which binds to the VEGF promoter [21]. VEGF can also be upregulated by the inflammatory cytokines TNF∀, IL-1 and IL-6, and by COX-2 [18, 22, 23]. PDGF-B, as well as EGF, TGF∀, IGF-1 and bFGF, has also been shown to upregulate VEGF in glioma cells [21]. Mutations in tumor suppressor genes, such as VHL and P53, during disease progression can regulate VEGF expression [7]. Glioma stem cell-like cells have also been shown to secrete high levels of VEGF relative to other tumor cells [7, 24]. Thus VEGF was proven to be a key growth factor in angiogenesis.

The VEGF gene family consists of six molecular subtypes: VEGF-A, VEGF-B, VEGF-C, VEGF-D, and VEGF-E, and placenta growth factor (PLGF) (PGF) [18, 21]. VEGF-A, referred to as VEGF, has four isoforms: VEGF121, VEGF165, VEGF189, VEGF206 [13, 18]. VEGF165, a basic, heparin-binding protein, is the most common and has the highest potency. This isoform is found in the soluble form or bound to the extracellular matrix (ECM). VEGF121 is freely diffusible, and VEGF 189 and 206 are completely sequestered in the ECM. Since VEGF 165 is the most common and most effective, this isoform is the target of most anti-VEGF therapies.

VEGF RECEPTORS

The VEGF ligand is able to bind to three tyrosine kinase VEGF receptors. VEGFR1 and 2 are expressed on endothelial cells and involved in tumor angiogenesis, while VEGFR3 is expressed on the lymphatic vasculature and responsible for lymphatic vessel activation [21]. VEGFR1 is also expressed in the soluble form. VEGFR1 is expressed on macrophages as well as endothelial cells, while VEGFR2 is expressed on hematopoietic stem cells, endothelial progenitor cells, platelets and blood vessel- associated endothelial cells [21]. Hypoxia upregulates VEGFR1 and VEGFR2 expression (21). Neuropilin-1, a transmembrane protein, is a co- receptor for VEGF165, and presents VEGF165 to VEGFR2 for optimal signaling [21]. Binding of VEGF to its receptor causes ligand-dependent receptor homodimerization and autophosphorylation of the tryosine kinase domains, resulting in the activation of specific signal-transduction pathways [15]. Activation of VEGFR2 (also referred to as KDR/flk) by VEGF leads to increased endothelial cell proliferation and migration, and is the predominant angiogenesis activation pathway [25]. Activation of VEGFR1 (also referred to as Flt-1) has inhibitory effects on angiogenesis [25]. Thus VEGFR1 functions as a negative regulator, while VEGFR2 functions as a positive angiogenic, growth promoter and permeability receptor [26]. VEGFR2 is responsible for migration, via activation of p38 MAPK, and phosphorylation of FAK resulting in stress fiber polymerization [16]. VEGF signaling pathway results in endothelial cell proliferation, migration, survival and mobilization of endothelial progenitor cells from the bone marrow.

BEVACIZUMAB AS AN ANTI-ANGIOGENIC THERAPY

One approach to decreasing angiogenesis through the VEGF pathway is to bind or functionally remove the VEGF ligand itself, thereby reducing the signaling through the VEGF receptor, at the tumor site. This was accomplished with the humanized monoclonal antibody to VEGF, bevacizumab (Avastin), formulated for intravenous administration. Bevacizumab was the first drug to be developed as an angiogenesis inhibitor and is currently approved by the FDA for treatment of glioma in conjunction with other chemotherapeutic agents, particularly CPT11 [27-29]. During Phase I trials in patients with rectal carcinoma, treatment with bevacizumab, in combination with chemotherapy showed significant reduction in tumor microvessel density, and tumor blood volume [29].

Bevacizumab has been shown to have a wide range of effects. The principle mechanism of action is the binding to soluble VEGF, thus reducing the activation of VEGF receptors and the subsequent signaling processes [13]. It is very important to emphasize that bevacizumab is an antibody, and therefore it would stay in the lumen of the blood vessel. How much bevacizumab is actually able to cross the brain tumor interface into the tumor itself is not really known. However, since the site of activity of this anti-VEGF agent is the endothelial cell layer, this antibody is effective on the vasculature of the brain, without crossing the brain tumor interface.

Blocking VEGF signaling could result in several events including: the inhibition of new vessel growth; the regression of newly formed blood vessels; and/or the alteration of the tumor vessel function. Inhibition of new blood vessel growth would cause a halt in tumor growth, rather than a decrease in tumor size [2, 15]. By reducing VEGF activity, bevacizumab has been shown to decrease endothelial cell survival, and thus sensitize endothelial cells to cytotoxic agents, such as radiation [29]. The mechanism of this sensitization, more specifically how the endothelial cells become chemosensitive is under investigation. Although VEGF is successful in inhibiting the endothelial cell growth and proliferation initially, continued long term exposure may result in a patient with a MRI scan suggestive of gliomatosis cerebri [30]. This response is most likely secondary to the fact that other angiogeneic factors (i.e., SDF1∀, IL8, bFGF, PDGF, IL-6) are all still active, and may play a larger role in stimulating greater blood vessel formation, even at sites distant to the original GBM [31,42].

High levels of VEGF cause edema, an accumulation of fluid around the tumor due to increased endothelial cell permeability, thereby compromising the blood-brain-barrier (BBB). Decreasing VEGF levels with bevacizumab has been shown to reverse this endothelial cell permeability [1]. This decrease in permeability actually restores the integrity of the BBB to some extent. It is proposed that this restoration of the BBB or "normalization" of the vasculature, results in a more functional vasculature [32]. Functional blood vessels would be more likely to effectively distribute the chemotherapy agents, thereby killing tumor cells resulting in reduced tumor growth [32]. Because bevacizumab may help close the normally leaky "blood tumor interface," the tumor may go from gadolinium enhancing to non-enhancing. Moreover, bevacizumab has actually been found to reduce the steroid dosage and dependency of patients using steroids on a long term basis [1]. Again, this effect is most likely secondary to the tightening of the blood tumor interface. Studies have shown that bevacizumab administration as monotherapy also reduced tumor size and vascularity, suggesting that other mechanisms may be operational [33]. Another hypothesis suggests that reducing VEGF causes a disruption to the perivascular cancer-stem cell niche, thereby reducing the cancer stem cell pool [32, 34]. Moreover, bevacizumab has now been used in patients with radiation necrosis to decrease the hypervascularity that is encountered in those patients. Since VEGF is responsible for so many functions of endothelial cells, it is likely that the effects observed with this drug are a sum total of several different properties of depletion of VEGF in tumors.

Clinical evidence has shown that the continuous administration of bevacizumab reduces new blood vessel formation and tumor growth. However, preclinical and clinical evidence shows that halting bevacizumab treatment for over 2 weeks causes a resurgence of blood vessel growth in the tumor [35, 36]. The mechanism of this rapid regrowth is not clear. Several studies have shown that blocking VEGF signaling in a highly vascularized tumor will result in the cessation of blood flow, endothelial cell death, pericyte migration and the appearance of empty basement membrane sleeves [35, 37]. When anti-VEGF treatment is stopped and VEGF is again available to activate the remaining endothelial cells, these sprouting endothelial cells use the empty basement membrane sleeves as a scaffold for rapid revascularization of the tumors [35]. This blood vessel regrowth may also be due to the over-compensation of other pro-angiogenic growth factors produced by tumors. Several of the pro-angiogenic factors (i.e., VEGF and IL-8) have somewhat redundant functions; thus, therapeutic agents temporarily eliminating one angiogenic factor will ultimately cause maximum angiogenesis because other proangiogenic factors are present and functional [31]. Therefore new anti-angiogenic therapies need to consider establishing a permanent or long term approach to blocking VEGF production and/or VEGF signaling in endothelial cells.

Treatment with VEGF has a serious side effect of hypertension [38]. This may be because VEGF is also responsible for the regulation of vascular tone. A decrease in VEGF causes vasoconstriction, which may be the result of either decreased nitric oxide or increased Et-1; these vasoregulatory agents are regulated by VEGF [39, 40]. Et-1 is a primary risk factor in hypertension [41]. Thus the hypertension resulting from VEGF treatment may be the result of the imbalance of these vasoregulatory agents. Another side effect of bevacizumab is an increased risk of thrombotic events. This may be the result of a decrease in the number of endothelial cells lining the basement membrane as a result of decreased endothelial cell survival. Since VEGF signaling is responsible for the expression of endothelial cell survival proteins, inhibition of VEGF results in endothelial cell apoptosis [15]. Exposure of subendothelial collagen leads to thrombotic events [15]. The reported problems with anti-VEGF therapy may be remedied with lower doses of drugs and changes in administration protocols.

CONCLUSION

The utilization, marketing, and use of bevacizumab in the treatment of malignant gliomas are really a story of bench to bedside. It has taken the theoretical understanding of VEGF, made a functional humanized monoclonal antibody, and applied it to the treatment of malignant gliomas with good success. There is unquestionable responsiveness to this drug, with many patients benefiting from treatment. Usage and adoption, however, have also brought understanding of the limitations and complications. This chapter characterizes bevacizumab activity from the translational perspective, attempting to understand and enhance the clinical results based on a thorough analysis of the function of this antibody in gliomas.

REFERENCES

[1]   Wen PY, Kesari S, Malignant gliomas in adults. N Engl J Med 2008; 359(5):492-507.

[2]   Folkman J. Angiogenesis: an organizing principle for drug discovery? Nat Rev Drug Discov 2007; 6(4):273-286.

[3]   Bergers G, and Benjamin LE. 2003. Tumorigenesis and the angiogenic switch. Nat Rev Cancer 2003; 3:401-410.

[4]   Carmeliet P. Mechanisms of angiogenesis and arteriogenesis. Nat Med 2000; 6: 389-395.

[5]   Kerbel R, and Folkman J. Clinical translation of angiogenesis inhibitors. Nat Rev Cancer 2002; 2(10):727-739.

[6]   Roybal CN, Yang S, Sun CW, *et al.* Homocysteine increases the expression of vascular endothelial growth factor by a mechanism involving endoplasmic reticulum stress and transcription factor ATF4. J Biol Chem 2004; 279(15):14844-14852.

[7]   Everson RG, Graner MW, Gromeier M, *et al.* Immunotherapy against angiogenesis-associated targets: evidence and implications for the treatment of malignant glioma.

[8]   Expert Rev Anticancer Ther. 2008; 8(5):717-732.

[9]   Carmeliet P, and Jain RK. Angiogenesis in cancer and other diseases. Nature 2000; 407(6801):249-257.

[10]   McDonald DM, and Choyke PL. Imaging of angiogenesis: from microscope to clinic. Nat Med 2003; 9(6):713-725.

[11]   Charalambous C, Hofman FM, Chen TC. Functional and phenotypic differences between glioblastoma multiforme-derived and normal human brain endothelial cells. J Neurosurg 2005; 102(4):699-705.

[12]   Charalambous C, Virrey J, Kardosh A, *et al.* Glioma-associated endothelial cells show evidence of replicative senescence. Exp Cell Res 2007; 313(6):1192-1202.

[13] Hlatky L, Hahnfeldt P, Folkman J. Clinical application of antiangiogenic therapy: microvessel density, what it does and doesn't tell us. J Nat Can Inst 2002; 94(12):883-893.

[14] Ferrara N. Role of vascular endothelial growth factor in regulation of physiological angiogenesis. Am J Physiol Cell Physiol. 2001; 280(6):C1358-C1366.

[15] Dvorak HF. Vascular permeability factor/vascular endothelial growth factor: a critical cytokine in tumor angiogenesis and a potential target for diagnosis and therapy. J Clin Oncol 2002; 20(21):4368-4380.

[16] Soltau J, and Drevs J. Mode of action and clinical impact of VEGF signaling inhibitors. Expert Rev Anticancer Ther. 2009; 9(5):649-662.

[17] Rousseau S, Houle F, Kotanides H, *et al.* Vascular endothelial growth factor (VEGF)-driven actin-based motility is mediated by VEGFR2 and requires concerted activation of stress-activated protein kinase 2 (SAPK2/p38) and geldanamycin-sensitive phosphorylation of focal adhesion kinase. J Biol Chem 2000; 275(14):10661-10672.

[18] Rousseau S, Houle F, and Huot J. Integrating the VEGF signals leading to actin-based motility in vascular endothelial cells. Trends Cardiovasc Med. 2000; 10(8):321-327

[19] Ferrara N, Gerber HP, and LeCouter J. The biology of VEGF and its receptors. Nat Med 2003: 9(6):669-676.

[20] Sennino B, Kuhnert F, ans Tabruyn SP, *et al.* Cellular source and amount of vascular endothelial growth factor and platelet-derived growth factor in tumors determine response to angiogenesis inhibitors. Cancer Res 2009; 69(10):4527-4536.

[21] Barbera-Guillem E, Nyhus JK, and Wolford CC, *et al.* VEGF Vascular endothelial growth factor secretion by tumor-infiltrating macrophages essentially supports tumor angiogenesis, and IgG immune complexes potentiate the process. Cancer Res 2002; 62(23):7042-7049.

[22] Argyriou AA, Giannopoulou E, and Kalofonos HP. Angiogenesis and anti-angiogenic molecularly targeted therapies in malignant gliomas. Oncology 2009; 77(1):1-11.

[23] Loeffler S, Fayard B, Weis J, *et al.* Interleukin-6 induces transcriptional activation of vascular endothelial growth factor (VEGF) in astrocytes *in vivo* and regulates VEGF promoter activity in glioblastoma cells via direct interaction between STAT3 and Sp1.

[24] Int J Can 2005; 115(2):202-213.

[25] Huang SP, Wu MS, Shun CT, *et al.* Cyclooxygenase-2 increases hypoxia-inducible factor-1 and vascular endothelial growth factor to promote angiogenesis in gastric carcinoma. J Biomed Sci 2005; 12(1):229-241.

[26] Folkins C, Man S, Xu P, *et al.* Anticancer therapies combining antiangiogenic and tumor cell cytotoxic effects reduce the tumor stem-like cell fraction in glioma xenograft tumors. Cancer Res 2007; 67(8):3560-3564.

[27] Zeng H, Dvorak HF, and Mukhopadhyay D. Vascular permeability factor (VPF)/vascular endothelial growth factor (VEGF) peceptor-1 down-modulates VPF/VEGF receptor-2-mediated endothelial cell proliferation, but not migration, through phosphatidylinositol 3-kinase-dependent pathways. J Biol Chem 2001; 276(29):26969-26979.

[28] Vosseler S, Mirancea N, Bohlen P, *et al.* Angiogenesis inhibition by vascular endothelial growth factor receptor-2 blockade reduces stromal matrix metalloproteinase expression, normalizes stromal tissue, and reverts epithelial tumor phenotype in surface heterotransplants. Cancer Res 2005; 65(4):1294-1305.

[29] Stupp R, Hegi ME, Gilbert MR, *et al.* Chemoradiotherapy in malignant glioma: standard of care and future directions. J Clin Oncol 2007; 25(26):4127-4136.

[30] Desjardins A, Reardon DA, Herndon JE 2nd, *et al.* Bevacizumab plus irinotecan in recurrent WHO grade 3 malignant gliomas. Clin Can Res 2008; 14(21):7068-7073.

[31] Ma J, and Waxman DJ. Combination of antiangiogenesis with chemotherapy for more effective cancer treatment. Mol Can Ther 2008; 7: 3670-3684.

[32] Lassman AB, Iwamoto FM, Gutin PH, *et al.* Patterns of relapse and prognosis after bevacizumab (BEV) failure in recurrent glioblastoma (GBM). *ASCO* 2008; abstract # 2028, Chicago, IL.

[33] LoRusso PM, and Eder JP. Therapeutic potential of novel selective-spectrum kinase inhibitors in oncology. Expert Opinion on Investigational Drugs 2008; 17(7):1013-1028.

[34] Jain RK, di Tomaso E, Duda DG, *et al.* Angiogenesis in brain tumours. Nat Rev Neurosci. 2007; 8(8):610-622.

[35] Yang JC, Hawaorht L, Sherry RM *et al.* A randomized trial of bevacizumab, an anti-vasculare endothelial growth factor antibody, for metastatic renal cancer. N.Eng. J. Med 2003; 349: 427-434.

[36] Folkins C, Shaked Y, Man S, *et al.* Glioma Tumor Stem-Like Cells Promote Tumor Angiogenesis and Vasculogenesis via Vascular Endothelial Growth Factor and Stromal-Derived Factor 1. Can Res 2009; 69(19):7243-7251.

[37] Mancuso MR, Davis R, Norberg SM, *et al.* Rapid vascular regrowth in tumors after reversal of VEGF inhibition. J Clin Invest 2006; 116(10):2610-2621.

[38] Zuniga RM, Torcuator R, Doyle T, *et al.* Retrospective analysis of patterns of recurrence seen on MRI in patients with recurrent glioblastoma multiforme treated with bevacizumab plus irinotecan. ASCO 2008 abstract #13013, Chicago, IL.

[39]   Baffert F, Le T, Sennino B, *et al.* Cellular changes in normal blood capillaries undergoing regression after inhibition of VEGF signaling. Am J Physiol Heart Circ Physiol. 2006; 290(2):H547-559.

[40]   Socinski MA. Bevacizumab as first-line treatment for advanced non-small cell lung cancer. Drugs Today (Barc). 2008; 44(4):293-301.

[41]   Drevs J, Siegert P, Medinger M, *et al.* Phase I clinical study of AZD2171, an oral vascular endothelial growth factor signaling inhibitor, in patients with advanced solid tumors. J Clin Oncol 2007; 25, 3045-3054.

[42]   Morgan B, Thomas AL, Drevs J, *et al.* Dynamic contrast-enhanced magnetic resonance imaging as a biomarker for the pharmacological response of PTK787/ZK 222584, an inhibitor of the vascular endothelial growth factor receptor tyrosine kinases, in patients with advanced colorectal cancer and liver metastases: results from two phase I studies. J Clin Oncol 2003; 21(21):3955-3964.

[43]   Pollock DM. Endothelin, angiotensin, and oxidative stress in hypertension.

[44]   Hypertension 2005; 45(4):477-480.

[45]   Xu L, Duda DG, di Tomaso E, *et al.* Direct Evidence that Bevacizumab, an Anti-VEGF Antibody, Up-regulates SDF1∀, CXCR4, CXCL6, and Neuropilin 1 in Tumors from Patients with Rectal Cancer. Cancer Res 2009; 69(20):7905-7910.

CHAPTER 2

Avastin for Recurrent Malignant Gliomas

Annick Desjardins* and James J. Vredenburgh

Duke University Medical Center, DUMC Box 3624, Durham, NC 27710

Abstract: Glioblastoma multiforme (GBM) is the most aggressive cancer and has the worst prognosis of all malignant gliomas at diagnosis. At the time of disease recurrence/progression, GBM has an even worse prognosis. Vascular proliferation is an important marker in the histological grading of gliomas. Malignant gliomas overexpress VEGF, the principal mediator of tumor angiogenesis, the levels of which correlate directly with tumor vascularity and grade, and inversely with prognosis. Bevacizumab is a humanized monoclonal antibody against VEGF. Bevacizumab with irinotecan has been approved by the US Food and Drug Administration (FDA) for colorectal cancer. Bevacizumab is also FDA approved as a first line treatment for non-small cell lung cancer in combination with carboplatin and paclitaxel, has obtained accelerated approval for metastatic HER2-negative breast cancer patients in combination with paclitaxel, and most recently, accelerated approval for recurrent glioblastoma multiforme as single agent. In the first FDA approved phase II trial for recurrent malignant glioma patients published patients received irinotecan [125 mg/m^2 for patients on non enzyme inducing antiepileptic drug (EIAED) or not on an antiepileptic drug, and 340 mg/m^2 for patients on EIAED] intravenously (IV) every two weeks in combination with bevacizumab 10 mg/kg IV every two weeks. Thirty-two patients were enrolled and a radiographic response rate of 63% was observed [1 complete response (CR) and 19 partial responses (PRs)]. A 6-month PFS of 38% for all patients and a 6-month overall survival of 72% were observed. Following these findings, multiple studies with irinotecan and other agents more commonly used in malignant gliomas were initiated to evaluate alternative bevacizumab-based regimens for recurrent malignant glioma patients. In the vast majority, all those studies showed an unprecedented increase in PFS and response rate in malignant glioma patients treated with bevacizumab as a single agent or in combination, as well a significant improvement in the quality of life of the patients exposed to bevacizumab. However, the utilization of a bevacizumab based regimen for recurrent malignant gliomas has opened a brand new field in neuro-oncology. Further study is needed to determine optimal managements and enhance the quality of life for these patients.

INTRODUCTION

Malignant gliomas represent less than 2% of all cancers, but their prognosis is very poor. Glioblastoma multiforme (GBM) is the most aggressive cancer and has the worst prognosis of all malignant gliomas at diagnosis. At the time of disease recurrence/progression, GBM has an even worse prognosis given that available systemic chemotherapies offer modest clinical benefit with a 6-month progression free survival (PFS) of less than 15% [1], and a median overall survival (OS) of 25 weeks from the time of recurrence [1]. In addition to the fatal prognosis, malignant gliomas affect many patients in their 40s and 50s, frequently terminating promising lives prematurely and depriving young families of parents and spouses. Clearly, more effective therapies are desperately needed for patients afflicted with these tumors.

Vascular proliferation is an important marker in the histological grading of gliomas [2-6]. The degree of vascularization is seen to correlate well with tumor grade and aggressiveness as tumors with a faster growth rate need an increased supply of oxygen and nutrients [7]. In malignant gliomas, rapid cellular proliferation results in hypoxic conditions within the tumor. The release of humoral factors that promote angiogenesis, such as vascular endothelial growth factor (VEGF), seem to play a particularly important role in the process of neovascularization [8-9]. Malignant gliomas utilize humoral factors to recruit new sources of blood supply to counter the hypoxic conditions resulting from the rapid proliferation of the tumor cells. This vicious cycle of proliferation causing hypoxia, which triggers angiogenesis leading to further proliferation, is a key feature of malignant gliomas [10]. Interruption of this cycle by inhibition of angiogenesis should have a direct impact on glioma growth and recurrence.

*****Address correspondence to the Annick Desjardins:** The Preston Robert Tisch Brain Tumor Center at Duke, Duke University Medical Center, Rm. 047, Baker House, Trent Drive, DUMC 3624, Durham, NC 27710; Tel: (919)668-2993; Fax: (919)684-6674; E-mail: desja002@mc.duke.edu

Thomas C. Chen (Ed)

Malignant gliomas overexpress VEGF, the principal mediator of tumor angiogenesis, the levels of which correlate directly with tumor vascularity and grade, and inversely with prognosis [3, 7, 11-16] pluripotent factor that has multiple effects on the vasculature, including induction of angiogenesis and enhancement of endothelial cell survival, the ability to induce vascular permeability, and production of a dilated and disorganized vascular network. This altered tumor vascular network leads to inefficient blood flow, which can theoretically be 'normalized' with anti-VEGF therapy, augmenting delivery of chemotherapy and oxygen [17]. Tumor-associated endothelial cells express VEGFR2, creating a paracrine loop of angiogenic activation, indicating that VEGF and its receptors are important therapeutic targets [3-4, 13].

Bevacizumab is a humanized monoclonal antibody against VEGF which binds to VEGF-A [14-15], prevents its interaction with the VEGF receptor tyrosine kinases VEGFR1 and VEGFR2, and inhibits the growth of human tumor cell lines in mice [8, 18]. VEGF is an important endothelial cell-specific mitogen that regulates vascular proliferation and permeability and functions as an antiapoptotic factor for newly formed blood vessels [19]. This therapeutic antibody targets the process of angiogenesis and the acquisition of new blood vessels by a tumor – a key process if a tumor is to grow and metastasize. It was initially believed that the VEGF receptors (VEGFRs) are present only on endothelial cells, but recent studies have demonstrated that VEGFRs are present on tumor cells [20-21]. So, another potential mechanism of action of anti-VEGF therapy is a direct effect on tumor cells, where it might inhibit processes involved in tumor progression and metastasis. Following early clinical trials showing that bevacizumab as a single agent was relatively non-toxic, and that it could be added to standard cytotoxic chemotherapy regimes, large clinical trials were initiated in several cancer types, including colorectal cancer [18].

Bevacizumab was generally well tolerated in these clinical trials; however, some serious and unusual toxicities were noted. In particular, bevacizumab was associated with gastrointestinal perforations and wound healing complications in about 2% of patients. Other adverse events associated with bevacizumab use include thromboembolic complications, hypertension, bleeding and proteinuria.

Given in combination with conventional chemotherapy, bevacizumab significantly improves the survival of patients with metastatic colorectal and lung cancer [16, 22] and PFS of patients with breast cancer [23]. Bevacizumab with irinotecan has been approved by the US Food and Drug Administration (FDA) for colorectal cancer. Bevacizumab is also FDA approved as a first line treatment for non-small cell lung cancer in combination with carboplatin and paclitaxel, has obtained accelerated approval for metastatic HER2-negative breast cancer patients in combination with paclitaxel, and most recently, accelerated approval for recurrent glioblastoma multiforme as single agent.

BEVACIZUMAB AND IRINOTECAN FOR MALIGNANT GLIOMAS

In the first FDA approved phase II trial for recurrent malignant glioma patients published [24] patients received irinotecan [125 mg/m^2 for patients on non enzyme inducing antiepileptic drug (EIAED) or not on an antiepileptic drug, and 340 mg/m^2 for patients on EIAED] intravenously (IV) every two weeks in combination with bevacizumab 10 mg/kg IV every two weeks. Thirty-two patients, 23 with WHO grade IV glioma and 9 with WHO grade III, were enrolled and a radiographic response rate of 63% was observed [1 complete response (CR) and 19 partial responses (PRs)]. A 6-month PFS of 38% for all patients (32% for GBM patients) and a 6-month overall survival of 72% were observed.

Due to the encouraging preliminary results observed, the initial trial was expanded to include a total of 68 patients with recurrent malignant glioma, 35 patients with a pathological diagnosis of GBM and 33 with an anaplastic glioma (WHO grade III). In the recurrent GBM cohort, a 6-month PFS of 46% (95% CI, 32% to 66%) was observed, as well as a 6-month overall survival (OS) of 77% (95% CI, 64% to 92%). A radiographic response (PR or CR) was observed in 20 of the 35 patients (57%; 95% CI, 39% to 74%). Adverse events included one patient with a CNS hemorrhage and four patients with thromboembolic complications (deep venous thrombosis and/or pulmonary emboli) [25]. In the recurrent anaplastic glioma cohort, the observed 6-month PFS was 55% (95% CI, 36% to 70%) and the 6-month OS was 79% (95% CI, 61% to 89%). Radiographic response was observed in 20 patients (61%). Significant adverse events included one patient with symptomatic CNS hemorrhage and one patient who developed thrombotic thrombocytopenic purpura (TTP). The patient with CNS hemorrhage required hospitalization and high-dose dexamethasone, but made a full recovery following rehabilitative therapy. The patient who developed TTP remains on peritoneal dialysis without sign of disease progression four years later [26]. Both studies showed a significant improvement in response rate, PFS and OS of malignant gliomas when compared to historical controls.

These findings led to a phase II, randomized, multicenter, non-comparative clinical trial of bevacizumab alone or in combination with irinotecan for GBM patients at first or second recurrence. In this trial, patients were randomized into two different groups; the bevacizumab alone group received bevacizumab dosed at 10 mg/kg IV every two weeks and the combination group received the same dose of bevacizumab plus irinotecan. Irinotecan was administered at 125 mg/m² for patients on non-EIAED or not on an antiepileptic drug, and 340 mg/m² for patients on EIAED. The preliminary results of this trial were first presented at the 2008 Association of Clinical Oncology Meeting (ASCO) [27]. Eighty-five patients were randomized to the bevacizumab alone group and 82 to the combination of bevacizumab plus irinotecan group. At the time of disease progression, patients in the bevacizumab alone group were allowed to receive the combination of bevacizumab and irinotecan at the discretion of the investigator. Median OS was comparable for both groups, 9.2 months (95% CI, 8.2-10.7 months) for the bevacizumab alone group and 8.7 months (95% CI, 7.8-10.9 months) for the combination group. However, the 6-month PFS was higher in the combination group (50.3%; 95% CI, 36.8- 63.9%) comparatively to the bevacizumab alone group (42.6%; 95% CI, 29.6-55.5%). Higher rate of grade 3 and higher toxicities were reported in the combination group, 65.8% vs 46.4% for the bevacizumab alone group, but grade 5 adverse events happened more frequently in the bevacizumab alone group (2.4% vs 1.3% for the combination group) [27].

ALTERNATIVE BEVACIZUMAB-BASED REGIMENS

Following these findings, multiple studies with agents more commonly used in malignant gliomas were initiated to evaluate alternative bevacizumab-based regimens for recurrent malignant glioma patients. A phase II study of etoposide plus bevacizumab in recurrent malignant glioma patients was conducted and etoposide was administered orally daily (50 mg/m2/day) for 21 days of a 28 day cycle and bevacizumab was dosed at 10 mg/kg IV every 2 weeks. Fifty-nine patients were enrolled on that study (27 GBM and 32 WHO grade III MG). A median OS of 46 weeks was observed for GBM. The 6-month PFS was 44% and 40.6% for GBM and WHO grade III, respectively. Radiographic responses were achieved in 23% of GBM and 22% WHO grade III malignant glioma patients. Adverse events were grade 2 in most cases, including neutropenia (48%), fatigue (33%) and infection (31%). One patient developed a grade 1 intracranial hemorrhage and one patient suffered a grade 4 GI perforation [28]. A phase II study combining daily temozolomide at 50 mg/m²/day with bevacizumab 10 mg/kg IV every 2 weeks was performed for patients with recurrent GBM. Thirty-two patients were enrolled. Twelve patients (37.5%) demonstrated a radiographic response and twelve patients (37.5%) demonstrated disease stabilization. Twenty-two percent of patients (7) remained progression free at 6 months (6-month PFS 22%) and the overall survival at 10 months was 47%. At the time of publication, four patients (12.5%) remained on treatment. No grade 3 or 4 hematologic toxicities were observed. One patient suffered *Pneumocystis carinii* pneumonia (grade 5), one patient pancreatitis (grade 4), one patient colitis with gastrointestinal bleed (grade 4) and one patient a hemorrhoidal bleed with diarrhea (grade 3) [29]. A phase II trial of erlotinib and bevacizumab for recurrent malignant glioma patients was also conducted. Erlotinib was administered orally daily at 200 mg/day for patients on non-EIAED or not on an antiepileptic drug and at 650 mg/day for patients on EIAED. Bevacizumab was dosed at 10 mg/kg intravenously every two weeks. Fifty-six malignant glioma patients were assessable for outcome (24 GBM and 32 WHO grade III). The 6-month PFS rates were 25% for GBM and 50% for WHO grade III MG. The most common side effect was a rash (54% grade 1-2 and 38% grade 3). Serious adverse events suffered by patients included two pulmonary embolisms, one intestinal perforation, one ischemic stroke, one gastric bleeding, and one nasal septum perforation [30]. We also have initiated a study combining bortezomib, the first proteasome inhibitor, and bevacizumab. Preliminary results on this study have not been published yet.

CONCLUSION

The unprecedented increase in PFS and response rate in malignant glioma patients treated with bevacizumab as a single agent or in combination, as well as the significant improvement in the quality of life of the patients exposed to bevacizumab, has stimulated research with bevacizumab as well as other VEGF-directed or antiangiogenic therapies (see Table **1**). Treatment with bevacizumab has not only improved the survival of the patients, but has also allowed a significant improvement in quality of life, decreasing intracranial edema and thus allowing decadron to be tapered and in some cases, discontinued. These patients are at less risk for developing steroid-induced hyperglycemia, osteoporosis, ulcerative disease, weight gain and steroid myopathy. However, the utilization of a bevacizumab based regimen for recurrent malignant gliomas has opened a brand new field in neuro-oncology. The radiographic responses, as well as the new patterns of progression on MRI is opening a new field in neuroradiology not only to define a new response criteria for malignant glioma patients treated with VEGF therapies, but also the need to develop new imaging techniques to help us determine more rapidly the patients who will benefit from such treatment as well as help us determine more quickly when they will progress. The advent of VEGF based therapies has also brought to light new resistance mechanisms for which additional research is necessary. Patients are surviving longer, some times at the price of significant neurologic and medical complications. Further study is needed to determine optimal managements and enhance the quality of life for these patients.

Table 1: Abbreviations: PFS: Progression-free survival; OS: Overall Survival.

Bevacizumab-based combination trials done at Duke					
	Number of patients	Radiographic Response Rate	6-month PFS	6-month OS	median OS
Irinotecan/bevacizumab grade III and grade IV	32	63%	38%	72%	
Irinotecan/bevacizumab grade IV	35	57%	46%	77%	
Irinotecan/bevacizumab grade III	33	61%	55%	79%	
Etoposide/bevacizumab grade III and grade IV	59		44%		
grade IV	27	23%	44%		46 weeks
grade III	32	22%	40.6%		
Daily temozolomide/bevacizumab grade IV	32	37.5%	22%		
Erlotinib/bevacizumab grade III and grade IV	56				
grade IV	24	25%			
grade III	32	50%			

REFERENCES

[1]   Wong ET, Hess KR, Gleason MJ, *et al.* Outcomes and prognostic factors in recurrent glioma patients enrolled onto phase II clinical trials. J Clin Oncol 1999; 17(8):2572-2578.

[2]   Daumas-Duport C, Scheithauer B, O'Fallon J, Kelly P. Grading of astrocytomas. A simple and reproducible method. Cancer 1988; 62:2152-2165.

[3]   Kleihues P, Cavenee WK. Pathology and Genetics Tumours of the Nervous System. IARC Press, Lyon, 2000; 314 pp.

[4]   Reijneveld JC, Voest EE, Taphoorn MJ. Angiogenesis in malignant primary and metastatic brain tumors. J Neurol 2000; 247:597-608.

[5]   Fukumura D, Xu L, Chen Y, Gohongi T, Seed B, Jain RK. Hypoxia and acidosis independently up-regulate vascular endothelial growth factor transcription in brain tumors in vivo. Cancer Res 2001; 61:6020-6024.

[6]   Lu H, Forbes RA, Verma A. Hypoxia-inducible factor 1 activation by aerobic glycolysis implicates the Warburg effect in carcinogenesis. J Biol Chem 2002; 277:23111-23115.

[7]   Plate KH, Breier G, Weich HA, Risau W. Vascular endothelial growth factor is a potential tumour angiogenesis factor in human gliomas *in vivo*. Nature 1992; 359:845-848.

[8]   Plate KH, Mennel HD. Vascular morphology and angiogenesis in glial tumors. Exp Toxicol Pathol 1995; 47:89-94.

[9]   Kurimoto M, Endo S, Hirashima Y, Nishijima M, Takaku A. Elevated plasma basic fibroblast growth factor in brain tumor patients. Neurol Med Chir (Tokyo) 1996; 36:865-868; discussion 869.

[10] Shweiki D, Neeman M, Itin A, Keshet E. Induction of vascular endothelial growth factor expression by hypoxia and by glucose deficiency in multicell spheroids: implications for tumor angiogenesis. Proc Natl Acad Sci USA 1995; 92:768-772.

[11] Xu L, Fukumura D, Jain RK. Acidic extracellular pH induces vascular endothelial growth factor (VEGF) in human glioblastoma cells via ERK1/2MAPK signalling pathway: mechanisms of low pH-induced VEGF. J Biol Chem 2002; 277:11368-11374.

[12] Wang D, Huang HJ, Kazlauskas A, Cavenee WK. Induction of vascular endothelial growth factor expression in endothelial cells by platelet-derived growth factor through the activation of phosphatidylinositol 3-kinase. Cancer Res 1999; 59:1464-1472.

[13] Sanchez-Elsner T, Botella LM, Velasco V, Corbi A, Attisano L, Bernabeu C. Synergistic cooperation between hypoxia and transforming growth factor-beta pathways on human vascular endothelial growth factor gene expression. J Biol Chem 2001; 276:38527-38535.

[14] Chaudhry IH, O'Donovan DG, Brenchley PE, Reid H, Roberts IS. Vascular endothelial growth factor expression correlates with tumour grade and vascularity in gliomas. Histopathology 2001; 39:409-415.

[15] Ke LD, Shi YX, Im SA, Chen X, Yung WK. The relevance of cell proliferation, vascular endothelial growth factor, and basic fibroblast growth factor production to angiogenesis and tumorigenicity I human glioma cell lines. Clin Cancer Res 2000; 6:2562-2572.

[16] Samoto K, Ikezaki K, Ono M, *et al.* Expression of vascular endothelial growth factor and its possible relation with neovascualarization in human brain tumors. Cancer Res 1995; 55:1189-1193.

[17] Jain RK. Normalization of tumor vasculature: an emerging concept in antiangiogenic therapy. Science 2005; 307:58-62.

[18] Ferrara N *et al.* Discovery and development of bevacizumab, an anti-VEGF antibody for treating cancer. Nature Rev Drug Discov 2004; 3:391-400.

[19] Rosen LS. Clinical experience with angiogenesis signalling inhibitors: focus on vascular endothelial growth factor (VEGF) blockers. Cancer Control 2002; 9(suppl):36-44.

[20] Dias S, *et al.* Autocrine stimulation of VEGFR-2 activates human leukemic cell growth and migration. J Clin Invest 2000; 106:511-521.

[21] Fan F, *et al.* Expression and function of vascular endothelial growth factor receptor-1 on human colorectal cancer cells. Oncogene 2005; 24:2647-2653.

[22] Kim KJ, Li B, Winer J, Armanini M, Gillett N, Phillips HS, Ferrara N. Inhibition of vascular endothelial growth factor-induced angiogenesis suppresses tumour growth in vivo. Nature 1993;362:841-844.

[23] Millauer B, Shawver LK, Plate KH, Risau W, Ullrich A. Glioblastoma growth inhibited *in vivo* by a dominant-negative Flk-1 mutant. Nature 1994; 367:576-579.

[24] Vredenburgh JJ, Desjardins A, Herndon JE, *et al.* Phase II trial of bevacizumab and irinotecan in recurrent malignant glioma. Clin Cancer Res, 2007;13(4):1253-1259.

[25] Vredenburgh J, Desjardins A, Herndon JE, *et al.*: Bevacizumab plus irinotecan in recurrent glioblastoma multiforme. J Clin Oncol 2007; 25:4722-4729.

[26] Desjardins A, Reardon DA, Herndon JE, *et al.* Bevacizumab plus irinotecan in recurrent WHO grade III malignant gliomas. Clin Cancer Res 2008 ; 14:7068-7073.

[27] Cloughesy TF, Prados MD, Wen PY, *et al.* A phase II, randomized, non-comparative clinical trial of the effect of bevacizumab (BV) alone or in combination with irinotecan (CPT) on 6-month progression free survival (PFS6) in recurrent, treatment-refractory glioblastoma (GBM). J Clin Oncol 2008; 26: May 20 suppl; abstr 2010b.

[28] Reardon D, Desjardins A, Vredenburgh JJ, Gururangan S, Peters KB, Norfleet JA. Bevacizumab plus etoposide among recurrent malignant glioma patients: Phase II study final results. J Clin Oncol 2009; 27:15s (suppl; abstr 2046).

[29] Maron R, Vredenburgh JJ, Desjardins A, et al. Bevacizumab and daily temozolomide for recurrent glioblastoma multiforme (GBM). J Clin Oncol 2008; 26:(May 20 suppl; abstr 2074).

[30] Sathornsumetee S, Vredenburgh JJ, Rich JN, et al. Phase II study of bevacizumab and erlotinib in patients with recurrent glioblastoma multiforme. J Clin Oncol 2008; 26: (May 20 suppl; abstr 13008).

CHAPTER 3

Avastin and Malignant Gliomas: Is there a Role?

Teri N. Kreisl*

Neuro-Oncology Branch – NCI, 9030 Old Georgetown Road, Bldg. 82, Rm. 243, Bethesda, MD 20892

Abstract: Bevacizumab is the first new drug approved for malignant glioma in a decade and demonstrates the potential for antiangiogenic therapy in the management of these patients. It has demonstrated improved radiographic response and progression free survival rates compared to historical controls as monotherapy. Bevacizumab has also been shown to improve patient symptoms of disease and decrease steroid requirements contributing to improved quality of life for glioma patients. Optimal combinations with other standard and targeted therapies are under investigation, as well as new imaging techniques to evaluate response to therapy, motivated in part by concerns over suspected increase potential for tumor invasion.

INTRODUCTION

Benefit from chemotherapy in the treatment of malignant glioma was only recently established in 2005 when a multicentered prospective randomized trial demonstrated a modest survival benefit for patients who added temozolomide to radiation for initial therapy [1]. Temozolomide had previously been approved for recurrent anaplastic astrocytoma and earned an indication for the treatment of newly diagnosed glioblastoma multiforme (GBM). Bevacizumab is the first new drug labeled for gliomas in the last decade after it received accelerated approval by the FDA in May 2009 based on improved response rates relative to historical controls. This provisional approval expedited patient access to an effective therapy for one of the most lethal and aggressive cancers.

Bevacizumab (Avastin, Genentech) is a humanized monoclonal antibody against vascular endothelial growth factor (VEGF) and is a potent angiogenesis inhibitor. The drug was originally developed for the treatment of metastatic colorectal cancer used in combination with standard therapy [2]. It was the first angiogenesis inhibitor approved as a cancer therapeutic and is used successfully in non-small cell lung and metastatic breast cancer as well [3, 4]. Bevacizumab is a logical drug to study in malignant gliomas which harbor the trademark histological feature of tumor neovasculature. Unlike for other solid tumors, a survival benefit has yet to be demonstrated for GBM patients. While clinical trials for initial therapy of GBM with bevacizumab are underway to investigate survival effects, patients receiving the drug as second line adjuvant treatment are gaining clinical benefit in terms of tumor response, decreased dependency on corticosteroids and improvement in symptoms of disease.

BEVACIZUMAB FOR RECURRENT MALIGNANT GLIOMA

Many groups have reported their experience with bevacizumab for recurrent malignant glioma in retrospective studies that demonstrate response rates from 11-79%, median progression free survival (mPFS) from 4.2 to 7.6 months, and median overall survival (mOS) from 4.6-12.6 months [5-14]. (Table **1**) Interpretation of these data is complicated because the studies often mix WHO grade III and IV tumors, and describe a variety of combinations with other cytotoxic drugs such as irinotecan, carboplatin, and temozolomide.

Vrendenburg *et al.* [15] published the first prospective trial data for bevacizumab in recurrent GBM patients. They reported 35 patients treated with two regimens of bevacizumab 10 mg/kg with irinotecan 125-340 mg/m2 given every two weeks, or bevacizumab 15 mg/kg every 3 weeks with irinotecan weekly for four out of every six weeks. Six month progression free survival (PFS6) was 46% [95%CI, 32-66%]. 57% of patients achieved at least a partial response to therapy. These results appeared to be dramatic improvements compared to historical controls which demonstrate PFS6 of only 9% and response rates of 7-9% [16-18]. Toxicity was notable in that 11/35 (31%) patients discontinued therapy due to toxicity and an additional four patients withdrew due to fatigue.

Address correspondence to Teri N. Kreisl: Neuro-Oncology Branch – NCI, 9030 Old Georgetown Road, Bldg. 82, Rm. 243, Bethesda, MD 20892; Tel: (301) 402-3423, Fax: (301) 480-2246, Email: kreislt@mail.nih.gov

Concomitantly, an industry sponsored multicentered trial was conducted as a non-comparative study of bevacizumab monotherapy and combination therapy with irinotecan [19]. The combination arm was similar to the previously described study where PFS6 was 50.2% [95%CI, 36.6-63.8] and response rate was 32.9% [95%CI, 23.4-43.5]. There were also higher rates of grade ≥ 3 toxicity and more patients discontinued due to adverse events when treated with irinotecan (13.9 vs. 3.5%). In this trial, bevacizumab 10 mg/kg was administered every two weeks either alone or in combination with 125-340 mg/m2 of irinotecan depending on use of enzyme inducing antiepileptic drugs.

The bevacizumab monotherapy experience comes from the single agent arm of the industry sponsored trial and a separate independent study conducted at the National Cancer Institute where patients were treated with bevacizumab 10 mg/kg every two weeks [20]. Patients who progressed were offered participation in a companion study where irinotecan 125-340 mg/m2 was immediately added to biweekly bevacizumab. The first 48 of the 56 patients enrolled in this study were reported with a response rate of 35% and PFS6 29% [95%CI, 18-48%]. This compared closely to the single agent arm of the multicentered trial where responses were seen in 20% [95%CI, 12.7-29.5] and PFS6 was 35.1% [95%CI, 23.2-47.0]. None of the patients in the NCI trial who were treated subsequently with irinotecan had a response after progression on bevacizumab alone, and there was no significant difference in PFS6 between both arms of the multicentered trial. Based on these data, bevacizumab received FDA approval as monotherapy for recurrent GBM.

The questionable utility of irinotecan weighed against the added toxicity did not warrant its approval for use in combination with bevacizumab. This comes of little surprise since single agent use of irinotecan in glioma patients has shown little efficacy in several prior clinical studies [21, 22]. Investigators, therefore, are studying combinations of bevacizumab and other therapies. Mohile *et al.* reported 12 patients who received bevacizumab with fractionated focal radiotherapy who achieved a 58% response rate and PFS6 76% in a very selected population of patients with small volume tumors [23]. Prospective trials of combinations with etoposide and erlotinib have been conducted [24, 25]. A key question is whether cytotoxic agents may be synergistic with an antiangiogenic drug as they are for other systemic solid tumors. Several groups have reviewed their experience with bevacizumab, given most often in combination with irinotecan, carboplatin, nitrosureas, temozolomide and etoposide. Narayana *et al.* found no significant difference in survival between 54 patients treated with irinotecan versus 7 with carboplatin in combination with bevacizumab [8]. Norden *et al.* identified 23 patients where the cytotoxic agent was switched after progression on initial combination bevacizumab therapy, where no cases of subsequent response were observed, but two patients had prolonged PFS of five and eight months [26]. Certain patients may benefit from added standard therapy, particularly those with significant non-enhancing tumor not likely controlled with antiangiogenic treatment alone. Currently, however, there is no "leader" in terms of optimal partnership with bevacizumab for malignant glioma. Clinicians are faced with a trial and error approach directed by the given patient's prior treatment history.

BEVACIZUMAB FOR NEWLY DIAGNOSED MALIGNANT GLIOMA

Since a survival benefit from bevacizumab for recurrent disease has not been established, and will not likely be a planned endpoint for future trials in the recurrent setting, investigators are conducting upfront studies for newly diagnosed GBM. Nicholas *et al.* presented preliminary results from a phase II study of bevacizumab added to the adjuvant phase of temozolomide chemotherapy after concurrent chemo radiation. Of the 42 patients enrolled, 26 received at least one full four week cycle of temozolomide 150-200 mg/m2 5/28 days with bevacizumab 10 mg/kg every 2 weeks. 14/42 (33%) patients had objective radiographic response. None of the patients removed for toxicity had unexpected adverse events and there was one incidence of gastrointestinal hemorrhage [27].

Other groups are initiating bevacizumab therapy during the chemo radiation phase of treatment. Lai *et al.* reported the first 10 in a series of 70 patients treated with bevacizumab 10 mg/kg every two weeks starting with involved field external beam radiation 60 Gy in 30 fractions and temozolomide 75 mg/m2 daily. After a two week post-radiation interval combination therapy with biweekly bevacizumab and monthly temozolomide was given. Isolated cases of retinal detachment and optic neuropathy were some unexpected observed adverse events.[28, 29] Narayana *et al.* reported their experience with a similar protocol in 15 patients. One year PFS and overall survival were 59.3% and 86.7% [30]. Gruber *et al.* used a slightly more dose intense schedule of adjuvant temozolomide and showed mPFS 17 months, PFS6 77%, and mOS 57% [31]. Genentech will sponsor a multicentered randomized trial to assess the survival benefit of adding bevacizumab to the standard upfront regimen for GBM.

CLINICAL BENEFIT FROM BEVACIZUMAB

In neuro-oncology, perhaps more so than other areas of cancer research, quality of life is an important measure of clinical efficacy due to high rates of neurological and functional disability suffered by glioma patients. For the first time, brain tumor patients and their doctors have at their disposal a drug other than dexamethasone that can improve the signs and symptoms of their disease. Bevacizumab has an effect on vascular permeability that confers a steroid like effect that can be observed quite early in treatment [32]. Both trials leading to the indication approval demonstrated a decreased dependence on corticosteroid for GBM patients treated with bevacizumab. In the NCI trial, 50% patients had decreased cerebral edema, 58% on steroids at the start of treatment were able to achieve an average dose reduction of 59%, and 52% had improved neurologic symptoms [20]. The industry sponsored trial showed a decrease in steroid use from an average of 7.3 mg/kg on day 1 to 3.1 mg/kg on day 84 of treatment for the bevacizumab alone arm. This trial also assessed cognitive function where the majority of patients demonstrated stable performance on a variety of tests at the six week follow-up and 18-25% had improved performance [33]. A separate series of 22 GBM patients treated with bevacizumab and irinotecan demonstrated improvement in Blessed Orientation Memory Concentration (BOMC) testing scores in 62% and a median improvement in Karnofsky Performance Status by 10 points [12]. Given the myriad side effects of high dose steroids and the high impact of brain tumors on quality of life, bevacizumab has a role in the management of malignant glioma patients independent of controversies over combination therapy and survival effects.

PATTERNS OF RECURRENCE AND INVASION

Bevacizumab is thought to be a breakthrough in the historically dismal practice of neuro-oncology. However, nihilism and pessimism are difficult habits to break. The early experience with bevacizumab in the community has raised concerns that the drug may be influencing the pattern of disease progression in treated patients, suggesting the drug may promote tumor invasion. Bevacizumab was shown to increase tumor invasion *in vitro* and *in vivo* by up regulating expression of invasion related genes such as MMP 9. Anti-VEGF therapy also upregulates other proangiogenic factors [34]. These observations are mirrored by the early experience in the clinic where progression of non-enhancing disease is observed with a seemingly higher frequency than prior to the introduction of bevacizumab.

Lassman *et al.* reported 21 patients who progressed on bevacizumab-based therapy where 14 (67%) recurred in a multifocal or gliomatosis cerebri pattern associated with an increase risk of death (Hazard Ratio 13; 95%CI 1.7-1-1, p=0.01).[35] Zuniga *et al.* also showed that 60% of cases of progression on bevacizumab were associated with development of disease distant from the original tumor, while others report a lower rate of infiltrative recurrence (20-30%).[8, 36] In one study, this infiltrative pattern was negatively associated with age [36]. It is difficult to discern whether anti-VEGF therapy actually accelerates or promotes tumor invasion or whether the natural course of disease is altered so that patients are alive long enough for us to observe this degree of tumor progression, unmasked by the effect bevacizumab has on gadolinium enhancement.

The effect on MRI contrast signal may not be as reliable a proxy for tumor as it is for cytotoxic therapy. The often dramatic radiographic changes seen after just a few doses of bevacizumab are not likely anti-tumor effects but changes in vascular permeability. Accordingly, several groups are looking at alternative imaging methods to assess tumor response such as dynamic susceptibility contrast enhanced MRI and apparent diffusion coefficient measures [37-39]. This issue further fuels the need to find rational and effective therapies to combine with bevacizumab, that either mitigate escape from VEGF mediated antiangiogenesis or provides more direct cytotoxic activity.

CONCLUSION

Is there a role for bevacizumab in the management of malignant glioma? Clearly, yes. While monotherapy has afforded encouraging results, it by no means approaches a cure or durable disease control for the majority of patients.   Continued efforts are needed to improve on this early success.   Trials are underway to combine bevacizumab with other targeted therapy in addition to investigating its role in the upfront treatment of glioma patients. Bevacizumab has also changed the face of therapeutic development for recurrent disease. Studies must use a new benchmark for efficacy. Comparison to historical controls of essentially ineffective therapies will no longer be appropriate for trial design. The post-bevacizumab era will prove to be a challenging environment for the neuro-oncology community, but one that for the first time may carry real hope.

Table 1: Bevacizumab (B) in the Treatment of Recurrent Malignant Glioma

Study	Patients	Regimen	Response Rate	mPFS	PFS6	mOS
Ali *et al.* [5]	13 MG[a]	(9) B 5mg/m2 q 2wks (4) B 10mg/m2 + I 125mg/m2 q3wks	10 (77%)		mTTP[b] 24wks	27wks
Cloughesy *et al.* [19]	167 GBM	(85) B[c] (82) B+I[d]	20% [95%CI 12.7-29.5] 32.9% [95%CI 23.4-43.5]		35.1% [23.2-47.0] 50.2 [36.6-63.8]	9.7 [8.2-11.8] 8.9 [7.8-11.9]
Desjardins *et al.* [40]	23 AG[e]	(9) B 10mg/kg + I q2wks (24) B 15mg/kg + I q3wks	20 (61%)		55% [36-70]	OS6 79% [61-89]
Dresemann *et al.* [41]	44 GBM	B 4mg/kg +I 80mg/m2 q2wks	22 (50%)			
Gil Gil *et al.* [6]	28 GBM 16 AG	B 10mg/kg + I 125mg/m2 q2wks	25 (57% [41-71.6])	7.4m [4.6-10.1]		9.8m [6.8-12.8]
Kang *et al.* [7]	27 MG	B + I		5.1m	46%	12.6m
Kreisl *et al.* [20]	48 GBM	B 10mg/kg q2wks	17 (35%)	16 wks [12-26]	29% [18-48]	31 wks [21-54]
Maron *et al.* [42]	32 GBM	TMZ[f] 50mg/m2 qd + B 10mg/kg q2wks	12 (37.5%)			
Mohile *et al.* [23]	10 GBM 2 AG	B 10mg/kg q2wks + IMRT 6Gy x5	7 (58%)		76%	
Narayana *et al.* [43]	37 GBM 24 AG	B 10mg/kg q2wks + I 125mg/m2 q2wks or carboplatin AUC6 q4wks	39/54 (72%)	5m [2.3-7.7]		9m [7.6-10.4]
Nghiemphu *et al.* [44]	44 GBM	B 5mg/kg q2wks + various		4.25m	41%	9.0m
Norden *et al.* [10]	33 GBM 22 AG	B 10mg/kg q2wks + various	34.1%	23.9w [17.7-28.3]	42% GBM 32% AG	35.7 wks [27.7-61.4]
Poulson *et al.* [11]	27 GBM 22 AG 3 other	B 10mg/kg + I q2wks	30% GBM 15% AG	22wks	40% GBM 33% AG	28 wks GBM 32 wks AG
Raizer *et al.* [45]	14 GBM 2 AO[g]	B 15mg/kg q2wks	2/9 (22%)			
Raval *et al.* [12]	22 GBM	B 5mg/kg _ I 125mg/m2 q2wks	16/21 (76%)	mTTP 3m		4.6m
Rich *et al.* [46]	27 GBM 26 AG	B 10mg/kg q2wks + etoposide 50mg/m2 qd 3/4wks	10/47 (21%)			
Sathornsumetee *et al.* [25]	24 GBM 32 AG	B 10mg/kg q2wks + erlotinib 200 or 500 mg/d			25% GBM 50% AG	
Stankewitz *et al.* [13]	35 GBM progressed after B + I	B 4mg/kg + I 80 mg/m2 q2wks + TMZ 20mg/d	4/35 (11%)			
Vrendenburgh *et al.* [15]	35 GBM	(23) B 10mg/kg + I q2wks (12) B 15mg/kg q3wks + I qwk 4/6wks	20 (57% [39-74])	24% [18-36]	46% [32-66]	42% [35-60]
Zuniga *et al.* [14]	37 GBM 14 AG	B 10mg/kg + I	25/37 (68%) GBM 11/14 (79%) AG	7.6m GBM 13.4m AG	63.7% GBM 78.6% AG	11.5m GBM NA AG

a=malignant glioma; b=bevacizumab 10 mg/kg every 2 weeks; c=median time to tumor progression; d=iriotecan 125-340 mg/m2 every 2 weeks ;e=anaplastic glioma ;f=temozolomide ;g=anaplastic oligodendroglioma

REFERENCES

[1]   Stupp R, Mason WP, van den Bent MJ, Weller M, Fisher B, Taphoorn MJ, *et al.* Radiotherapy plus concomitant and adjuvant temozolomide for glioblastoma. N Engl J Med 2005 Mar 10;352(10):987-96.

[2]   Kabbinavar FF, Hambleton J, Mass RD, Hurwitz HI, Bergsland E, Sarkar S. Combined analysis of efficacy: the addition of bevacizumab to fluorouracil/leucovorin improves survival for patients with metastatic colorectal cancer. J Clin Oncol 2005 Jun 1;23(16):3706-12.

[3]   Sandler A, Gray R, Perry MC, Brahmer J, Schiller JH, Dowlati A, *et al.* Paclitaxel-carboplatin alone or with bevacizumab for non-small-cell lung cancer. N Engl J Med 2006 Dec 14;355(24):2542-50.

[4]   Miller K, Wang M, Gralow J, Dickler M, Cobleigh M, Perez EA, *et al.* Paclitaxel plus bevacizumab versus paclitaxel alone for metastatic breast cancer. N Engl J Med 2007 Dec 27;357(26):2666-76.

[5]   Ali SA, McHayleh WM, Ahmad A, Sehgal R, Braffet M, Rahman M, *et al.* Bevacizumab and irinotecan therapy in glioblastoma multiforme: a series of 13 cases. J Neurosurg 2008 Aug;109(2):268-72.

[6]   Gil Gil Sr MJ, Martinez-Garcia M, Reynes G, Costas E, Fernandez-Chacon C, Pernas S, *et al.* Combination of bevacizumab plus irinotecan in recurrent malignant gliomas (MG): A retrospective study of efficacy and safety. ASCO Meeting Abstracts 2008 May 20, 2008;26(15_suppl):13011.

[7]   Kang T, Jin T, Peereboom D. Irinotecan and bevacizumab in progressive primary brain tumors: The Cleveland Clinic experience. ASCO Meeting Abstracts 2007 June 20, 2007; 25(18_suppl):2077.

[8]   Narayana A, Kelly P, Golfinos J, Parker E, Johnson G, Knopp E, *et al.* Antiangiogenic therapy using bevacizumab in recurrent high-grade glioma: impact on local control and patient survival. J Neurosurg 2009 Jan;110(1):173-80.

[9]   Nghiemphu P, Graham C, Liu W, Than T, Lai A, Green R, *et al.* A retrospective single institutional analysis of bevacizumab and chemotherapy versus non-bevacizumab treatments for recurrent glioblastoma. ASCO Meeting Abstracts 2008 May 20, 2008; 26(15_suppl):2023.

[10]   Norden AD, Drappatz J, Muzikansky A, David K, Gerard M, McNamara MB, *et al.* An exploratory survival analysis of anti-angiogenic therapy for recurrent malignant glioma. J Neurooncol 2009 Apr 92(2):149-55.

[11]   Poulsen HS, Grunnet K, Sorensen M, Olsen P, Hasselbalch B, Nelausen K, *et al.* Bevacizumab plus irinotecan in the treatment patients with progressive recurrent malignant brain tumours. Acta Oncol 2009 48(1):52-8.

[12]   Raval S, Hwang S, Dorsett L. Bevacizumab and irinotecan in patients (pts) with recurrent glioblastoma multiforme (GBM). ASCO Meeting Abstracts 2007 June 20, 2007;25(18_suppl):2078.

[13]   Stankewitz S, Dresemann G. Addition of continuous low dose temozolomide (T) to bevacizumab (Bev) plus irinotecan (Iri) after bevacizumab plus irinotecan failure in heavily pretreated glioblastoma multiforme (GBM). ASCO Meeting Abstracts 2009 May 20, 2009;27(15S):e13015.

[14]   Zuniga RM, Torcuator R, Jain R, Anderson J, Doyle T, Ellika S, *et al.* Efficacy, safety and patterns of response and recurrence in patients with recurrent high-grade gliomas treated with bevacizumab plus irinotecan. J Neurooncol 2009 Feb;91(3):329-36.

[15]   Vredenburgh JJ, Desjardins A, Herndon JE, II, Marcello J, Reardon DA, Quinn JA, *et al.* Bevacizumab Plus Irinotecan in Recurrent Glioblastoma Multiforme. J Clin Oncol 2007 October 20, 2007;25(30):4722-9.

[16]   Ballman KV, Buckner JC, Brown PD, Giannini C, Flynn PJ, LaPlant BR, *et al.* The relationship between six-month progression-free survival and 12-month overall survival end points for phase II trials in patients with glioblastoma multiforme. Neuro Oncol 2007 Jan;9(1):29-38.

[17]   Lamborn KR, Yung WK, Chang SM, Wen PY, Cloughesy TF, DeAngelis LM, *et al.* Progression-free survival: an important end point in evaluating therapy for recurrent high-grade gliomas. Neuro Oncol 2008 Apr;10(2):162-70.

[18]   Wong ET, Hess KR, Gleason MJ, Jaeckle KA, Kyritsis AP, Prados MD, *et al.* Outcomes and prognostic factors in recurrent glioma patients enrolled onto phase II clinical trials. J Clin Oncol 1999 Aug;17(8):2572-8.

[19]   Cloughesy TF, Prados MD, Wen PY, Mikkelsen T, Abrey LE, Schiff D, *et al.* A phase II, randomized, non-comparative clinical trial of the effect of bevacizumab (BV) alone or in combination with irinotecan (CPT) on 6-month progression free survival (PFS6) in recurrent, treatment-refractory glioblastoma (GBM). ASCO Meeting Abstracts 2008 May 20, 2008;26(15_suppl):2010b.

[20]   Kreisl TN, Kim L, Moore K, Duic P, Royce C, Stroud I, *et al.* Phase II Trial of Single-Agent Bevacizumab Followed by Bevacizumab Plus Irinotecan at Tumor Progression in Recurrent Glioblastoma. J Clin Oncol 2009 February 10, 2009;27(5):740-5.

[21]   Batchelor TT, Gilbert MR, Supko JG, Carson KA, Nabors LB, Grossman SA, *et al.* Phase 2 study of weekly irinotecan in adults with recurrent malignant glioma: final report of NABTT 97-11. Neuro Oncol 2004 Jan;6(1):21-7.

[22]   Prados MD, Lamborn K, Yung WK, Jaeckle K, Robins HI, Mehta M, *et al.* A phase 2 trial of irinotecan (CPT-11) in patients with recurrent malignant glioma: a North American Brain Tumor Consortium study. Neuro Oncol 2006 Apr;8(2):189-93.

[23]   Mohile NA, Abrey LE, Lymberis SC, Karimi S, Hou BL, Gutin PH. A pilot study of bevacizumab and stereotactic intensity modulated re-irradiation for recurrent high grade gliomas. ASCO Meeting Abstracts 2007 June 20, 2007;25(18_suppl):2028.

[24]   Rossi A, Torri V, Gridelli C. Paclitaxel plus bevacizumab for metastatic breast cancer. N Engl J Med 2008 Apr 10;358(15):1637; author reply -8.

[25]   Sathornsumetee S, Desjardins A, Vredenburgh JJ, Rich JN, Gururangan S, Friedman AH, *et al.* Phase II study of bevacizumab plus erlotinib for recurrent malignant gliomas. ASCO Meeting Abstracts 2009 May 20, 2009;27(15S):2045.

[26]   Norden AD, Young GS, Setayesh K, Muzikansky A, Klufas R, Ross GL, *et al.* Bevacizumab for recurrent malignant gliomas: efficacy, toxicity, and patterns of recurrence. Neurology 2008 Mar 4;70(10):779-87.

[27]   Nicholas MK, Lucas RV, Arzbaecher J, Paleologos N, Krouwer H, Malkin M, *et al.* Bevacizumab in combination with temozolomide in the adjuvant treatment of newly diagnosed glioblastoma multiforme: Preliminary results of a phase II study. ASCO Meeting Abstracts 2009 May 20, 2009;27(15S):2016.

[28]   Lai A, Filka E, McGibbon B, Nghiemphu PL, Graham C, Yong WH, *et al.* Phase II pilot study of bevacizumab in combination with temozolomide and regional radiation therapy for up-front treatment of patients with newly diagnosed glioblastoma multiforme: interim analysis of safety and tolerability. Int J Radiat Oncol Biol Phys 2008 Aug 1;71(5):1372-80.

[29]   Lai A, Nghiemphu P, Green R, Spier L, Peak S, Phuphanich S, *et al.* Phase II trial of bevacizumab in combination with temozolomide and regional radiation therapy for up-front treatment of patients with newly diagnosed glioblastoma multiforme. ASCO Meeting Abstracts 2009 May 20, 2009;27(15S):2000.

[30]   Narayana A, Golfinos JG, Fischer I, Raza S, Kelly P, Parker E, *et al.* Feasibility of using bevacizumab with radiation therapy and temozolomide in newly diagnosed high-grade glioma. Int J Radiat Oncol Biol Phys 2008 Oct 1;72(2):383-9.

[31]   Gruber ML, Raza S, Gruber D, Narayana A. Bevacizumab in combination with radiotherapy plus concomitant and adjuvant temozolomide for newly diagnosed glioblastoma: Update progression-free survival, overall survival, and toxicity. ASCO Meeting Abstracts 2009 May 20, 2009;27(15S):2017.

[32]   Ananthnarayan S, Bahng J, Roring J, Nghiemphu P, Lai A, Cloughesy T, *et al.* Time course of imaging changes of GBM during extended bevacizumab treatment. J Neurooncol 2008 Jul;88(3):339-47.

[33]   Wefel JS, Cloughesy T, Zazzali J, Yi J, Friedman HS, for the BI. Neurocognitive function in patients with glioblastoma multiforme in first or second relapse treated with bevacizumab in the BRAIN study. ASCO Meeting Abstracts 2009 May 20, 2009;27(15S):2056.

[34]   Lucio-Eterovic AK, Piao Y, de Groot JF. Mediators of glioblastoma resistance and invasion during antivascular endothelial growth factor therapy. Clin Cancer Res 2009 Jul 15;15(14):4589-99.

[35]   Lassman AB, Iwamoto FM, Gutin PH, Abrey LE. Patterns of relapse and prognosis after bevacizumab (BEV) failure in recurrent glioblastoma (GBM). ASCO Meeting Abstracts 2008 May 20, 2008;26(15_suppl):2028.

[36]   Potthast L, Chowdhary S, Pan E, Yu D, Zhu W, Brem S. The infiltrative, diffuse pattern of recurrence in patients with malignant gliomas treated with bevacizumab. ASCO Meeting Abstracts 2009 May 20, 2009;27(15S):2057.

[37]   Desjardins A, Barboriak DP, Herndon JE, II, Reardon DA, Quinn JA, Rich JN, *et al.* Dynamic contrast-enhanced magnetic resonance imaging (DCE-MRI) evaluation in glioblastoma (GBM) patients treated with bevacizumab (BEV) and irinotecan (CPT-11). ASCO Meeting Abstracts 2007 June 20, 2007;25(18_suppl):2029.

[38]   Paldino M, Desjardins A, Friedman HS, Vredenburgh JJ, Barboriak DP. Prognostic significance of early changes in the apparent diffusion coefficient that occurs after treatment of patients with glioblastoma multiforme with bevacizumab. ASCO Meeting Abstracts 2009 May 20, 2009;27(15S):2058.

[39]   Pope WB, Kim HJ, Huo J, Alger J, Brown MS, Gjertson D, *et al.* Recurrent glioblastoma multiforme: ADC histogram analysis predicts response to bevacizumab treatment. Radiology 2009 Jul;252(1):182-9.

[40]   Desjardins A, Reardon DA, Herndon JE, 2nd, Marcello J, Quinn JA, Rich JN, *et al.* Bevacizumab plus irinotecan in recurrent WHO grade 3 malignant gliomas. Clin Cancer Res 2008 Nov 1;14(21):7068-73.

[41]   Dresemann A, Hobbold A, Dresemann G. Bevacizumab (B) plus irinotecan (I) in progressive multiple pretreated and temozolomide (T) refractory glioblastoma multiforme (GBM): A single center experience using a low dose regimen. ASCO Meeting Abstracts 2008 May 20, 2008;26(15_suppl):13007.

[42]   Maron R, Vredenburgh JJ, Desjardins A, Reardon DA, Quinn JA, Rich JN, *et al.* Bevacizumab and daily temozolomide for recurrent glioblastoma multiforme (GBM). ASCO Meeting Abstracts 2008 May 20, 2008;26(15_suppl):2074.

[43]   Narayana A, Chheang S, Knopp E, Peccerelli N, Babb J, Johnson G, *et al.* Comparing cerebral blood volume and vascular permeability measurements with tumor volume measurements following anti-angiogenesis therapy in recurrent gliomas. ASCO Meeting Abstracts 2007 June 20, 2007;25(18_suppl):2030.

[44]   Nghiemphu PL, Liu W, Lee Y, Than T, Graham C, Lai A, *et al.* Bevacizumab and chemotherapy for recurrent glioblastoma: a single-institution experience. Neurology 2009 Apr 7;72(14):1217-22.

[45]   Raizer JJ, Gallot L, Cohn R, Chandler J, Levy R, Getch C, *et al.* A phase II safety study of bevacizumab in patients with multiple recurrent or progressive malignant gliomas. ASCO Meeting Abstracts 2007 June 20, 2007;25(18_suppl):2079.

[46]   Rich JN, Desjardins A, Sathornsumetee S, Vredenburgh JJ, Quinn JA, Gururangan S, *et al.* Phase II study of bevacizumab and etoposide in patients with recurrent malignant glioma. ASCO Meeting Abstracts 2008 May 20, 2008;26(15_suppl):2022

Bevacizumab with Hypofractionated Stereotactic Irradiation for Recurrent Malignant Gliomas

Fabio M. Iwamoto[1] and Philip H. Gutin[2,3,4,*]

[1]*Neuro-Oncology Branch, National Cancer Institute, National Institute of Neurological Disorders and Stroke, National Institutes of Health, Bethesda, Maryland,* [2]*The Brain Tumor Center and* [3]*Department of Neurosurgery, Memorial Sloan-Kettering Cancer Center;* [4]*Department of Neurological Surgery, Weill Medical College of Cornell University, New York, New York*

Abstract: Bevacizumab, a monoclonal antibody against vascular endothelial growth factor (VEGF), recently received accelerated approval by the US Federal and Drug Adminstration as single-agent for recurrent glioblastomas (GBM). Preclinical studies suggest that inhibition of VEGF and radiotherapy (RT) have a synergistic effect in gliomas. We recently conducted a pilot study of bevacizumab and hypo-fractionated stereotactic RT for patients with recurrent GBM and anaplastic gliomas (AG). Patients received bevacizumab (10 mg/kg IV) every 2 weeks of 28-day cycle and 30 Gy of hypofractionated stereotactic RT in 5 fractions after the first cycle of bevacizumab. Twenty-five patients (20 GBM and 5 AG) were included. For the GBM cohort, overall response rate was 50%, 6-month progression free survival was 65% and median overall survival was 12.5 months. Bevacizumab with hypofractionated RT is an active regimen in malignant gliomas and is currently being studied in newly-diagnosed glioblastomas in combination with temozolomide.

INTRODUCTION

Malignant gliomas, the most common primary brain tumors in adults, are associated with significant morbidity and mortality. The median survival from the initial diagnosis is approximately 15 months for protocol eligible glioblastomas (GBM) or grade IV gliomas and 2 to 5 years for anaplastic or grade III gliomas [1]. Despite aggressive treatment including maximal safe resection, radiotherapy (RT) and temozolomide, most patients with malignant gliomas develop progressive or recurrent tumor [2]. At time of progression, GBM patients have a median progression-free survival (PFS) time of only 9 weeks and median overall survival (OS) of 25 weeks, while anaplastic gliomas have a median PFS of 13 weeks and median OS of 47 weeks [3].

Malignant gliomas are highly vascular tumors with increased expression of vascular endothelial growth factor (VEGF) [4-6], which is a principal driver of tumor angiogenesis [7]. VEGF binds to VEGF receptor-2 (VEGFR-2) and induces endothelial cell proliferation, migration, and tumor angiogenesis [8]. Bevacizumab, a humanized monoclonal antibody that inhibits VEGF, recently received Food and Drug Administration (FDA) accelerated approval as single-agent for recurrent or progressive GBM based on two phase II clinical trials. The approval was based on demonstration of durable objective response rates observed in the bevacizumab monotherapy arm of a multicenter trial [9] and the National Cancer Institute intramural trial [10]. These trials have validated the VEGF pathway as an important therapeutic target in GBM but most patients develop tumor progression while on bevacizumab and median duration of response was approximately 4 months. Phase II studies combining bevacizumab with other agents such as irinotecan [9, 11], etoposide [12], erlotinib [13] and metronomic temozolomide [14] have not shown significant more activity than single-agent bevacizumab in recurrent GBM patients [9, 10].

RATIONALE FOR THE COMBINATION OF BEVACIZUMAB AND RADIOTHERAPY IN MALIGNANT GLIOMAS

Despite intrinsic glioma radioresistance and the limited radiation tolerance of surrounding normal brain, RT continues to be the most effective adjuvant treatment for malignant gliomas [15, 16]. The conventional explanation

*Address correspondence to Philip H. Gutin: Department of Neurosurgery, Memorial Sloan-Kettering Cancer Center, Tel: 212-639-8556, Fax: 212-717-3231, E-mail: gutinp@mskcc.org

Thomas C. Chen (Ed)

for the clinical utility of radiotherapy is that tumor cells are the main target of ionizing radiation, which damages tumor DNA causing glioma cells to undergo apoptosis [17]. However, there is increasing evidence that the radiosensitivity of the tumor as a whole is highly dependent on the sensitivity of the tumor vasculature to radiotherapy. Garcia-Barros and colleagues used knockout *asmase*[-/-] mice, which do not produce the pro-apoptotic lipid ceramide and thus have radiation-resistant endothelium, and showed that overall tumor response to radiation was highly dependent on endothelial cell apoptosis [18]. Moreover, tumor xenografts, including U87 gliomas, induce vascular endothelial growth factor (VEGF) expression in response to irradiation, which protects the tumor endothelium and decreases the RT efficacy [19, 20].

In fact, blocking angiogenesis can dramatically increase the radiosensitivity of tumor vasculature and as a result, increase overall tumor responsiveness to radiotherapy [19]. For example, the combination of angiostatin, a proteolytic fragment of plasminogen with known antiangiogenic activity, with radiation had synergistic anti-tumor effect in multiple cancer models, including gliomas [21]. Also, blockade of the VEGF receptor-2 by the monoclonal antibody DC101 can lower the dose of radiation needed to control tumor xenografts, including glioma U87 [22].

Malignant gliomas are innately hypoxic tumors and inhibition of angiogenesis could lead to increased hypoxia and further increase resistance to RT. However, experimental models have shown that anti-angiogenic drugs improve, at least temporarily, tumor oxygenation and thus response to RT [23, 24]. This paradoxal response is explained by the ability of anti-angiogenic drugs to 'normalize' the abnormal tumor vasculature, resulting in a more efficient oxygen delivery through redistribution of blood flow to hypoxic zones of tumor [25]. Winkler and colleagues studied U87 glioma animal models and showed that DC101 treatment markedly increased pericyte recruitment to tumor vessels, consequently 'normalizing' leaky, dilated tumor vessels and increasing tumor oxygenation. This temporary tumor vessel normalization and increased tumor oxygenation provide another rational basis for combining anti-angiogenic drugs with radiation [26].

In addition, recent evidence points to a population of glioma stem cells residing within vascular niches. These vascular niches, formed by abnormal tumor vessels, contribute directly to the maintenance of glioma stem cells and consequently tumor growth. These glioma stem cells are radioresistant [27] and may be a nidus for regrowth following RT. However, RT directed at endothelial cells and anti-angiogenic agents can disrupt this vascular niche, kill glioma stem cells, and consequently provide long-term tumor control [28, 29].

Because malignant gliomas usually relapse in their original tumor bed [30], anti-angiogenic treatment in the post-irradiation period may help to prevent recovery of the tumor bed. RT is known to damage the tumor stroma and delays regrowth, in part by the inability of the damaged bed to provide adequate vascularity [31]. Revascularization after RT depends upon both sprouting of local vessels and the incorporation of bone marrow-derived VEGFR-2-positive endothelial progenitor cells and perivascular infiltration of VEGFR-1-positive myelomonocytic cells [32, 33]. All of these mechanisms are suppressed by anti-VEGF therapies [33-35]. As examples, daily endostatin administered after radiation has been shown to block xenograft revascularization in mice, prolonging disease free survival.[36] Also, the growth rate of lung cancer xenografts, recurrent after irradiation, is slower in animals treated with DC101.[37]

In summary, reasons to combine bevacizumab and RT include the 1) ability of antiangiogenic agents to sensitize tumor endothelium to RT by depletion of VEGF and reduction of its pro-survival signaling, 2) potential tumor vessel normalization and improvement in tumor oxygenation and consequently reduced hypoxia-induced radioresistance, 3) potential ability to disrupt glioma stem cell vascular niches and 4) prevention of tumor vasculature recovery after RT by continuing anti-angiogenic treatment.

PILOT STUDY OF BEVACIZUMAB WITH HYPOFRACTIONATED STEREOTACTIC IRRADIATION FOR RECURRENT MALIGNANT GLIOMAS

We conducted a pilot study of bevacizumab and hypofractionated stereotactic irradiation in adult patients with recurrent or progressive malignant glioma who had failed prior RT [38]. The maximum tumor size allowed was ≤ 3.5 cm in its largest diameter. Patients received bevacizumab 10 mg/kg every 14 days on days 1 and 15 of 28-day cycles. After completion of the first cycle of bevacizumab, patients underwent a total dose of 30 Gy (6 Gy x 5 fractions), starting on day 7-10 of cycle 2 and delivered over a two and half week period.

Twenty-five patients with histologically confirmed malignant glioma (20 GBM, 5 AG) were enrolled in this single institution trial at Memorial Sloan-Kettering Cancer Center. The median age of patients was 56 years and median Karnofsky performance scale was 80. Only one patient did not undergo hypofractionated stereotactic RT because overlap with prior RT would exceed the safe dose allowed to the optic chiasm. Of the 24 patients who received radiation therapy all had re-irradiation to the same region that was previously treated to 60 Gy except for one patient who had a recurrence outside of their initial field; the median planning target volume was 34 cm^3 (range 2 to 62 cm^3).

Overall the combination of bevacizumab and re-irradiation was well tolerated. Three patients discontinued treatment due to toxicity; one patient had a grade 3 CNS intratumoral hemorrhage, one had bowel perforation in the setting of chronic dexamethasone, and one patient who had undergone craniotomy for tumor resection four weeks prior to starting bevacizumab developed wound dehiscence. In fact, bevacizumab appeared to have improved the therapeutic ratio of radiation with a lower than expected side effects and no cases of radionecrosis. Moreover, patients did not require additional corticosteroid use during or after RT and most patients were able to discontinue or decrease dexamethasone during the clinical trial.

Thirteen patients (52%) had an objective radiographic response (ORR), including complete response in five and partial response in eight. Fifty percent of patients with GBM and 60% of patients with AG had an ORR. Twelve patients (48%) had stable disease for a median of 4.6 months. The 6-month PFS was 65% for GBM and 60% for AG patients. The median PFS was 7.3 months for GBM and 7.5 months for AG patients. Median OS was 12.5 months for GBM and 16.5 months for the AG patients.

These results compare favorably to historical controls even considering selection of smaller tumors and patients with good performance status. For example, Vordermark and his coworkers [39] re-irradiated patients with recurrent malignant gliomas with hypofractionated regimens similar to the one we adopted and the median OS for GBM was 7.9 months. Moreover, our 6-month PFS of 65% in recurrent GBM also seemed better than patients treated with single-agent bevacizumab (6-month PFS of 29% to 42.6%) [9, 10], suggesting that addition of re-irradiation to bevacizumab was beneficial to this patient population (Table).

LIMITATIONS OF CURRENT STUDY AND FUTURE DIRECTIONS

Although these initial results of combining hypofractionated stereotactic irradiation with bevacizumab for recurrent malignant gliomas seem promising, our sample size was relatively small and the selection of smaller tumors may explain at least part of our favorable findings. Moreover, the radiation dose necessary to induce endothelial cell apoptosis in humans is still unknown. We used an aggressive radiation regimen but experimental studies suggest that fractions as high as 8 to 10 Gy may be necessary to cause endothelial apoptosis [18]. Moreover, the ideal timing to combine radiation with antiangiogenic drugs in humans in unclear but future studies should try to take advantage of tumor vessel normalization and increased tumor oxygenation, which consequently enhances response to RT [40].

Bevacizumab with hypofractionated radiotherapy was well tolerated suggesting that it is reasonable to treat larger tumors with this regimen and also to export this approach to a newly diagnosed patient population. A phase II trial of hypofractionated RT with bevacizumab and temozolomide for newly-diagnosed GBM is ongoing at Memorial Sloan-Kettering Cancer Center and allows tumor volume up to 60 cm^3 or approximately 5 cm in maximum diameter.

Table 1: Prospective Studies of Bevacizumab for Recurrent Glioblastoma

Study	N patients	Median Age	Median KPS	Median prior recurrences	Radiographic response rate	6-month PFS	Median PFS (months)	Median OS (months)
Bevacizumab single agent [10]	48	53	90	2	35%	29%	3.7	7.2
Bevacizumab single agent [9]	85	54	80	1	28.2%	42.6%	4.2	9.2

Bevacizumab plus irinotecan [9]	82	57	80	1	37.8%	50.3%	5.6	8.7
Bevacizumab plus irinotecan [11]	35	48	80	2	57%	46%	5.6	9.8
Bevacizumab plus re-irradiation [38]	20	56	80	1	50%	65%	7.3	12.5
Bevacizumab plus etoposide [12]	27	NA	NA	NA	NA	44%	NA	10.7
Bevacizumab plus erlotinib [13]	25	NA	NA	NA	48%	24%	NA	NA
Bevacizumab plus daily temozolomide [14]	32	NA	NA	NA	37.5%	NA	NA	NA

KPS = Karnofsky performance scale; PFS = progression-free survival; OS = overall survival; NA = not available.

REFERENCES

[1] Wen PY, Kesari S. Malignant gliomas in adults. N Engl J Med 2008 Jul 31;359(5):492-507.

[2] Stupp R, Mason WP, van den Bent MJ, Weller M, Fisher B, Taphoorn MJ, *et al.* Radiotherapy plus concomitant and adjuvant temozolomide for glioblastoma. N Engl J Med 2005 Mar 10;352(10):987-96.

[3] Wong ET, Hess KR, Gleason MJ, Jaeckle KA, Kyritsis AP, Prados MD, *et al.* Outcomes and prognostic factors in recurrent glioma patients enrolled onto phase II clinical trials. J Clin Oncol 1999 Aug;17(8):2572-8.

[4] Plate KH, Breier G, Weich HA, Risau W. Vascular endothelial growth factor is a potential tumour angiogenesis factor in human gliomas in vivo. Nature 1992 Oct 29;359(6398):845-8.

[5] Lamszus K, Ulbricht U, Matschke J, Brockmann MA, Fillbrandt R, Westphal M. Levels of soluble vascular endothelial growth factor (VEGF) receptor 1 in astrocytic tumors and its relation to malignancy, vascularity, and VEGF-A. Clin Cancer Res 2003 Apr;9(4):1399-405.

[6] Samoto K, Ikezaki K, Ono M, Shono T, Kohno K, Kuwano M, *et al.* Expression of vascular endothelial growth factor and its possible relation with neovascularization in human brain tumors. Cancer Res 1995 Mar 1;55(5):1189-93.

[7] Millauer B, Shawver LK, Plate KH, Risau W, Ullrich A. Glioblastoma growth inhibited *in vivo* by a dominant-negative Flk-1 mutant. Nature 1994 Feb 10;367(6463):576-9.

[8] Ferrara N, Gerber HP, LeCouter J. The biology of VEGF and its receptors. Nat Med 2003 Jun;9(6):669-76.

[9] Friedman HS, Prados MD, Wen PY, Mikkelsen T, Schiff D, Abrey LE, *et al.* Bevacizumab Alone and in Combination With Irinotecan in Recurrent Glioblastoma. J Clin Oncol 2009 Aug 31.

[10] Kreisl TN, Kim L, Moore K, Duic P, Royce C, Stroud I, *et al.* Phase II trial of single-agent bevacizumab followed by bevacizumab plus irinotecan at tumor progression in recurrent glioblastoma. J Clin Oncol 2009 Feb 10;27(5):740-5.

[11] Vredenburgh JJ, Desjardins A, Herndon JE, 2nd, Marcello J, Reardon DA, Quinn JA, *et al.* Bevacizumab plus irinotecan in recurrent glioblastoma multiforme. J Clin Oncol 2007 Oct 20;25(30):4722-9.

[12] Reardon D, Desjardins A, Vredenburgh JJ, Gururangan S, Peters KB, Norfleet JA. Bevacizumab plus etoposide among recurrent malignant glioma patients: Phase II study final results. J Clin Oncol (Meeting Abstracts) 2009 May 20, 2009;27(15S):2046-.

[13] Sathornsumetee S, Desjardins A, Vredenburgh JJ, Rich JN, Gururangan S, Friedman AH, *et al.* Phase II study of bevacizumab plus erlotinib for recurrent malignant gliomas. J Clin Oncol (Meeting Abstracts) 2009 May 20, 2009;27(15S):2045-.

[14] Maron R, Vredenburgh JJ, Desjardins A, Reardon DA, Quinn JA, Rich JN, *et al.* Bevacizumab and daily temozolomide for recurrent glioblastoma multiforme (GBM). J Clin Oncol (Meeting Abstracts) 2008 May 20, 2008;26(15_suppl):2074-.

[15] Sheline GE, Wara WM, Smith V. Therapeutic irradiation and brain injury. Int J Radiat Oncol Biol Phys 1980 Sep;6(9):1215-28.

[16] Walker MD, Strike TA, Sheline GE. An analysis of dose-effect relationship in the radiotherapy of malignant gliomas. Int J Radiat Oncol Biol Phys 1979 Oct;5(10):1725-

[17] Folkman J, Camphausen K. Cancer. What does radiotherapy do to endothelial cells? Science 2001 Jul 13;293(5528):227-8.

[18] Garcia-Barros M, Paris F, Cordon-Cardo C, Lyden D, Rafii S, Haimovitz-Friedman A, *et al.* Tumor response to radiotherapy regulated by endothelial cell apoptosis. Science 2003 May 16;300(5622):1155-9.

[19] Gorski DH, Beckett MA, Jaskowiak NT, Calvin DP, Mauceri HJ, Salloum RM, *et al.* Blockage of the vascular endothelial growth factor stress response increases the antitumor effects of ionizing radiation. Cancer Res 1999 Jul 15;59(14):3374-8.

[20] Moeller BJ, Cao Y, Li CY, Dewhirst MW. Radiation activates HIF-1 to regulate vascular radiosensitivity in tumors: role of reoxygenation, free radicals, and stress granules. Cancer Cell 2004 May;5(5):429-41.

[21] Mauceri HJ, Hanna NN, Beckett MA, Gorski DH, Staba MJ, Stellato KA, *et al.* Combined effects of angiostatin and ionizing radiation in antitumour therapy. Nature 1998 Jul 16;394(6690):287-91.

[22] Kozin SV, Boucher Y, Hicklin DJ, Bohlen P, Jain RK, Suit HD. Vascular endothelial growth factor receptor-2-blocking antibody potentiates radiation-induced long-term control of human tumor xenografts. Cancer Res 2001 Jan 1;61(1):39-44.

[23] Teicher BA, Holden SA, Ara G, Dupuis NP, Liu F, Yuan J, *et al.* Influence of an anti-angiogenic treatment on 9L gliosarcoma: oxygenation and response to cytotoxic therapy. Int J Cancer 1995 May 29;61(5):732-7.

[24] Griffin RJ, Williams BW, Wild R, Cherrington JM, Park H, Song CW. Simultaneous inhibition of the receptor kinase activity of vascular endothelial, fibroblast, and platelet-derived growth factors suppresses tumor growth and enhances tumor radiation response. Cancer Res 2002 Mar 15;62(6):1702-6.

[25] Jain RK. Normalization of tumor vasculature: an emerging concept in antiangiogenic therapy. Science 2005 Jan 7;307(5706):58-62.

[26] Winkler F, Kozin SV, Tong RT, Chae SS, Booth MF, Garkavtsev I, *et al.* Kinetics of vascular normalization by VEGFR2 blockade governs brain tumor response to radiation: role of oxygenation, angiopoietin-1, and matrix metalloproteinases. Cancer Cell 2004 Dec;6(6):553-63.

[27] Bao S, Wu Q, McLendon RE, Hao Y, Shi Q, Hjelmeland AB, *et al.* Glioma stem cells promote radioresistance by preferential activation of the DNA damage response. Nature 2006 Dec 7;444(7120):756-60.

[28] Bao S, Wu Q, Sathornsumetee S, Hao Y, Li Z, Hjelmeland AB, *et al.* Stem cell-like glioma cells promote tumor angiogenesis through vascular endothelial growth factor. Cancer Res 2006 Aug 15;66(16):7843-8.

[29] Calabrese C, Poppleton H, Kocak M, Hogg TL, Fuller C, Hamner B, *et al.* A perivascular niche for brain tumor stem cells. Cancer Cell 2007 Jan;11(1):69-82.

[30] Hochberg FH, Pruitt A. Assumptions in the radiotherapy of glioblastoma. Neurology 1980 Sep;30(9):907-11.

[31] Milas L, Ito H, Hunter N, Jones S, Peters LJ. Retardation of tumor growth in mice caused by radiation-induced injury of tumor bed stroma: dependency on tumor type. Cancer Res 1986 Feb;46(2):723-7.

[32] Ahn GO, Brown JM. Matrix metalloproteinase-9 is required for tumor vasculogenesis but not for angiogenesis: role of bone marrow-derived myelomonocytic cells. Cancer Cell 2008 Mar;13(3):193-205.

[33] Rafii S, Lyden D, Benezra R, Hattori K, Heissig B. Vascular and haematopoietic stem cells: novel targets for anti-angiogenesis therapy? Nat Rev Cancer 2002 Nov;2(11):826-35.

[34] Batchelor TT, Sorensen AG, di Tomaso E, Zhang WT, Duda DG, Cohen KS, *et al.* AZD2171, a pan-VEGF receptor tyrosine kinase inhibitor, normalizes tumor vasculature and alleviates edema in glioblastoma patients. Cancer Cell 2007 Jan;11(1):83-95.

[35] Kerbel RS. Tumor angiogenesis. N Engl J Med 2008 May 8;358(19):2039-49.

[36] Itasaka S, Komaki R, Herbst RS, Shibuya K, Shintani T, Hunter NR, *et al.* Endostatin improves radioresponse and blocks tumor revascularization after radiation therapy for A431 xenografts in mice. Int J Radiat Oncol Biol Phys 2007 Mar 1;67(3):870-8.

[37] Kozin SV, Winkler F, Garkavtsev I, Hicklin DJ, Jain RK, Boucher Y. Human tumor xenografts recurring after radiotherapy are more sensitive to anti-vascular endothelial growth factor receptor-2 treatment than treatment-naive tumors. Cancer Res 2007 Jun 1;67(11):5076-82.

[38] Gutin PH, Iwamoto FM, Beal K, Mohile NA, Karimi S, Hou BL, *et al.* Safety and efficacy of bevacizumab with hypofractionated stereotactic irradiation for recurrent malignant gliomas. Int J Radiat Oncol Biol Phys 2009 Sep 1;75(1):156-63.

[39] Vordermark D, Kolbl O, Ruprecht K, Vince GH, Bratengeier K, Flentje M. Hypofractionated stereotactic re-irradiation: treatment option in recurrent malignant glioma. BMC Cancer 2005;5:55.

[40] Ou G, Itasaka S, Zeng L, Shibuya K, Yi J, Harada H, *et al.* Usefulness of HIF-1 imaging for determining optimal timing of combining bevacizumab and radiotherapy. Int J Radiat Oncol Biol Phys 2009 Oct 1;75(2):463-7

CHAPTER 5

Bevacizumab Failure in Patients with Recurrent Malignant Glioma

Andrew D. Norden[*]

Brigham and Women's Hospital, Dana-Farber/Brigham and Women's Cancer Center, Harvard Medical School, Boston MA 02115

Abstract: In patients with recurrent malignant glioma, bevacizumab therapy achieves high response rates, prolonged progression-free survival, and reduced corticosteroid requirements. However, progressive disease during bevacizumab therapy is the rule. Resistance to bevacizumab may be mediated by upregulation of alternative pro-angiogenic factors or an infiltrative tumor growth pattern characterized by vascular co-option. Clinically, bevacizumab failure is often followed by rapid progression and death. In patients with progressive disease despite bevacizumab monotherapy, adding cytotoxic chemotherapy has not proven beneficial. Similarly, when patients develop progressive disease despite bevacizumab and chemotherapy, continuing bevacizumab and changing the concurrent chemotherapy agent is not effective. Combining bevacizumab with anti-invasion therapies is an appealing approach that has yet to be investigated in clinical trials. Additional research into mechanisms of resistance to anti-angiogenic therapy is needed in order to develop other promising strategies.

INTRODUCTION

The introduction of bevacizumab into the therapeutic armamentarium for malignant gliomas is among the most important advances in malignant gliomas therapy of the past decade. The benefits of bevacizumab therapy have been demonstrated by several retrospective series [1-4] and prospective clinical trials [5-8]. These include high radiographic response rates, prolongation of progression-free survival (PFS), and reduced corticosteroid requirements for the majority of patients. Other purported but as yet unsubstantiated benefits include improved quality-of-life and prolonged overall survival. Toxicity is mild in most cases, although bevacizumab therapy is associated with rare, catastrophic or life-threatening complications. Unfortunately, neither bevacizumab nor other anti-angiogenic therapies are curative, and patients go on to develop progressive disease which ultimately proves fatal. The management of progressive disease after bevacizumab failure is challenging. As yet, no effective therapy for this scenario has emerged. Recent pre-clinical and clinical reports suggest potential avenues that should be explored in attempting to identify an effective salvage regimen.

Limited data suggest that failure of anti-angiogenic therapy may correlate with upregulation of alternative pro-angiogenic factors such as basic fibroblast growth factor (bFGF) [9], stromal-derived factor-1α (SDF1α) [9], the angiopoietin receptor tie2, and placental growth factor (PlGF) [10], or with mobilization of circulating endothelial cells or their bone marrow-derived precursor cells [9, 11]. Older pre-clinical data suggested that anti-angiogenic therapy might promote an infiltrative tumor growth pattern characterized by co-option of existing cerebral blood vessels [12-16]. In an orthotopic mouse model of glioblastoma (GBM), genetic deletion of vascular endothelial growth factor (VEGF) or other pro-angiogenic molecules increased vascular co-option [17]. The findings were corroborated in the same murine tumor model by blocking VEGF receptors with two different inhibitors; in each case, increased infiltration of tumor cells along existing vasculature was observed [18]. Additionally, the authors showed in a model of pancreatic neuroendocrine cancer that anti-angiogenic therapy increased the likelihood of metastasis [18]. These changes in tumor phenotype may reflect attempts on the part of individual tumor cells to access new sources of nutrients and oxygen and to eliminate cellular waste products, even when neoangiogenesis is inhibited. These pre-clinical findings are consistent with the observation in recurrent bevacizumab-treated malignant glioma patients that there is an increased risk of infiltrative, non-enhancing tumor growth observed on MRI scans, as shown in (Fig. **1**) [2, 19-21].

Perhaps in part because of increased infiltrative growth, tumors that progress during bevacizumab therapy cannot be

---
*Address correspondence to this Andrew D. Norden: Brigham and Women's Hospital, Dana-Farber/Brigham and Women's Cancer Center, Harvard Medical School, Boston MA 02115, Tel: 617-632-4773, Fax: 617-632-2166; Email: ANORDEN@PARTNERS.ORG

satisfactorily treated in most circumstances. Though not formally reported in the literature, many neuro-oncologists observe that withdrawal of bevacizumab results in rapid emergence of peri-tumoral edema and associated neurologic symptoms. When patients are continued on bevacizumab, progressive clinical deterioration and death frequently occur. The best way to treat patients whose tumors progress despite anti-angiogenic therapy is unclear. In a retrospective series of 54 recurrent malignant glioma patients who were treated with bevacizumab in combination with cytotoxic chemotherapy, continuing bevacizumab and changing to an alternative chemotherapeutic at recurrence was ineffective. This approach provided a median PFS of approximately 6 weeks, and a single patient achieved 6-month PFS [22]. There were no radiographic responders. In a phase II study of 48 recurrent GBM patients treated with bevacizumab monotherapy, 19 patients went on to receive combination therapy with bevacizumab and irinotecan at recurrence [6]. Standard doses were used (bevacizumab 10 mg/kg every 2 weeks and irinotecan 125 or 340 mg/m^2 every 2 weeks, depending on enzyme-inducing anti-epileptic drug status). Despite an encouraging median PFS of 16 weeks for patients treated with bevacizumab monotherapy, the median PFS for patients who recurred again and were treated with the combination had a median PFS of only 30 days. There were no radiographic responses using standard Macdonald criteria [23].

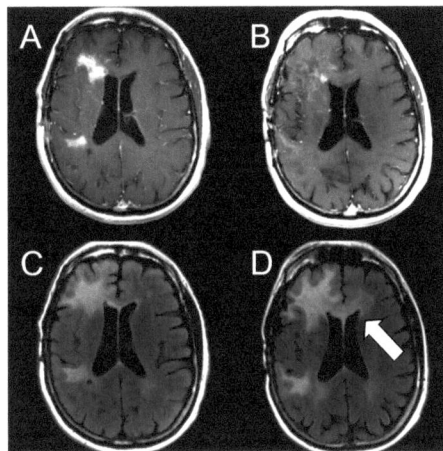

Figure 1: T1 post-gadolinium (A) and fluid-attenuated inversion recovery (FLAIR; C) MRI scan in a patient with recurrent glioblastoma prior to bevacizumab therapy, showing multifocal enhancing disease with surrounding FLAIR hyperintensity. After 8 months of treatment with bevacizumab 10 mg/kg every 2 weeks, contrast enhancement remains well controlled on the T1 post-gadolinium image (B). However, there is increasing FLAIR hyperintensity in the genu of the corpus callosum (arrow, D), suggestive of progressive non-enhancing tumor growth.

Thus, it appears that combining bevacizumab with cytotoxic chemotherapy after failure of bevacizumab monotherapy or combination therapy is not an effective approach. An open question is whether changing from bevacizumab to an alternative anti-angiogenic or targeted molecular drug may be worthwhile. In a phase II study of 46 recurrent GBM patients treated with the VEGF receptor and c-Met inhibitor XL184 at a dose of 175 mg by mouth daily, 11 patients had been previously treated with other anti-angiogenic therapies (8 bevacizumab, 2 vandetanib, 1 aflibercept [VEGF-Trap]) [24]. Of these, 9 patients were evaluable for efficacy, and 3 of the 9 had measurable tumor shrinkage. One achieved partial response. The median PFS for this small cohort was 55 days. Because of toxicity, primarily including fatigue and palmar-plantar erythrodysesthesia, dosing interruptions occurred frequently. The phase II study has recently re-opened with a number of changes intended to minimize toxicity-related treatment interruptions. Although most enrolled patients will be naïve to anti-angiogenic therapy, 20 of the 100 planned accruals will be patients whose tumors have progressed on bevacizumab.

No other clinical data have been reported in malignant glioma patients who have failed bevacizumab therapy. In light of the pre-clinical data reported above, which suggests invasive growth and vascular co-option as important mechanisms of resistance to bevacizumab and other anti-VEGF targeted therapies, combining bevacizumab with anti-invasive strategies may prove fruitful. Thus far, only a small number of anti-invasive therapeutics have been developed for malignant glioma. Targets of potential interest include NF-κB, hepatocyte growth factor/scatter factor (HGF/SF), stromal derived factor-1α (SDF-1α), focal adhesion kinase (FAK), matrix metalloproteinases 2 and 9 (MMP-2, MMP-9), Akt, transforming growth factor-β (TGF-β), tenascin, integrins, and src, among many others

[25]. Drugs that inhibit several of these targets have been evaluated in early trials in malignant glioma. None have yet been combined in clinical trials with anti-angiogenic therapies, nor used in patients following failure of anti-angiogenic therapies. A phase I clinical trial that is currently in development in the Adult Brain Tumor Consortium (ABTC) will evaluate the combination of the pan-VEGF receptor inhibitor cediranib with the $\alpha v \beta 3$ and $\alpha v \beta 5$ integrin inhibitor cilengitide for recurrent malignant glioma. Both drugs have shown promising results in phase II monotherapy trials for recurrent GBM [9, 26]. The cediranib-cilengitide trial will represent an important proof-of-principle for combination anti-angiogenesis/anti-invasion therapy.

Although bevacizumab represents an important step forward in malignant glioma therapy, resistance to therapy inevitably emerges, distressingly often after only a few months of treatment. Pre-clinical and human imaging data suggest that the addition of effective anti-invasion therapy to bevacizumab could dramatically improve outcomes. However, our understanding of the mechanisms of resistance to bevacizumab in glioma therapy is relatively limited. As scientists further unravel the means by which glioma cells overcome bevacizumab's potent anti-angiogenic effect, important new therapeutic targets are likely to emerge.

REFERENCES

[1]   Guiu S, Taillibert S, Chinot O, *et al.* [Bevacizumab/Irinotecan. An active treatment for recurrent high grade gliomas: Preliminary results of an ANOCEF Multicenter Study.]. Rev Neurol (Paris). 2008 June - July;164(6-7):588-94.

[2]   Norden AD, Young GS, Setayesh K, *et al.* Bevacizumab for recurrent malignant gliomas: efficacy, toxicity, and patterns of recurrence. Neurology. 2008 Mar 4;70(10):779-87.

[3]   Pope WB, Lai A, Nghiemphu P, Mischel P, Cloughesy TF. MRI in patients with high-grade gliomas treated with bevacizumab and chemotherapy. Neurology. 2006 Apr 25;66(8):1258-60.

[4]   Stark Vance V. Bevacizumab (Avastin®) and CPT-11 (Camptosar®) in the Treatment of Relapsed Malignant Glioma. World Federation of Neuro-Oncology Second Quadrennial Meeting; 2005 May 5-8; Edinburgh, Scotland. 2005.

[5]   Cloughesy TF, Prados MD, Mikkelsen T, *et al.* A phase II, randomized, non-comparative clinical trial of the effect of bevacizumab (BV) alone or in combination with irinotecan (CPT) on 6-month progression free survival (PFS6) in recurrent, treatment-refractory glioblastoma (GBM). American Society of Clinical Oncology 44th Annual Meeting; 2008 May 30 - Jun 3; Chicago. 2008.

[6]   Kreisl TN, Kim L, Moore K, *et al.* Phase II trial of single-agent bevacizumab followed by bevacizumab plus irinotecan at tumor progression in recurrent glioblastoma. J Clin Oncol. 2009 Feb 10;27(5):740-5.

[7]   Vredenburgh JJ, Desjardins A, Herndon JE, 2nd, *et al.* Phase II trial of bevacizumab and irinotecan in recurrent malignant glioma. Clin Cancer Res. 2007 Feb 15;13(4):1253-9.

[8]   Vredenburgh JJ, Desjardins A, Herndon JE, 2nd, *et al.* Bevacizumab plus irinotecan in recurrent glioblastoma multiforme. J Clin Oncol. 2007 Oct 20;25(30):4722-9.

[9]   Batchelor TT, Sorensen AG, di Tomaso E, *et al.* AZD2171, a pan-VEGF receptor tyrosine kinase inhibitor, normalizes tumor vasculature and alleviates edema in glioblastoma patients. Cancer Cell. 2007 Jan;11(1):83-95.

[10]   Willett CG, Boucher Y, Duda DG, *et al.* Surrogate markers for antiangiogenic therapy and dose-limiting toxicities for bevacizumab with radiation and chemotherapy: continued experience of a phase I trial in rectal cancer patients. J Clin Oncol. 2005 Nov 1;23(31):8136-9.

[11]   Kerbel RS. Tumor angiogenesis. N Engl J Med. 2008 May 8;358(19):2039-49.

[12]   Chi A, Norden AD, Wen PY. Inhibition of angiogenesis and invasion in malignant gliomas. Expert Rev Anticancer Ther. 2007 Nov;7(11):1537-60.

[13]   Holash J, Maisonpierre PC, Compton D, *et al.* Vessel cooption, regression, and growth in tumors mediated by angiopoietins and VEGF. Science. 1999 Jun 18;284(5422):1994-8.

[14]   Kunkel P, Ulbricht U, Bohlen P, *et al.* Inhibition of glioma angiogenesis and growth *in vivo* by systemic treatment with a monoclonal antibody against vascular endothelial growth factor receptor-2. Cancer Res. 2001 Sep 15;61(18):6624-8.

[15]   Lamszus K, Kunkel P, Westphal M. Invasion as limitation to anti-angiogenic glioma therapy. Acta Neurochir Suppl. 2003;88:169-77.

[16]   Rubenstein JL, Kim J, Ozawa T, *et al.* Anti-VEGF antibody treatment of glioblastoma prolongs survival but results in increased vascular cooption. Neoplasia. 2000 Jul-Aug;2(4):306-14.

[17]   Du R, Lu KV, Petritsch C, *et al.* HIF1alpha induces the recruitment of bone marrow-derived vascular modulatory cells to regulate tumor angiogenesis and invasion. Cancer Cell. 2008 Mar;13(3):206-20.

[18]   Paez-Ribes M, Allen E, Hudock J, *et al.* Antiangiogenic therapy elicits malignant progression of tumors to increased local invasion and distant metastasis. Cancer Cell. 2009 Mar 3;15(3):220-31.

[19]   Lassman AB, Iwamoto FM, Gutin PH, Abrey LE. Patterns of relapse and prognosis after bevacizumab (BEV) failure in recurrent glioblastoma (GBM). American Society of Clinical Oncology 44th Annual Meeting; 2008 May 30 - Jun 3; Chicago. 2008.

[20]   Narayana A, Kelly P, Golfinos J, *et al.* Antiangiogenic therapy using bevacizumab in recurrent high-grade glioma: impact on local control and patient survival. J Neurosurg. 2009 Jan;110(1):173-80.

[21]   Zuniga RM, Torcuator R, Doyle T, *et al.* Retrospective analysis of patterns of recurrence seen on MRI in patients with recurrent glioblastoma multiforme treated with bevacizumab plus irinotecan. American Society of Clinical Oncology 44th Annual Meeting; 2008 May 30 - Jun 3; Chicago. 2008.

[22]   Quant E, Norden AD, Drappatz J, *et al.* Role of a second chemotherapy in recurrent malignant glioma patients who progress on a bevacizumab-containing regimen [abstract]. J Clin Oncol. 2008;26:2008.

[23]   Macdonald DR, Cascino TL, Schold SC, Jr., Cairncross JG. Response criteria for phase II studies of supratentorial malignant glioma. J Clin Oncol. 1990 Jul;8(7):1277-80.

[24]   De Groot J, Prados M, Urquhart T, *et al.* A Phase 2 Study of XL184 in Patients with Progressive Glioblastoma Multiforme. American Society of Clinical Oncology 45th Annual Meeting; 2009; Orlando. 2009.

[25]   Drappatz J, Norden AD, Wen PY. Therapeutic strategies for inhibiting invasion in glioblastoma. Expert Rev Neurother. 2009 Apr;9(4):519-34.

[26]   Reardon DA, Fink KL, Mikkelsen T, *et al.* Randomized phase II study of cilengitide, an integrin-targeting arginine-glycine-aspartic acid peptide, in recurrent glioblastoma multiforme. J Clin Oncol. 2008 Dec 1;26(34):5610-7.

CHAPTER 6

An Update on the Role of Anti-Angiogenic Therapy for Newly Diagnosed Glioblastoma

David A. Reardon[1, 2,*], Sith Sathornsumetee[4] and James V. Vredenburgh[3]

[1]*Departments of Surgery,* [2]*Pediatrics, and* [3]*Medicine, The Preston Robert Tisch Brain Tumor Center, Duke University Medical Center, Durham, NC 27710,* [4]*Director, Neuro-Oncology Program, Department of Medicine, Faculty of Medicine Siriraj Hospital, Mahidol University, Bangkok, Thailand*

Abstract: Given the marked upregulation of angiogenesis in glioblastoma, the integration of anti-angiogenic agents into treatment approaches is a highly attractive consideration. Preclinical data support an anti-tumor benefit with anti-angiogenic agents in GBM models. However, translation of these agents into the clinic was initially tempered by concern that anti-angiogenics may be associated with severe complications in brain tumor patients including hemorrhages and strokes. Extensive clinical experience to date provides reassurance that such complications are rare and that anti-angiogenics can be safely administered to brain tumor patients. Furthermore, clinical trials conducted among recurrent GBM patients using either bevacizumab, a humanized monoclonal antibody against the primary mediator of tumor angiogenesis, vascular endothelial growth factor (VEGF), or VEGF-receptor tyrosine kinase inhibitors such as cediranib, demonstrate encouraging evidence of anti-tumor benefit. In particular, durable radiographic responses observed among recurrent GBM patients were sufficiently frequent to lead to accelerated approval by the U.S. Food and Drug Administration for bevacizumab in May, 2009. Ongoing efforts are evaluating additional strategies to augment the anti-tumor benefit of anti-angiogenic agents for recurrent patients as well as the safety and efficacy of these agents among newly diagnosed GBM patients.

INTRODUCTION

Malignant gliomas, including the most common subtype, glioblastoma (GBM), remain highly lethal tumors despite current, multi-modality therapy [1]. Although temozolomide given during and after radiotherapy provides a modest increment to improve outcome compared to radiation alone, recurrence is essentially universal [2,3]. Furthermore, recent meta-analyses of salvage therapies evaluated in cooperative group studies reveal negligible anti-tumor benefit which is as poor or worse, than that achieved historically [4-6].

Dysregulated, prominent angiogenesis, driven primarily by hypoxia-dependent and independent VEGF overexpression is a hallmark of malignant gliomas [7-12]. Preclinical studies confirm substantial anti-tumor benefit of targeting VEGF in malignant glioma animal models [13,14]. Initial clinical studies of bevacizumab among recurrent patients yielded dramatic radiographic responses and less impressive, yet encouraging, PFS and OS benefit [15-18]. Bevacizumab subsequently received FDA accelerated approval in May 2009 for recurrent GBM based on durable response rates [19,20]. Analogously, preliminary results with VEGFR tyrosine kinase inhibitors have also yielded encouraging results, and a phase 3 randomized registration study of the pan-VEGFR TKI cediranib for recurrent GBM is nearing completion [21].

Although significant angst regarding risks, particularly hemorrhage and stroke, initially delayed undertaking anti-VEGF therapy clinical trials for primary CNS tumor patients, a substantial accumulated body of clinical data now supports a comparable toxicity profile among these patients to that of other cancer populations. Specifically, among recurrent malignant glioma patients treated on prospective studies with bevacizumab monotherapy (n=132), the incidence of wound dehiscence, GI perforation, CNS hemorrhage and grade ≥ 3 thrombosis are 1.5%, 0.8%, 0, and 7.8% [19,20]. These complications vary slightly following bevacizumab plus the topoisomerase-1 inhibitor irinotecan (n=204): 0.5%, 0.5%, 2.5% and 11.8%, respectively [15,16,19,22]. Data regarding toxicities following VEGFR tyrosine kinase inhibitor therapy are limited due to small patient numbers reported on prospective studies to date. However, preliminary analysis of a phase 2 study revealed no episodes of wound dehiscence, GI perforation, CNS hemorrhage or thrombosis among recurrent GBM patients treated with cediranib [21].

[2]**Address correspondence to David A. Reardon:** The Preston Robert Tisch Brain Tumor Center at Duke, Duke University Medical Center, Box 3624, Durham, NC 27710; Tel: 919.668.2650; Fax: 919.668.2485; Email: reard003@mc.duke.edu

RATIONALE

Several factors support the evaluation of anti-angiogenic therapy among newly diagnosed GBM patients. First, as discussed above, substantial accumulated data confirms the benefit as well as safety of these agents among recurrent patients. Second, preclinical models suggest that anti-VEGF therapy may enhance the anti-glioma activity of radiation and chemotherapy [23-25]. At least three possible mechanisms may underlie such an augmentation. First, radiation can induce transient hypoxia which can stimulate VEGF and VEGFR-2 expression by tumor cells as well as upregulation of the nitric oxide pathway in tumor endothelial cells [26-30]. Second, anti-VEGF therapy may transiently normalize tumor vasculature leading to improved blood flow within the tumor which may improve tumor oxygenation as well as chemotherapy delivery [31-33]. Supportive clinical data for the normalization hypothesis have emerged in colorectal cancer as well as GBM [21,34]. Third, anti-VEGF therapy has been shown to target glioma-associated stem cells, which appear to contribute to radiation resistance [35,36].

ONGOING EFFORTS

Based on the above rationale, clinical application of anti-angiogenic therapies for newly diagnosed GBM patients are underway. Specifically, interim results of single-arm phase 2 studies incorporating bevacizumab into standard therapy for newly diagnosed GBM patients were recently reported and phase 3 studies randomizing newly diagnosed GBM patients to standard temozolomide chemoradiation +/- bevacizumab have recently been initiated. In addition, single-arm phase 2 studies evaluating VEGFR tyrosine kinase inhibitors with standard therapy have begun.

A major consideration of these efforts is patient safety. In addition to toxicities commonly associated with anti-angiogenic agents, impaired wound healing is a particularly relevant focus given that many newly diagnosed patients have recently undergone craniotomy and are also on prolonged corticosteroids which can further slow wound healing. Although an initial assessment of ten patients suggested that bevacizumab may enhance toxicity of standard radiation and temozolomide [37], recent reports of larger, ongoing studies with longer follow-up reveal an acceptable safety profile of this combination [38,39]. In fact, data to date suggests that common toxicities of these agents, including hypertension, proteinuria and fatigue, as well as more serious complications such as wound dehiscence, GI perforation, intra-tumoral hemorrhage and thromboses, impact brain tumor patients comparably to patients with other malignancies. Among 70 newly diagnosed GBM patients who began bevacizumab with XRT and daily temozolomide within 3-5 weeks of initial surgery followed by monthly cycles of temozolomide and bi-weekly bevacizumab, Lai reported wound dehiscence in 4 patients (5.7%) while ischemic stroke, CNS hemorrhage, GI perforation and grade $\geq$ 3 thrombosis occurred in 2 (2.9%), 1 (1.4%), 2 (2.9%) and 8 (11.4%) patients, respectively [38]. Among 75 patients treated with bevacizumab plus radiation and daily temozolomide followed by monthly cycles of temozolomide and bi-weekly bevacizumab and irinotecan, Vredenburgh noted no episodes of wound dehiscence or GI perforation, while CNS hemorrhage and grade $\geq$ 3 thrombosis were observed in only 3 patients (4%) and 1 patient (1.3%), respectively [39]. Unlike the Lai study, the Vredenburgh study required a minimum of four weeks from initial surgery to bevacizumab initiation.

With regard to anti-tumor activity, data from these two studies are preliminary as treatment is ongoing and overall follow-up is limited. Nonetheless, initial outcome data are encouraging. The median and 6-month PFS reported by Lai were 13 months and 89% respectively compared to 8.1 months and 64% for historical, institutional controls treated with standard radiation and temozolomide [38]. In the Vredenburgh study, with a median follow-up of nine months, 81% of patients remain alive and progression-free [39]. In contrast, only 54% of patients treated with standard temozolomide chemoradiation remained progression-free at six months on the EORTC/NCIC study [3]. Currently two, multi-national, randomized, placebo-controlled, blinded, registration phase 3 studies are ongoing to further evaluate the safety and anti-tumor efficacy of standard temozolomide chemoradiation +/- bevacizumab for newly diagnosed GBM tumors (Fig. **1**). Although both studies share a common backbone, there are important differences between the studies including stratification criteria for randomization, timing of randomization, number of post-radiation temozolomide cycles and incorporation of a monotherapy phase following completion of monthly temozolomide cycles.

	Concurrent Phase (6 weeks)	Maintenance Phase (6 months)	Monotherapy Phase (until PD)

Surgery

Randomize
(stratify by RPA class and region)

N=460 → RT 2 Gy 5 days/ wk X 6 wks / TMZ 75 mg/m2/qd / Placebo 10 mg/kg IV q 2wks → TMZ 150-200 mg/m2/qd d 1-5 q 28 d / Placebo 10 mg/kg IV q 2wks → Placebo 15 mg/kg IV q 3wks

N=460 → RT 2 Gy 5 days/ wk X 6 wks / TMZ 75 mg/m2/qd / BV 10 mg/kg IV q 2wks → TMZ 150-200 mg/m2/qd d 1-5 q 28 d / BV 10 mg/kg IV q 2wks → BV 15 mg/kg IV q 3wks

Primary endpoints: OS and PFS
Secondary endpoints: OS at 1 and 2 yrs; safety; HRQOL

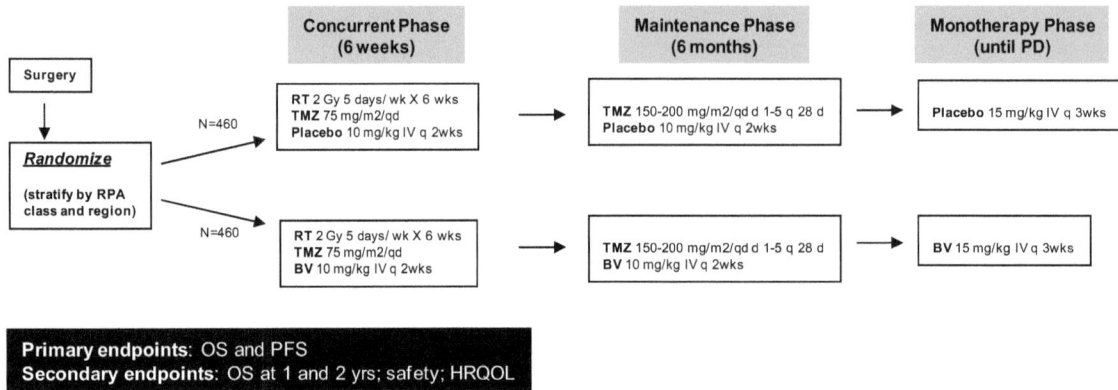

Figure 1b. RTOG 0825

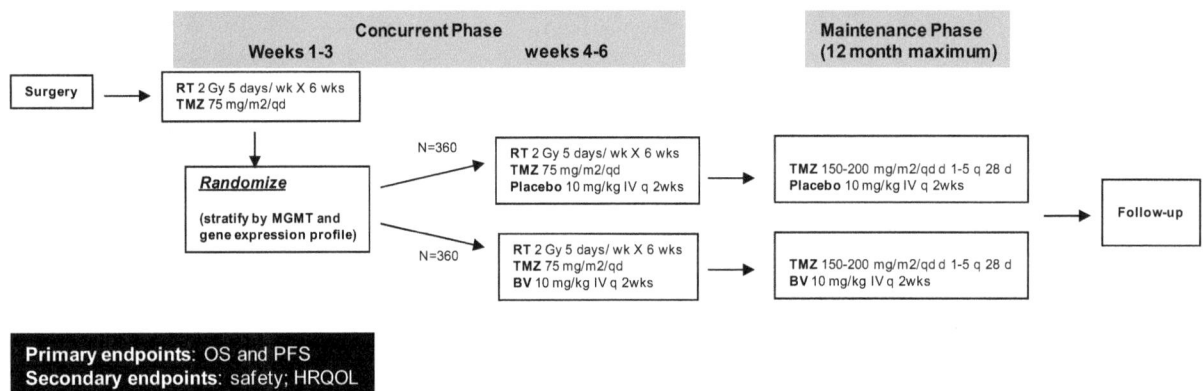

	Concurrent Phase — Weeks 1-3 ... weeks 4-6	Maintenance Phase (12 month maximum)

Surgery → RT 2 Gy 5 days/ wk X 6 wks / TMZ 75 mg/m2/qd

Randomize
(stratify by MGMT and gene expression profile)

N=360 → RT 2 Gy 5 days/ wk X 6 wks / TMZ 75 mg/m2/qd / Placebo 10 mg/kg IV q 2wks → TMZ 150-200 mg/m2/qd d 1-5 q 28 d / Placebo 10 mg/kg IV q 2wks → Follow-up

N=360 → RT 2 Gy 5 days/ wk X 6 wks / TMZ 75 mg/m2/qd / BV 10 mg/kg IV q 2wks → TMZ 150-200 mg/m2/qd d 1-5 q 28 d / BV 10 mg/kg IV q 2wks

Primary endpoints: OS and PFS
Secondary endpoints: safety; HRQOL

Figure 1a. AVGLIO Study (Roche Phase III, protocol B021990)

FUTURE CHALLENGES

Although anti-angiogenic agents are now recognized as an important class of therapeutics for malignant glioma patients, several challenges have emerged. First, an understanding of factors underlying failure of these agents as well as the development of resistance is critical. A recent review suggests that a number of tumor and host factors may be responsible [40]. Second, a more widespread and distant pattern of failure has been noted among some patients [41-43], suggesting that anti-angiogenic therapy may select for a more infiltrative and invasive tumor subpopulation. Some preclinical studies support these observations [44]. Third, salvage therapy following progression on bevacizumab-based therapy has been markedly limited and to date, no effective therapy has been identified for such patients [45]. Fourth, further study to determine which combinatorial regimens may optimize the anti-tumor benefit associated with anti-angiogenic strategies is a key priority. With ongoing preclinical and clinical investigation to effectively address these and other challenges, the full potential of anti-angiogenic therapy for malignant glioma patients is an exciting prospect.

REFERENCES

[1]   Wen PY, Kesari S. Malignant gliomas in adults. N Engl J Med 359:492-507, 2008

[2]   Stupp R, Hegi ME, Mason WP, *et al.* Effects of radiotherapy with concomitant and adjuvant temozolomide versus radiotherapy alone on survival in glioblastoma in a randomised phase III study: 5-year analysis of the EORTC-NCIC trial. Lancet Oncol 10:459-66, 2009

[3]   Stupp R, Mason WP, van den Bent MJ, *et al.* Radiotherapy plus concomitant and adjuvant temozolomide for glioblastoma. N Engl J Med 352:987-96, 2005

[4]   Ballman KV, Buckner JC, Brown PD, *et al.* The relationship between six-month progression-free survival and 12-month overall survival end points for phase II trials in patients with glioblastoma multiforme. Neuro Oncol 9:29-38, 2007

[5]   Lamborn KR, Yung WK, Chang SM, *et al.* Progression-free survival: An important end point in evaluating therapy for recurrent high-grade gliomas. Neuro Oncol 10:162-170, 2008

[6]   Wong ET, Hess KR, Gleason MJ, *et al.* Outcomes and prognostic factors in recurrent glioma patients enrolled onto phase II clinical trials. J Clin Oncol 17:2572-8, 1999

[7]   Chaudhry IH, O'Donovan DG, Brenchley PE, *et al.* Vascular endothelial growth factor expression correlates with tumour grade and vascularity in gliomas. Histopathology 39:409-15, 2001

[8]   Plate KH, Breier G, Millauer B, *et al.* Up-regulation of vascular endothelial growth factor and its cognate receptors in a rat glioma model of tumor angiogenesis. Cancer Res 53:5822-7, 1993

[9]   Salmaggi A, Eoli M, Frigerio S, *et al.* Intracavitary VEGF, bFGF, IL-8, IL-12 levels in primary and recurrent malignant glioma. J Neurooncol 62:297-303, 2003

[10]   Zhou YH, Tan F, Hess KR, *et al.* The expression of PAX6, PTEN, vascular endothelial growth factor, and epidermal growth factor receptor in gliomas: relationship to tumor grade and survival. Clin Cancer Res 9:3369-75, 2003

[11]   Shweiki D, Itin A, Soffer D, *et al.* Vascular endothelial growth factor induced by hypoxia may mediate hypoxia-initiated angiogenesis. Nature 359:843-5, 1992

[12]   Johansson M, Brannstrom T, Bergenheim AT, *et al.* Spatial expression of VEGF-A in human glioma. J Neurooncol 59:1-6, 2002

[13]   Kim KJ, Li B, Winer J, *et al.* Inhibition of vascular endothelial growth factor-induced angiogenesis suppresses tumour growth in vivo. Nature 362:841-4, 1993

[14]   Millauer B, Shawver LK, Plate KH, *et al.* Glioblastoma growth inhibited *in vivo* by a dominant-negative Flk-1 mutant. Nature 367:576-9, 1994

[15]   Desjardins A, Reardon DA, Herndon JE, 2nd, *et al.* Bevacizumab plus irinotecan in recurrent WHO grade 3 malignant gliomas. Clin Cancer Res 14:7068-73, 2008

[16]   Vredenburgh JJ, Desjardins A, Herndon JE, 2nd, *et al.* Phase II trial of bevacizumab and irinotecan in recurrent malignant glioma. Clin Cancer Res 13:1253-9, 2007

[17]   Vredenburgh JJ, Desjardins A, Herndon JE, 2nd, *et al.* Bevacizumab plus irinotecan in recurrent glioblastoma multiforme. J Clin Oncol 25:4722-9, 2007

[18]   Starks-Vance V: Bevacizumab and CPT-11 in the treatment of relapsed malignant glioma., World Federation of Neuro-Oncology Meeting, 2005

[19]   Friedman HS, Prados MD, Wen PY, *et al.* Bevacizumab alone and in combination with irinotecan in recurrent glioblastoma. J Clin Oncol 2009 Aug 31 [Epub ahead of print]

[20]   Kreisl TN, Kim L, Moore K, *et al.* Phase II trial of single-agent bevacizumab followed by bevacizumab plus irinotecan at tumor progression in recurrent glioblastoma. J Clin Oncol 27:740-5, 2009

[21]   Batchelor TT, Sorensen AG, di Tomaso E, *et al.* AZD2171, a Pan-VEGF Receptor Tyrosine Kinase Inhibitor, Normalizes Tumor Vasculature and Alleviates Edema in Glioblastoma Patients. Cancer Cell 11:83-95, 2007

[22]   Gilbert MR, Wang M, Aldape K, *et al.* RTOG 0625: A phase II study of bevacizumab with irinotecan in recurrent glioblastoma (GBM), 2009 ASCO Annual Meeting Proceedings, 2009, pp 89s

[23]   Lee CG, Heijn M, di Tomaso E, *et al.* Anti-Vascular endothelial growth factor treatment augments tumor radiation response under normoxic or hypoxic conditions. Cancer Res 60:5565-70, 2000

[24]   Takano S, Tsuboi K, Matsumura A, *et al.* Anti-vascular endothelial growth factor antibody and nimustine as combined therapy: effects on tumour growth and angiogenesis in human glioblastoma xenografts. Neuro Oncol 5:1-7, 2003

[25]   Mathieu V, De Neve N, Le Mercier M, *et al.* Combining bevacizumab with temozolomide increases the antitumor efficacy of temozolomide in a human glioblastoma orthotopic xenograft model. Neoplasia 10:1383-92, 2008

[26]   Gorski DH, Beckett MA, Jaskowiak NT, *et al.* Blockage of the vascular endothelial growth factor stress response increases the antitumor effects of ionizing radiation. Cancer Res 59:3374-8, 1999

[27]   Abdollahi A, Lipson KE, Han X, *et al.* SU5416 and SU6668 attenuate the angiogenic effects of radiation-induced tumor cell growth factor production and amplify the direct anti-endothelial action of radiation in vitro. Cancer Res 63:3755-63, 2003

[28]   Kermani P, Leclerc G, Martel R, *et al.* Effect of ionizing radiation on thymidine uptake, differentiation, and VEGFR2 receptor expression in endothelial cells: the role of VEGF(165). Int J Radiat Oncol Biol Phys 50:213-20, 2001

[29]   Gaffney DK, Haslam D, Tsodikov A, *et al.* Epidermal growth factor receptor (EGFR) and vascular endothelial growth factor (VEGF) negatively affect overall survival in carcinoma of the cervix treated with radiotherapy. Int J Radiat Oncol Biol Phys 56:922-8, 2003

[30]   Sonveaux P, Brouet A, Havaux X, *et al*. Irradiation-induced angiogenesis through the up-regulation of the nitric oxide pathway: implications for tumor radiotherapy. Cancer Res 63:1012-9, 2003

[31]   Jain RK: Normalizing tumor vasculature with anti-angiogenic therapy: a new paradigm for combination therapy. Nat Med 7:987-9, 2001

[32]   Jain RK: Normalization of tumor vasculature: an emerging concept in antiangiogenic therapy. Science 307:58-62, 2005

[33]   Jain RK, Tong RT, Munn LL. Effect of vascular normalization by antiangiogenic therapy on interstitial hypertension, peritumor edema, and lymphatic metastasis: insights from a mathematical model. Cancer Res 67:2729-35, 2007

[34]   Willett CG, Boucher Y, di Tomaso E, *et al*. Direct evidence that the VEGF-specific antibody bevacizumab has antivascular effects in human rectal cancer. Nat Med 10:145-7, 2004

[35]   Bao S, Wu Q, McLendon RE, *et al*. Glioma stem cells promote radioresistance by preferential activation of the DNA damage response. Nature 444:756-60, 2006

[36]   Bao S, Wu Q, Sathornsumetee S, *et al*. Stem cell-like glioma cells promote tumor angiogenesis through vascular endothelial growth factor. Cancer Res 66:7843-8, 2006

[37]   Lai A, Filka E, McGibbon B, *et al*. Phase II pilot study of bevacizumab in combination with temozolomide and regional radiation therapy for up-front treatment of patients with newly diagnosed glioblastoma multiforme: interim analysis of safety and tolerability. Int J Radiat Oncol Biol Phys 71:1372-80, 2008

[38]   Lai A, Nghiemphu P, Green R, *et al*. Phase II trial of bevacizumab in combination with temozolomide and regional radiation therapy for up-front treatment of patients with newly diagnosed glioblastoma multiforme, 2009 ASCO Annual Meeting Proceedings. Orlando, FL, 2009, pp 87s

[39]   Vredenburgh JJ, Desjardins A, Reardon DA, *et al*. Safety and efficacy of the addition of bevacizumab (BV) to temozolomide (TMZ) and radiation therapy (RT) followed by BV, TMZ, and irinotecan (CPT-11) for newly diagnosed glioblastoma multiforme (GBM) American Society of Clinical Oncology Annual Meeting Proceedings, 2009, pp 90s

[40]   Ebos JM, Lee CR, Kerbel RS. Tumor and host-mediated pathways of resistance and disease progression in response to antiangiogenic therapy. Clin Cancer Res 15:5020-5, 2009

[41]   Norden AD, Young GS, Setayesh K, *et al*. Bevacizumab for recurrent malignant gliomas: efficacy, toxicity, and patterns of recurrence. Neurology 70:779-87, 2008

[42]   Narayana A, Kelly P, Golfinos J, *et al*. Antiangiogenic therapy using bevacizumab in recurrent high-grade glioma: impact on local control and patient survival. J Neurosurg 110:173-80, 2009

[43]   Fischer I, Cunliffe CH, Bollo RJ, *et al*. High-grade glioma before and after treatment with radiation and Avastin: initial observations. Neuro Oncol 10:700-8, 2008

[44]   Rubenstein JL, Kim J, Ozawa T, *et al*. Anti-VEGF antibody treatment of glioblastoma prolongs survival but results in increased vascular cooption. Neoplasia 2:306-14, 2000

[45]   Quant E, Norden AD, Drappatz J, *et al*. Role of a second chemotherapy in recurrent malignant glioma patients who progress on a bevacizumab-containing regimen. Neuro-Oncol 2009 Mar 30 [Epub ahead of print].

CHAPTER 7

Bevacizumab Plus Radiotherapy in Malignant Gliomas: Is there a Role?

Minesh Mehta[1,*], Disha Patel[2] and Arnab Chakravarti[2]

[1] University of Wisconsin, Madison, WI and [2] Ohio State University, Columbus, Ohio

Abstract: Malignant gliomas are one the most aggressive form of brain tumors and the current standard of care, combination chemoradiotherapy, prolongs survival to slightly more than a year after treatment. Current chemotherapeutic strategies produce limited benefit due to the rapid emergence of resistance. New strategies, among other things, are looking to target the prolific vascularization that supports the rapid growth of these malignant brain tumors. Several anti-angiogenic agents are in clinical testing, primarily as "salvage" therapies, after initial disease progression, and among these, the most mature data are for bevacizumab (Avastin), recently approved for salvage by the FDA, having shown success in a few Phase I/II trials. A small number of phase II trials have also provided very preliminary results with the up-front use of this agent, and at least two large Phase III trials are underway to determine whether bevacizumab will provide added benefit to patients with glioblastoma, when added to the initial chemoradiotherapy regimen. This paper lays out the rationale behind using bevacizumab in combination with radiotherapy, and discusses the up-front trials.

INTRODUCTION

Glioblastoma (GBM), a WHO grade IV glioma, is the most common type of malignant glioma. The current standard of care, which includes resection, radiation therapy, and treatment with temozolomide, has prolonged median survival to slightly more than one year [1]. GBMs are among the most highly vascularized tumors, with a significant pro-angiogenic molecular profile. Brain tumor angiogenesis is associated with tumor aggressiveness and recurrence [2]. These observations have led to the logical pursuit of anti-angiogenic therapies in this disease.

In gliomas, most new blood vessels form from existing vessels and these tend to be more permeable ("leakier') and lead to unequal distribution of chemotherapeutic drugs [3]. In spite of substantial vascularization, the functionally less competent vessels further promote hypoxia, leading to hypoxia-inducible factor (HIF) oversecretion, and subsequent upregulation of several pro-angiogenic factors, including vascular endothelial growth factor (VEGF), stimulating further angiogenesis [3, 4, 5]. This constant presence of hypoxia has been proposed as a major cause of radiation resistance of GBM, and putatively, reversal of such hypoxia could "sensitize" GBM to radiotherapy.

THE VASCULAR ENDOTHELIAL GROWTH FACTOR PATHWAY:

In GBM, theory would suggest that targeting VEGF would stop new blood vessels from forming and cause the tumor vasculature to "normalize," the so-called vascular-normalization hypothesis. Such normalization would reduce vascular leakage, thereby reducing interstitial edema, and its consequential effect of increased intracranial pressure (both of which induce further hypoxia) [6]. It is also thought that cancer stem cells (CSCs) grow in the hypoxic niches created by angiogenesis in the brain. Antiangiogenic therapies might reverse/reduce such hypoxia, which has at least three hypothetical advantages: 1. A reduction in HIF-1 transcription factor, and decrease in VEGF synthesis, thereby decreasing further tumor angiogenesis, which would reduce the rate of tumor growth; 2. "Vascular normalization" might reduce tumor hypoxia, thereby increasing tumor susceptibility to radiotherapy; and 3. Decrease the ability of CSCs to utilize hypoxic niches as a growth environment [2, 5, 7].

It is important to note that angiogenesis is not seen to the same extent in low grade gliomas but is very characteristic of high grade gliomas, suggesting that pro-angiogenic pathways might be crucial in the low-high grade transformation of gliomas [8]. Furthermore, VEGF is not the only molecule that promotes endothelial cell growth. Epidermal growth factor (EGF), platelet derived growth factor (PDGF), and basic fibroblast growth factors (BFGF) are also involved in angiogenesis [8]. The interactions of these pathways may also lead to treatment resistance.

Address correspondence to: **Minesh P Mehta,** 600 Highland Ave, Madison, WI, 53792, Email: Mehta@humonc.wisc.edu; Dr. Minesh Mehta serves as a consultant for Schering Plough, Genentech, Adnexus and Tomotherapy, and is on the Board of Directors of Pharmacyclics

BEVACIZUMAB (AVASTIN)

There are many targeted agents directed against VEGF or VEGF receptors in tumors. One of the current antiangiogenic therapies that is being investigated in clinical trials is bevacizumab (Avastin, Genentech, Inc.), which is a monoclonal antibody targeting VEGF-A, known to be over-secreted by glioma cells and a strong promoter of angiogenesis [7]. Bevacizumab has shown promise in other cancers, including colorectal, renal, breast, and non-small cell lung carcinomas [9], and was approved by the FDA after a Phase III trial showed a significant increase in OS in metastatic colorectal patients when used in combination with irinotecan, 5-fluorouracil, or leucovorin [10]. Other Phase III trials showed improved PFS, median survival, or OS in patients with metastatic breast cancer, nonsquamous and non-small cell lung cancer, and advanced colorectal cancer, respectively, when bevacizumab was used in combination with another standard therapy [10]. In none of these settings has bevacizumab alone yielded dramatic clinical improvement, and therefore it has been suggested that the drug, through the process of "vascular normalization" might in fact helps improve drug delivery to the tumor, explaining the efficacy of combination therapy, and lack thereof of monotherapy.

Stark-Vance was one of the first show the activity of this agent, using a combinatorial regimen in recurrent malignant glioma; subsequent studies by Desjardins *et al.* (combination therapy of Avastin and irinotecan), Nghiemphu *et al.*, and others showed improvement in progression free survival (PFS) and also in overall survival (OS), compared to historic controls [11, 12]. More recently, a non-comparative phase II randomized trial, treated patients with recurrent GBM with either bevacizumab alone or in combination with Irinotecan. The trial included 167 patients with recurrent glioblastoma and results were presented at the 2008 annual meeting of the American Society of Clinical Oncology. The overall survival, progression-free survival, and response rates for both groups were significantly superior to historic controls. The median overall survival for the bevacizumab-only group was 9.2 months, and 8.7 months for the combination group. Based on these results, the FDA recently granted approval for the use of bevacizumab as monotherapy for recurrent GBM [13].

BEVACIZUMAB (AVASTIN) AND RADIOTHERAPY: PRECLINICAL RATIONALE

Historically, there was considerable reluctance in combining antiangiogenic therapies with radiation, with the belief that antiangiogenic therapy would reduce tumor vasculature, and hence create more hypoxic regions, thereby increasing radioresistance, since hypoxic tumors are well known to exhibit radioresistance; one of the earliest pre-clinical experiments to dispel this "myth" was conducted by the Weichselbaum laboratory. The purpose of this study was to evaluate whether endostatin, an antiangiogenic cleavage fragment of collagen XVIII, enhances the antitumor effects of ionizing radiation. Endostatin was injected to coincide with fractionated radiotherapy. Xenografts of radioresistant SQ-20B tumor cells were established in athymic nude mice. Separately, Lewis lung carcinoma cells were injected into C57Bl/6 mice to create xenografts. Mice bearing SQ-20B xenografts were injected intraperitoneally with 2.5 mg/kg/day of murine recombinant endostatin 5 times per week for 2 weeks 3 hours before radiation treatment (total dose 50 Gy). Mice bearing Lewis lung carcinoma tumors were injected intraperitoneally with endostatin (2.5 mg/kg/day) four times; the first injection was given 24 hours before the first radiation dose (15 Gy) and then 3 hours before radiation (15 Gy/day) for 3 consecutive days. Microvascular density was assessed on tumor tissue sections by use of CD31 immunohistochemistry and light microscopy. In SQ-20B xenografts, combined treatment with endostatin and radiation produced tumor growth inhibition that was most pronounced at the nadir of regression (day 21). By day 35, tumors receiving combined treatment with endostatin and IR were 47% smaller than tumors treated with endostatin alone. Interactive cytotoxic treatment effects between endostatin and IR were also demonstrated in mice bearing Lewis lung carcinoma tumors. Significant tumor growth inhibition was observed in the endostatin/radiation group at days 11 and 13 compared with radiation alone.

Histologic analyses demonstrated a reduction in microvascular density after combined treatment with endostatin and radiation compared with endostatin treatment alone. The tumor regression observed after combined treatment with endostatin and radiation suggests additive antitumor effects in both human and murine tumors. Importantly, the concentrations of endostatin employed produced little tumor regression when endostatin was employed as a single agent. The results from the clonogenic and apoptosis assays of endothelial cells, also conducted as part of this work support the hypothesis that the endothelial compartment is the target for the endostatin/IR interaction [14].

Another significant reason to combine anti-angiogenic agents with radiation therapy is the well-known phenomenon of tumor xenografts, including U87 gliomas, inducing VEGF expression in response to irradiation, which may serve to protect their endothelium, or induce radioresistance. Furthermore, adding VEGF to cultures of human umbilical endothelial cells enhances radioresistance [15,16]. Therefore, the addition of anti-VEGF agents in this context is hypothesized to abrogate this source of radioresistance.

Other preclinical reasons to combine bevacizumab and RT include the ability of antiangiogenic agents to sensitize tumor endothelium to RT by depletion of VEGF and reduction of its pro-survival signaling [16,17]. It is known that blockade of the VEGF receptor-2 by the monoclonal antibody DC101 can lower the dose of radiation needed to control 50% of tumor xenografts, including the glioblastoma U87 [18].

Recent evidence points to a population of radioresistant glioma stem cells residing within vascular niches. These stem cells may be a nidus for regrowth following RT, but, promisingly, this niche can be disrupted by bevacizumab in xenograft brain tumor models[19,20]. Garcia-Barros *et al.* have found that at a single dose threshold of approximately 8–10 Gy, the endothelium in tumor xenografts undergoes apoptosis, legitimizing tumor endothelium as an additional target for radiotherapy [21], and putatively suggesting a role for hypofractionated large-fraction radiation strategies, including radiosurgery.

Several other preclinical studies have since validated this concept of synergy between antiangiogenic agents and radiotherapy. Lee *et al.* found that the addition of a VEGF antibody to irradiation significantly lengthened the growth delay of U87 (glioblastoma) tumors in both normoxic and hypoxic conditions[22]. Gupta *et al.* found that tumors in VEGF null mice showed much greater growth delay after exposure to ionizing radiation [23]. Furthermore, human tumor xenografts treated with a VEGF antibody alone did not result in an anti-tumor effect, but in combination with radiation, there was a very pronounced delay in tumor growth [23]. Other studies, using VEGF receptor (VEGFR) inhibitors, have also shown promise. For example, the inhibition of VEGFR-2 also enhances sensitivity to ionizing radiation, similar to the synergy seen with VEGF inhibitors [24,25]. Collectively, these preclinical studies imply that VEGF inhibition improves response to radiotherapy, and although the exact mechanisms have not been elucidated, a reduction in tumor hypoxia could putatively represent one mechanism explaining this synergy. Another potential explanation is that tumor response to radiotherapy might be mediated by endothelial cell apoptosis.

BEVACIZUMAB (AVASTIN) AND RADIOTHERAPY: EARLY CLINICAL DATA

One of the earliest attempts at incorporating bevacizumab with radiotherapy for malignant glioma was reported by Gutin *et al*, in 2009. Their objectives were to study the safety and efficacy of concurrent bevacizumab with brain irradiation in malignant gliomas. After prior treatment with standard radiation therapy patients with recurrent glioblastoma (GBM) and anaplastic gliomas (AG) received bevacizumab (10 mg/kg intravenous) every 2 weeks of a 28-day cycle until tumor progression. Patients also received 30 Gy of hypofractionated stereotactic radiotherapy (HFSRT) in five fractions after the first cycle of bevacizumab. Twenty-five patients (20 GBM, 5 AG; median age 56 years; median Karnofsky Performance Status 90) received a median of seven cycles of bevacizumab. One patient did not undergo HFSRT because overlap with prior radiotherapy would exceed the safe dose allowed to the optic chiasm. Three patients discontinued treatment because of Grade 3 central nervous system intratumoral hemorrhage, wound dehiscence, and bowel perforation. Other non-hematologic and hematologic toxicities were transient. Most notably, no radiation necrosis was seen in these previously irradiated patients. For the GBM cohort, overall response rate was 50%, 6-month progression-free survival was 65%; median overall survival was 12.5 months, and 1-year survival was 54% [26].

This trial highlights several important observations; first, bevacizumab with HFSRT is safe and well tolerated; radiographic responses, duration of disease control, and survival suggest that this regimen is active in recurrent malignant glioma. Such high response rates have previously not been reported in a re-treatment setting with radiotherapy. Most intriguingly, however, the trial was characterized by complete lack of radiation necrosis; in a cohort of patients having received prior full dose radiotherapy, the subsequent use of HFSRT would be expected to yield a reasonably high incidence of radiation necrosis! What does the absence of this toxicity imply? The 1-year survival rate was 54%, and therefore early deaths alone cannot explain this finding! A more intriguing possibility is that bevacizumab provided "vascular stabilization" in the face of repeat radiotherapy, controlling peritumoral edema, and also preventing the overt emergence of necrosis. This finding is of crucial significance, because if correct, it would imply the possibility of significant radiation dose-escalation with bevacizumab, in the up-front context, and indeed, such a trial is being formulated by us.

Bevacizumab has been successfully used in patients undergoing radiotherapy and chemotherapy for solid tumors, including glioblastoma [27-30]. In the last 18-24 months, preliminary results from clinical trials utilizing up-front radiotherapy plus TMZ plus bevacizumab have started becoming available. Lai *et al.* and Narayana *et al.* each treated 10 newly diagnosed GBM patients with RT, TMZ, and bevacizumab[29,30]. Lai *et al*, reported results from a phase II study, which treated ten newly diagnosed GBM patients with bevacizumab in combination with TMZ and radiation therapy, found that the addition of bevacizumab looked promising in terms of PFS [29], consistent with the observations in the setting of recurrent GBM [31].

In an ongoing up-front trial in GBM patients of TMZ, radiotherapy and Bevacizumab, the UCLA group has observed no "pseudo-progression" events (personal communication, T Cloughsey). Pseudo-progression is an entity that is now described in up to 30% of GBM patients treated with radiotherapy and TMZ, and likely represents blood-brain barrier disruption, leaky vasculature, and consequential edema, mass effect and worsening T1 MR contrast enhancement in patients whose tumors are actually not progressing[32-34]; most likely, this represents vascular injury from TMZ and radiotherapy, and if indeed bevacizumab abrogates this, it would further support the observation made by the Memorial group that retreatment is not associated with necrosis, possibly because of vascular stabilization; once again, this opens up the opportunity to test radiation dose-escalation in the up-front context in GBM, when combined with bevacizumab.

Currently, two major prospective phase III trials are ongoing, attempting to define the role of bevacizumab in the up-front setting, in conjunction with radiotherapy and TMZ. One is a trial sponsored by Roche/Genentech, and is primarily being performed in Europe; the second trial, an intergroup effort, focusing on N. America is led by the Radiation Therapy Oncology Group (RTOG). In this trial, patients with histopathologically confirmed, newly diagnosed GBM will initially be treated with 3 weeks of TMZ and radiation (30Gy in 2Gy doses) and undergo MGMT methylation and molecular profile analysis. Then the patients will be stratified by MGMT methylation status (methylated vs. unmethylated vs. invalid) and molecular profile (favorable vs. unfavorable vs. undetermined). After stratification, these patients will be assigned to one of two treatments arms. Patients in Arm 1 will be given their final 3 weeks of concurrent TMZ and radiation (30Gy in 2Gy doses) with the addition of a placebo for 2 weeks and receive additional TMZ and placebo 4 weeks after the completion of chemoradiation. Patients in Arm 2 will be given their final 3 weeks of concurrent TMZ and radiation (30Gy in 2Gy doses) with the addition of bevacizumab for 2 weeks and receive additional TMZ and bevacizumab 4 weeks after the completion of chemoradiation. This study will primarily assess whether the addition of bevacizumab to the standard of care improves PFS or OS. Also, this study will look at whether certain molecular profiles are associated with an increased benefit from the addition of bevacizumab and compare the toxicities between the two regimens [35].

As with any other targeted agent, bevacizumab does have side effects. Common toxicities related to bevacizumab include hemorrhage, hypertension, wound healing complications, and fatigue [35,36]. Other toxicities that are rare include gastrointestinal perforation, arterial thromboembolism, congestive heart failure, proteinuria, reversible posterior leukoencephalopathy [10, 29]. It is important to note that patients who have any preexisting conditions or histories of these types of symptoms are at greater risk of toxicity when taking bevacizumab.

CONCLUSION

Preclinical investigations have shown that VEGF plays a major role in tumor vascularization and both chemo- and radio-resistance. However targeting VEGF alone is not enough. Anti-VEGF therapies have shown the most promise when used in combination with other chemotherapies or ionizing radiation. Many of these studies have shown remarkable tumor growth delay when combining anti-VEGF therapies with ionizing radiation. Ongoing clinical trials are investigating the use of bevacizumab in conjunction with other chemotherapies and radiation therapy in the setting of glioblastoma (Table **1**, 37) and other cancers. The outcome of the prospective Phase III trials led by

Roche/Genentech and RTOG will determine whether the standard of care for newly diagnosed GBM patients will change with the addition of bevacizumab.

Table 1: Current Clinical Trials Using Bevacizumab and Radiation Therapy (RT) in Newly Diagnosed Glioblastoma

Phase	Treatment Regimen	Status	Sponsor	Endpoints
II	Bevacizumab+ RT+ Temozolomide (TMZ)	Recruiting	Memorial Sloan Kattering Cancer Center, Genetech	Safety, OS, PFS
II	Bevacizumab+Everolimus+ TMZ+ RT	Recruiting	Sarah Cannon Research Inst., Genetech, Novartis	PFS
II	Bevacizumab+ RT+ Irinotecan vs. Bevacizumab + RT+ TMZ	Recruiting	Rigshospitalet, Denmark	Objective Response rate, PFS
II	Bevacizumab+ Erlotinib+ RT+ TMZ	Recruiting	Robert H. Lurie Cancer Center, National Cancer Institute (NCI)	OS
II	Bevacizumab+ Temodar+ Tarceva+ RT	Recruiting	University of California, San Francisco	OS, PFS
III	Bevacizumab+ TMZ +RT vs. Placebo+ TMZ+ RT	Recruiting	RTOG	OS, PFS

Other ongoing studies are investigating the use of tyrosine kinase inhibitors that target VEGF receptors, rather than VEGF itself. What remains to be found are crucial biomarkers that show the efficacy if anti-VEGF therapy. These biomarkers are needed also to validate mechanistic hypotheses, identify treatment response, and determine optimal doses [4, 12]. Ideally, these biomarkers will help determine which subset of patients will derive the greatest benefit from antiangiogenic therapies and predict treatment response. Future studies will also have to investigate the molecular pathways involved in mediating resistance to anti-VEGF therapy.

REFERENCES

[1]   El-Jawahri A, Patel D, Zhang M, *et al.* Biomarkers of Clinical Responsiveness in Brain Tumor Patients: progress and potential. *Mol Diag Ther.* 2008; 12: 199-208.

[2]   Fischer I, Gagner JP, Law M, *et al.* Angiogenesis in Gliomas: biology and molecular pathophysiology. *Brain Pathol.* 2005; 15: 297-310.

[3]   Jain RK, di Tomaso E, Duda DG, *et al.* Angiogenesis in brain tumours. *Nature* 2007; 8: 610-622.

[4]   Duda DG, Jain RK, Willett CG. Antiangiogenics: the potential role of integrating this novel treatment modality with chemoradiation for solid cancers. *J Clin Oncol.* 2007; 25: 4033-4042.

[5]   Sathornsumetee S, Rich JN. Antiangiogenic therapy in malignant glioma: promise and challenge. *Curr Pharm Des.* 2007; 13:3545-3558.

[6]   Norden AD, Drappatz J, Wen, PY. Novel anti-angiogenic therapies for malignant gliomas. *Lancet Neurol.* 2008; 7: 1152-1160.

[7]   Gerstner ER, Sorensen AG, Jain RK, *et al.* Anti-vascular endothelial growth factor therapy for malignant glioma. *Curr Neurol Neurosci Rep.* 2009; 9:254-262.

[8]   Jensen, RL. Growth Factor-Mediated Angiogenesis in the Malignant Progression of Glial Tumors: a review. *Surg Neurol.* 1998; 49: 189-196.

[9]   Idbaih A, Ducray F, Sierra Del Rio M, *et al.* Therapeutic Application on Noncytotoxic Molecular Targeted Therapy in Gliomas: growth factor receptors and angiogenesis inhibitors. *The Oncologist* 2008; 13: 978-992.

[10]   Jain RK, Duda DG, Clark JW, *et al.* Lessons from phase III clinical trials on anti-VEGF therapy for cancer. *Nat Clin Pract Oncol.* 2006; 3: 24-40.

[11]   Nghiemphu PL, Liu W, Lee Y, *et al.* Bevacizumab and chemotherapy for recurrent glioblastoma: a single institution experience. *Neurology.* 2009; 72: 1217-1222.

[12]   Desjardins A, Reardon DA, Herndon J, *et al.* Bevacizumab plus irinotecan in recurrent WHO grade 3 malignant gliomas. *Clin Cancer Res.* 2008; 14: 7068-7073.

[13]   Cloughesy T, *et al.* A Phase II, randomized, non-comparative clinical trial of the effect of bevacizumab (BV) alone or in combination with irinotecan (CPT) on 6-month progression free survival (PFS6) in recurrent, treatment-refractory glioblastoma (GBM). *J Clin Oncol.* 26: 2008; May 20 suppl; Abstract 2010b.

[14]   Hanna NN, Seetharam S, Mauceri HJ, *et al.* Antitumor interaction of short-course endostatin and ionizing radiation. *Cancer J.* 2000; 6: 287-93.

[15]   Gorski DH, Beckett MA, Jaskowiak NT, *et al.* Blockage of the vascular endothelial growth factor stress response increases the antitumor effects of ionizing radiation. *Cancer Res* 1999; 59: 3374–3378.

[16]   Moeller BJ, Cao Y, Li CY, *et al.* Radiation activates HIF-1 to regulate vascular radiosensivity in tumors: Role of reoxygenation, free radicals, and stress granules. *Cancer Cell* 2004; 5: 429–441.

[17]   Ahn GO, Brown JM. Matrix metalloproteinase-9 is required for tumor vasculogenesis but not for angiogenesis: Role of bone-marrow derived myelomocytic cells. *Cancer Cell* 2008; 13: 193-205.

[18]   Kozin SV, Boucher Y, Hicklin DJ, *et al.* Vascular endothelial growth factor receptor-2-blocking antibody potentiates radiation-induced long-term control of human tumor xenografts. *Cancer Res* 2001; 61: 39–44.

[19]   Bao S, Wu Q, Sathornsumetee S, *et al.* Stem cell-like glioma cells promote tumor angiogenesis through vascular endothelial growth factor. *Cancer Res* 2006; 66: 7843–7848.

[20]   Calabrese C, Poppleton H, Kocak M, *et al.* A perivascular niche for brain tumor stem cells. *Cancer Cell* 2007; 11: 69–82.

[21]   Garcia-Barros M, Paris F, Cordon-Cardo C, *et al.* Tumor response to radiotherapy regulated by endothelial cell apoptosis. *Science* 2003; 300:1155–1159.

[22]   Lee CG, Heijn M, di Tomaso E, *et al.* Anti-Vascular Endothelial Growth Factor Treatment Augments Tumor Radiation Response under Normoxic or Hypoxic Conditions. *Cancer Res* 2000; 60: 5565-5570.

[23]   Gupta VK, Jaskowiak NT, Beckett MA, *et al.* Vascular Endothelial Growth Factor Enhances Endothelial Cell Survival and Tumor Radioresistance. *Cancer J* 2002; 8: 47-54.

[24]   Winkler F, Kozin SV, Tong RT, *et al.* Kinetics of vascular normalization by VEGFR2 blockade governs brain tumor response to radiation: Role of oxygenation, angiopoietin-1, and matrix metalloproteinases. *Cancer Cell* 2004; 6: 553-563.

[25]   Fenton BM, Paoni SF, Ding I. Pathophysiological Effects of Vascular Endothelial Growth Factor Receptor-2- Blocking Antibody plus Fractionated Radiotherapy on Murine Mammary Tumors. *Cancer Res* 2004; 64: 5712-5719.

[26]   Gutin PH, Iwamoto FM, Beal K, Mohile NA, Karimi S Hou BL, Lymberis S, Yamada Y, Chang J, Abrey LE: safety and efficacy of bevacizumab with hypofractionated stereotactic irradiation for recurrent malignant gliomas; Int J Radiat Oncol Biol Phys, 2009 (in press).

[27]   Czito BG, Bendell JC, Willett CG, *et al.* Bevacizumab, oxaliplatin, and capecitabine with radiation therapy in rectal cancer: Phase I trial results. *Int J Radiat Oncol Biol Phys* 2007; 68: 472–478.

[28]   Willett CG, Boucher Y, Duda DG, *et al.* Surrogate markers for antiangiogenic therapy and dose-limiting toxicities for bevacizumab with radiation and chemotherapy: Continued experience of a Phase I trial in rectal cancer patients. *J Clin Oncol* 2005;23: 8136–8139.

[29]   Lai A, Filka E, McGibbon B, *et al.* Phase II pilot study of bevacizumab in combination with temozolomide and regional radiation therapy for up-front treatment of patients with newly diagnosed glioblastoma multiforme: interim analysis of safety and tolerability. *Int J Radiat Oncol Biol Phys.* 2008; 71: 1372-1380.

[30]   Narayana A, Golfinos J, Knopp E, *et al.* Feasibility of using bevacizumab with radiation therapy in high grade gliomas. *Int J Radiat Oncol Biol Phys* 2007;69: S51–S51.

[31]   Buie LW, Valgus JM. Bevacizumab: A treatment option for recurrent glioblastoma multiforme. *Ann of Pharmacother.* 2008; 42: 1486-1490.

[32]   Brandes A, Franceschi E, Tosoni A, *et al. MGMT* Promoter Methylation Status Can Predict the Incidence and Outcome of Pseudoprogression After Concomitant Radiochemotherapy in Newly Diagnosed Glioblastoma Patients. *J Clin Oncol.* 2008; 26: 2192-2197.

[33]   Brandes A, Tosoni A, Spagnolli F, *et al.* Disease progression or pseudoprogression after concomitant radiochemotherapy treatment: pitfalls in neurooncology. *Neuro-Oncology* 2008; 10: 361-367.

[34]   Chamberlain M. Pseudoprogression in Glioblastoma. *J Clin Oncol (Correspondence).* 2008; 26: 4359.

[35]   Radiation Therapy Oncology Group (RTOG) website. http://www.rtog.org/ (accessed August 25, 2009).

[36]   Gressett SM, Shah SR. Intricacies of bevacizumab-induced toxicities and their management. *Annals Pharma.* 2009; 43: 490-501.

[37]   Data for Tables 1&2 collected from National Cancer Institute website. http://clinicaltrials.gov/ct2/home (accessed Aug. 26, 2009).

CHAPTER 8

Bevacizumab and Malignant Glioma: Is there a Role for Upfront Therapy?

Jing Wu* and Mark R. Gilbert

M.D. Anderson Cancer Center

Abstract: Angiogenesis, largely driven by vascular endothelial growth factor (VEGF) is essential to the growth of glioblastoma (GBM). Furthermore, a mesenchymal gene signature related to vascular proliferation has been identified in a subset of poor prognosis GBM patients suggesting that a proangiogenic phenotype negatively influences survival. Therefore, disruption of the angiogenic cascade is a logical therapeutic target. Recently, anti-angiogenic therapy using bevacizumab, a VEGF targeting antibody, has shown promise against recurrent GBMs. A Phase III double blind placebo-controlled trial, RTOG 0825 was recently launched to compare conventional concurrent chemoradiation and adjuvant temozolomide plus bevacizumab versus treatment without bevacizumab in patients with newly diagnosed glioblastoma. MGMT methylation status and molecular profile are incorporated into the stratification design. This will not only balance the two treatment arms for these prognostic factors, but also may lead to prospective determination of optimal, individualized therapy based on tumor specific molecular profiles.

INTRODUCTION

Glioblastoma (GBM), the most common adult glioma, is associated with a dismal prognosis. In United State, there were 21, 810 new cases of primary brain tumor estimated in 2008 and about 13,070 deaths from this primary brain tumor [1]. Histologically, GBM displays a high mitotic index, cellular pleomorphism, extensive vascular proliferation and necrosis. They are characterized by their intrinsic heterogeneity and despite only rarely spreading outside the central nervous system, the high degree of tumor invasiveness leads to high morbidity and mortality. Despite aggressive multimodality treatment approaches in surgery, radiation therapy and cytotoxic chemotherapeutic agents, the prognosis of patients with newly diagnosed GBM is only approximately 15 months [2]. Once recurrent, GBM has proven to be quite refractory to salvage therapy and most studies report a median overall survival (OS) of ~25 weeks [3] and a corresponding 6-month progression free survival rate (PFS6) of only 15%. Therefore, there is a clear need to find new therapies for patients with GBM, both to improve the initial therapies and enhance salvage regimens. Interrogation of our increasing knowledge of the molecular biology of the disease, particularly focusing on important signaling pathways that are involved in gliomagenesis and tumor biology, are thought to be most likely to uncover effective treatments.

ANGIOGENESIS IN GBM

Since the concept of tumor angiogenesis was postulated by Dr. J. Folkman in 1971 [4], angiogenesis has been studied widely. Most solid tumors are angiogenesis-dependent [5] and angiogenesis is a key feature in GBM [6]. Furthermore, several gene profiling studies found a mesenchymal/angiogenic gene expression signature in the poor prognosis subclass of GBM patients [7,8]. The GBM subpopulation that is classified as "proneural" frequently shifts to mesenchymal classification at the time of tumor recurrence [7]. This concept that the mesenchymal/angiogenic genotype is prognostic has been supported by recent molecular profiling studies. Colman and colleagues, compiling data from gene expression profiles from four distinct institutions, were able to identify a robust prognostic 38-gene profile. The profile pattern associated with mesenchymal/angiogenesis genes showed a highly significant association with poor prognosis in a patient cohort treated with standard chemoradiation and therefore was able to accurately predict survival in GBM [9.10]. This gene set was subsequently narrowed down to a 9-gene set which when expressed as a meta gene score was confirmed to be independent predictor of outcome in GBM (K. Aldape, personal communication). The identification of a mesenchymal/angiogenic phenotype in GBM supports the concept that angiogenesis plays a key role in tumor progression and treatment resistance.

*Address correspondence to Jing Wu:** Dept of Neuro-Oncology, M. D. Anderson Cancer Center, 1515 Holcombe Blvd., Unit 431, Houston, Texas 77030; Tel: 713- 792- 2883, Fax: 713- 794- 4999, Email: JWu1@mdanderson.org

Thomas C. Chen (Ed)

VASCULAR ENDOTHELIAL GROWTH FACTOR (VEGF) IN GBM ANGIOGENESIS

Angiogenesis in GBM is largely driven by a critical cytokine, VEGF. The VEGF family consists of 5 glycoproteins, which are named as VEGFA, VEGFB, VEGFC, VEGFD, and placenta growth factor (PLGF) [11]. The receptors of VEGF are 3 tyrosine kinase receptors which are VEGFR1, 2 and 3. VEGFR2 is the key mediator of VEGF induced angiogenesis. VEGF is exclusively required in the normal CNS development during embryonic stage, but the same degrees of dependency are not persisted into adult life [12]. However, both VEGF (particularly VEGFA) and VEGFR are up-regulated in GBM [13]. Higher expression of VEGF is associated with higher grade of glioma and worse prognosis [14]. VEGF is produced by tumor cells and stromal cells. VEGF mRNA was shown to be increased 50-fold in the pallisading cells in necrotic area of GBM by an in situ hybridization study [15]. Several studies demonstrated that VEGFRs are up-regulated in the endothelial cells in developing vasculature of GBM and normal brain tissues adjacent to the tumor, but not in the established vessels in the normal brain tissues [16-18]. Aberrant expression of VEGF, along with other growth factors, such as fibroblast growth factor (FGF), platelet derived growth factor (PDGF), epidermal growth factor (EGF), continuously stimulate proliferation of endothelium which results in profound angiogenesis. Nonetheless, VEGF also stimulates the up-regulation of integrins, which are expressed on the surface of endothelial cells and is important for cell-cell interaction and attachment to the matrix [19]. In summary, VEGF is a key regulator of angiogenesis in GBMs.

ANTI-ANGIOGENIC THERAPY IN GBM

Given the importance of angiogenesis in GBM, anti-angiogenic therapy is a promising strategy for improving survival of GBM patients. Bevacizumab, a humanized IgG1 monoclonal antibody against VEGF, has been the most extensively studied. It binds all isoforms of VEGF and results in inhibition of VEGF-induced proliferation and migration of endothelial cells. It was the first angiogenesis inhibitor approved against cancer by FDA based on improved survival of patients with advanced colon cancer.

Clinical studies of bevacizumab either as a single agent or in combination with irinotecan have demonstrated a significant improvement in objective response rate and progression-free survival compared to historical agents. In a Phase II trial by Duke University Medical Center, 35 patients with recurrent GBM were treated with bevacizumab and irinotecan. The objective response rate (ORR) was 57%; PFS6 was 46%; median OS was 42 weeks [20]. A subsequent Phase II, open-label, multi-center, randomized, non-comparative study, evaluated the efficacy and safety of bevacizumab alone, or in combination with irinotecan in 167 GBM patients with progressive diseases following tumor progression after initial treatment with temozolomide and radiation therapy. The primary endpoints were PFS6 and ORR. In the cohort of 85 patients received bevacizumab as single agent, ORR was 28.2% and median response time was 5.6 months. PFS6 and median OS were 42.6% and 9.2 months, respectively. Time-to-progression was not reported in this study but median PFS was 4.2 months. In the arm received bevacizumab and irinotecan, ORR was 37.8% and PFS6 was 50.3%. Based on these data, bevacizumab as a single agent was approved by the FDA for the treatment of GBM with progressive disease following prior therapy.

Data from the most of studies testing efficacy and safety of bevacizumab alone and in combination of cytotoxic agents suggested that the overall response rate and progression free rate are better in the combination treatment, although a true comparative study has not been completed. The mechanisms of this synergistic effect are not completely known at this time. However, there are several lines of potential explanation. First, removal of circulating VEGF by bevacizumab may cause apoptosis of endothelial cells within the tumor. Secondly, bevacizumab selectively inhibits the neovasculature, causing "normalization" of the vasculature, reducing intratumoral pressure and thus improve drug delivery and perfusion in the tumor tissue. Thirdly, bevacizumab treatment may cause resistance to anti-angiogenic therapy and the combined therapy may improve survival rate when compared to a single agent application. Lastly, unlike cytotoxic agents, bevacizumab cannot kill the tumor cells directly, but do more indirectly. Therefore, combination therapy with cytotoxic drugs could synergistically improve the response rate.

Other anti-angiogenic agents have also been tested in order to further explore the efficacy of agents with a different therapeutic target. For example, cediranib, an oral pan-VEGF receptor tyrosine kinase inhibitor, was tested in a Phase II study [21]. 31 patients with recurrent GBM were enrolled to the study. The study reported that daily treatment with cediranib reduced the tumor volume in 56% of patients. PFS6 and median OS were 28% and 7.4 months, respectively.

UP-FRONT TREATMENT WITH BEVACIZUMAB IN NEWLY DIAGNOSED GBM

Until recently, most of the clinical trials were designed to determine the efficacy and safety of bevacizumab in patients with recurrent GBM after failing the standard concurrent chemoradiation therapy with temozolomide. However, this leads to the question of whether bevacizumab has a role in the treatment of newly diagnosed GBM, particularly determining if bevacizumab will add further benefits to the current standard chemoradiation therapy. This is clearly the next step in exploring the efficacy of anti-angiogenic therapy in this malignant, poor prognostic and eventually fatal disease.

A Phase II trial of bevacizumab in combination with temozolomide and radiation therapy in patients with newly diagnosed GBM was initiated by Lai and colleagues [22]. 70 patients were enrolled to the study from 8/2006 to 11/2008. All eligible patients received bevacizumab infusion every 2 weeks start from day 1, together with temozolomide and concurrent radiation therapy, and continued every 2 weeks after completion of chemoradiation therapy. Patients with newly diagnosed GBM receiving concurrent chemoradiation therapy with temozolomide, who were enrolled at UCLA/Kaiser system from 1/2005 to 6/2007, and the published EORTC-NCIC data [2] from 8/2000 to 3/2002 were used as a control group. All patients were stratified by recursive partitioning analysis (RPA) as established by the RTOG [23]. The PFS6 was 89.1% in the treatment group compared to 64.4% and 54% in the control groups. Median OS was 25 months compared to 14.6 months in the control group from the EORTC-NCIC study and 21 months in the UCLA/Kasier control group. After data was analyzed based on RPA stratification, bevacizumab was found to improve OS and PFS in PRA Class V/VI, but not in the better prognosis Class III/VI group. These results suggest that GBM patients with poor prognosis may benefit more from up-front treatment with bevacizumab compared to those with better prognosis, although comparison with a non-randomized historical control may be misleading.

To further determine the benefit of this up-front therapy with bevacizumab in addition to the conventional concurrent chemoradiation therapy, the Radiation Therapy Oncology Group (RTOG) recently launched a Phase III, double-blind placebo-controlled trial of conventional concurrent chemoradiation and adjuvant temozolomide plus bevacizumab versus conventional concurrent chemoradiation and adjuvant temozolomide in patients with newly diagnosed GBM (RTOG 0825, Fig. **1**).

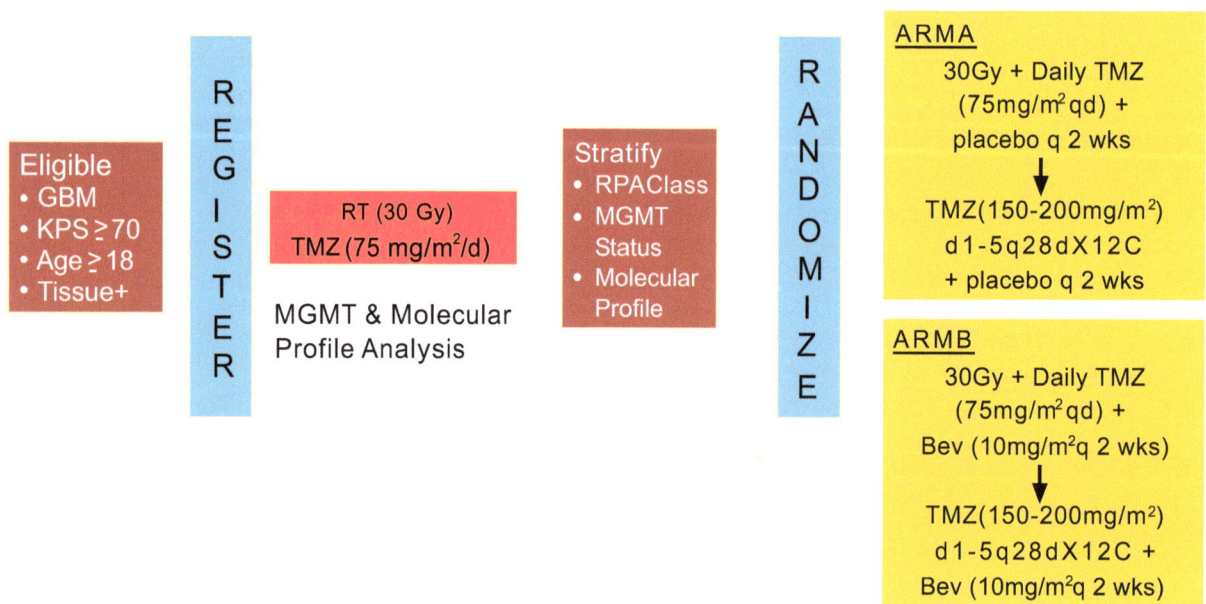

Figure1: RTOG 0825 Schema

RTOG 0825

This clinical trial is designed to determine whether the addition of bevacizumab to temozolomide and radiation therapy in patients with newly diagnosed GBM improves overall and progression free survival; and to determine whether molecular profile of GBM with and without angiogenic/mesenchymal signature is associated with a selective benefit from this up-front therapy. The acute effects, neurocognitive functions and health-related quality of life issues associated with the addition of bevacizumab to convention chemoradiation therapy will also be evaluated in an effort to determine the full impact of the addition of bevacizumab to standard chemoradiation.

The study is designed as a double-blind randomized placebo-controlled trial. Before the randomization step, there are 2 steps of registration. At the time of step 1 registration, patients with histological confirmed GBM or gliosarcoma (WHO grade IV) must provide tumor tissue blocks which are sufficient for MGMT analysis and molecular profiling. Step 2 registration occurs after the central pathology tissue screening that confirms adequate tumor tissue. Patients then undergo an initial 3 weeks of chemoradiation treatment (75mg/m2 daily and radiation 30 Gy in 2 Gy fraction). Upon step 2 registration, the analysis of molecular profile and MGMT status is performed and used as stratification factors for randomization. In addition to clinical factors, RPA class and extent of tumor resection, patients will be stratified by MGMT methylation status (methylated vs. unmethylated vs. invalid) and by the tumor molecular profile (meta-gene score: favorable vs. unfavorable vs. undetermined). The patient allocation schema described by Zelen [24] is used to balance patients' factors. Each patient with known MGMT status and molecular profile will be randomized to one of the two arms to receive bevacizumab or placebo. Temozolomide and radiation treatment will continue with the same regimen for another 21 days. Bevacizumab or placebo will be administered on day 1 and 15 of each 28-day cycle at the beginning of the 4th week of radiation therapy. Temozolomide will restart at 4 weeks after completion of radiation therapy on 5 days every 28-day cycle for total of 12 cycles. Bevacizumab/placebo will be continuously administered once every 2 weeks till the completion of 12 cycles of adjuvant temozolomide.

Overall survival and progression free survival are the primary endpoints, as well as the endpoints for the molecular correlative studies. The effect of molecular profile on OS and PFS will be identified. The differences in OS and PFS will be tested in favorable and unfavorable risk groups by univariate analysis. The multivariate analysis for both outcomes will determine whether the molecular profile is an independent prognostic factor and a predictive factor for the up-front use of bevacizumab. In the multi-variate analysis, the covariates are used are assigned protocol treatment, MGMT methylation status, molecular profiles, RPA risk class, and interactions of treatments with the methylation status, molecular profile and RPA class. In addition to these analyses, the two treatments, temozolomide and radiation with and without bevacizumab, are also going to be compared in two subsets of patients: one subset of patients with both unmethylated MGMT status and unfavorable molecular profile, and another subset of patients with methylated MGMT status and favorable molecular profile.

WHAT CAN WE LEARN FROM RTOG 0825?

The report by Stupp and colleagues proved to be one of seminal studies in the field of neuro-oncology, demonstrating that the addition of temozolomide to radiation therapy improves progression free survival, overall survival and the two-year survival rate [2]. This treatment has now been accepted as the standard of care for newly diagnosed GBM. Additionally, a correlative study was performed using the tumor tissue from patients enrolled on this study and it demonstrated a correlation between the status of MGMT gene methylation and overall outcome. The prognosis of patients with tumors containing a methylated MGMT promoter region was statistically significantly improved as measured by median OS and 2-year survival rate compared with patients whose tumor has an unmethylated promoter region [25].

As described above, RTOG 0825 will test bevacizumab as an upfront treatment for patients with newly diagnosed GBM. Stratification by molecular factors is an important component of the study, potentially enabling identification of the optimal patient population for this combined modality treatment. In addition to the well established MGMT methylation determination, the use of a novel 9 gene assay may be particularly useful in defining optimal patient populations for the upfront treatment with bevacizumab. Validation studies indicate that the 9 gene assay generates a meta-gene score that is highly correlated with prognosis [10]. Furthermore, a high percentage of the genes in the panel are associated with the mesenchymal and/or angiogenic pathway [7].

The rationale for the use of bevacizumab in newly diagnosed GBM stems from the prominent angiogenesis in these tumors, bolstered by the recent studies suggesting that anti-angiogenic treatment may paradoxically improve tumor perfusion through "vascular normalization" [26]. This would improve delivery of both chemotherapy and oxygen, which potentially will enhance radiation response. Bevacizumab is also expected to sequester the increased production of VEGF induced by radiation therapy as the concurrent chemoradiation therapy is initiated. However, the upfront treatment with bevacizumab may not benefit all patients with GBM, but the molecular profile studies may help define the optimal patient population for this early anti-angiogenic strategy.

In summary, RTOG 0825 is a phase III clinical trial that will determine whether the addition of bevacizumab to standard chemoradiation will improve OS and PFS. Additionally, it will test the hypothesis that molecular profiling will better define tumors more or less likely to benefit from this treatment regimen. The use of a placebo control design should minimize investigator and patient bias and provide a true assessment of the risks and benefits of this combination regimen.

REFERENCES

[1]   Gurney JG, Kadan-Lottick N. Brain and other central nervous system tumors: rates, trends, and epidemiology. Curr Opin Oncol. 2001 May;13(3):160-6.

[2]   Stupp R, Mason WP, van den Bent MJ, *et al.* Radiotherapy plus concomitant and adjuvant temozolomide for glioblastoma. N Engl J Med. 2005 Mar 10;352(10):987-96.

[3]   Wong ET, Hess KR, Gleason MJ, *et al.* Outcomes and prognostic factors in recurrent glioma patients enrolled onto phase II clinical trials. J Clin Oncol. 1999 Aug;17(8):2572-8.

[4]   Folkman J. Tumor angiogenesis: therapeutic implications. N Engl J Med. 1971 Nov 18;285(21):1182-6.

[5]   Folkman J. Angiogenesis. Annu Rev Med. 2006;57:1-18.

[6]   Jain RK, di Tomaso E, Duda DG, *et al.* Angiogenesis in brain tumours. Nat Rev Neurosci. 2007 Aug;8(8):610-22.

[7]   Phillips HS, Kharbanda S, Chen R, *et al.* Molecular subclasses of high-grade glioma predict prognosis, delineate a pattern of disease progression, and resemble stages in neurogenesis. Cancer Cell. 2006 Mar;9(3):157-73.

[8]   Tso CL, Shintaku P, Chen J, *et al.* Primary glioblastomas express mesenchymal stem-like properties. Mol Cancer Res. 2006 Sep;4(9):607-19.

[9]   Colman H MJ, popoff S, Zhang L, *et al.* A robust multigene classifier predictive of survival inptietns with newly diagnosed glioblastoma. AACR annual meeting; 2007.

[10]   Colman H ZL, sulman E, McDonald M, *et al.* A multipredictor of outcome in glioblastoma. Neurooncology. 2009;In Press.

[11]   Hicklin DJ, Ellis LM. Role of the vascular endothelial growth factor pathway in tumor growth and angiogenesis. J Clin Oncol. 2005 Feb 10;23(5):1011-27.

[12]   Kamba T, McDonald DM. Mechanisms of adverse effects of anti-VEGF therapy for cancer. Br J Cancer. 2007 Jun 18;96(12):1788-95.

[13]   Berkman RA, Merrill MJ, Reinhold WC, *et al.* Expression of the vascular permeability factor/vascular endothelial growth factor gene in central nervous system neoplasms. J Clin Invest. 1993 Jan;91(1):153-9.

[14]   Yao Y, Kubota T, Sato K, *et al.* Prognostic value of vascular endothelial growth factor and its receptors Flt-1 and Flk-1 in astrocytic tumours. Acta Neurochir (Wien). 2001;143(2):159-66.

[15]   Shweiki D, Itin A, Soffer D, *et al.* Vascular endothelial growth factor induced by hypoxia may mediate hypoxia-initiated angiogenesis. Nature. 1992 Oct 29;359(6398):843-5.

[16]   Plate KH, Breier G, Weich HA, *at al.* Vascular endothelial growth factor and glioma angiogenesis: coordinate induction of VEGF receptors, distribution of VEGF protein and possible *in vivo* regulatory mechanisms. Int J Cancer. 1994 Nov 15;59(4):520-9.

[17]   Carroll RS, Zhang J, Bello L, *et al.* KDR activation in astrocytic neoplasms. Cancer. 1999 Oct 1;86(7):1335-41.

[18]   Hatva E, Kaipainen A, Mentula P, *et al.* Expression of endothelial cell-specific receptor tyrosine kinases and growth factors in human brain tumors. Am J Pathol. 1995 Feb;146(2):368-78.

[19]   Friedlander M, Brooks PC, Shaffer RW, *et al.* Definition of two angiogenic pathways by distinct alpha v integrins. Science. 1995 Dec 1;270(5241):1500-2.

[20]   Vredenburgh JJ, Desjardins A, Herndon JE, 2nd, *et al.* Bevacizumab plus irinotecan in recurrent glioblastoma multiforme. J Clin Oncol. 2007 Oct 20;25(30):4722-9.

[21]   Batchelor T SA, Ancukiewicz M, Duda DG, *et al.* A phase II trial of AZD2171 (cediranib), an oral pan-VEGF receptor tyrosin kinase inhibitor, in patients with recurrent glioblastoma. ASCO Annual Meeting proceedings; 2007. 2007 American Society of Clinical Oncology.

[22]   Lai A, Filka E, McGibbon B, *et al.* Phase II pilot study of bevacizumab in combination with temozolomide and regional radiation therapy for up-front treatment of patients with newly diagnosed glioblastoma multiforme: interim analysis of safety and tolerability. Int J Radiat Oncol Biol Phys. 2008 Aug 1;71(5):1372-80.

[23]   Scott CB, Scarantino C, Urtasun R, *et al.* Validation and predictive power of Radiation Therapy Oncology Group (RTOG) recursive partitioning analysis classes for malignant glioma patients: a report using RTOG 90-06. Int J Radiat Oncol Biol Phys. 1998 Jan 1;40(1):51-5.

[24]   Zelen M. The randomization and stratification of patients to clinical trials. J Chronic Dis. 1974 Sep;27(7-8):365-75.

[25]   Hegi ME, Diserens AC, Gorlia T, *et al.* MGMT gene silencing and benefit from temozolomide in glioblastoma. N Engl J Med. 2005 Mar 10;352(10):997-1003.

[26]   Jain RK. Normalization of tumor vasculature: an emerging concept in antiangiogenic therapy. Science. 2005 Jan 7;307(5706):58-62

CHAPTER 9

Bevacizumab Toxicity in Glioblastoma

Dawit Aregawi[1] and David Schiff[2] *

[1]*University of Michigan, Hematology/Oncology, C369 Med Inn Building, 1500 E Medical Center Dr., SPC 5848, Ann Arbor, MI 48109-5848,* [2]*University of Virginia, Health System, Box 800432, Charlottesville VA 22908-0432*

Abstract: Bevacizumab recently received approval from the United States Food and Drug Administration for use in recurrent glioblastoma. Although, most patients tolerate bevacizumab with tolerable side effects, occasional patients sustain life-threatening complications and many others require medical management in order to continue on the drug. This chapter reviews the spectrum of bevacizumab complications in patients with malignant glioma, including mechanism when known as well as management.

INTRODUCTION

Vascular endothelial growth factor (VEGF) has a crucial role in tumor growth, progression, and metastasis by promoting angiogenesis [1,2]. Disruption of signaling of VEGF is a major focus of new cancer therapeutics [3]. Bevacizumab is a potent inhibitor of VEGF function, disrupting angiogenesis, normalizing pathologic tumor vasculature and allowing more efficient delivery of chemotherapeutic agents to the tumor [4-7].

Bevacizumab has demonstrated significant clinical activity in phase II single-arm studies both as a single agent as well as in combination with cytotoxic agents in recurrent glioblastoma (GBM) [8-10]. It received U.S. Food and Drug Administration approval in May 2009 for the treatment of recurrent GBM. It is the best known and most widely used VEGF inhibitor and it has been approved for many cancer types since 2004.

Bevacizumab is generally well tolerated. Frequently observed adverse effects include hypertension, proteinuria, and delayed wound healing. However, it is also associated with a small risk of life-threatening complications including thromboembolism, hemorrhage, gastrointestinal perforation, and posterior reversible encephalopathy syndrome (PRES). For an exhaustive list, the interested reader is referred to the product package insert.

BEVACIZUMAB AND HYPERTENSION

Hypertension is a known complication of bevacizumab therapy with an incidence ranging from 11%-43% of patients [10-14]. It is likely to be more prominent and clinically significant in patients with preexisting hypertension [15].

The mechanism of elevated blood pressure in patients treated with bevacizumab is likely multifactorial. One of the leading theories is the inhibition of nitric oxide, a potent vasodilator, which also plays a direct function in sodium handling by the kidney [16-18].

Most cases of bevacizumab induced hypertension are mild and can be managed with standard antihypertensives. Most clinicians use angiotensin converting enzyme inhibitors (ACEIs) and angiotensin II receptor blockers (ARBs), which have a dual effect of lowering proteinuria as well. Patients with hypertensive crisis and those who develop PRES should permanently discontinue bevacizumab.

BEVACIZUMAB AND PROTEINURIA

Proteinuria is one of the most common side effects of bevacizumab, with an incidence in the range of 21% to 64%. Most proteinuria is grade I-II. Nephrotic-range proteinuria implies structural damage to the glomerular filtration barrier and occurs in 1% to 2% [8-10,19,20]. Bevacizumab-related proteinuria is likely due to inhibition of VEGF at

---

*Address correspondence to David Schiff: University of Virginia, Health System, Box 800432, Charlottesville VA 22908-0432; Tel: (434) 982-4415, Fax: (434) 982-4467, Email: davidschiff@virginia.edu

Thomas C. Chen (Ed)

the glomerular level, or increased intraglomerular pressure in the presence of hypertension [20,21]. Like hypertension, bevacizumab- related proteinuria is usually temporary, as it resolves with drug discontinuation and is not generally associated with permanent renal dysfunction. ACEIs and ARBs play a salutary role in reducing proteinuria.

BEVACIZUMAB AND THROMBOEMBOLIC EVENTS

Bevacizumab appears to increase incidence of both venous and arterial thromboembolic events [8-10,12,22-24], although the data are more compelling for arterial events. Stroke and myocardial infarction are the chief types of arterial thromboembolism [12,22,23]. The most common venous thromboembolic events reported include deep venous thrombosis, pulmonary embolism, mesenteric venous thrombosis, and axillary venous thrombosis. A putative mechanism involves VEGF inhibition by bevacizumab causing exposure of the highly prothrombotic endothelial basement membrane and loss of integrity of the endothelium with subsequent thrombosis [11].

The risk of venous thromboembolism in recurrent GBM patients receiving bevacizumab is in the range of 3.6% to 10.4%; whether this is increased over the already high background rate of venous thromboembolism in this population remains uncertain [9,10,25]. The arterial thromboembolism rate may be as high as 4.8% [9,10]. Age > 65 and history of arterial thromboembolism increase the risk for arterial thromboembolism in patients with cancer receiving bevacizumab [26]. For such patients the relative risks and benefits of bevacizumab should be carefully considered and discussed.

Daily aspirin is suitable prophylaxis for patients on bevacizumab who are at high risk of developing thromboembolism and does not appear to increase the risk of bleeding significantly [26]. Any form of arterial thromboembolism warrants discontinuation of bevacizumab.

BEVACIZUMAB AND BLEEDING

Minor bleeding is a common complication of bevacizumab therapy, occurring in 27% of recurrent GBM patients; serious hemorrhage is unusual. Although concerns of precipitating intratumoral bleeding delayed the study of bevacizumab in malignant gliomas, initial results do not suggest a marked elevation of intracranial hemorrhage rates. In the largest GBM study to date, 3% of patients sustained intratumoral bleeding with grade 3+ intratumoral bleeding affecting < 1% [10]. As many patients with GBM require anticoagulation for venous thromboembolic disease, investigators initially excluded patients requiring anticoagulation from bevacizumab trials [8]. Fortunately, data suggest that the combination of full-dose anticoagulation with bevacizumab does not significantly increase the risk of serious intratumoral hemorrhage [27].

GASTROINTESTINAL PERFORATION WITH BEVACIZUMAB

Bevacizumab predisposes to gastrointestinal perforation. Proposed risk factors for GI perforation in patients treated with bevacizumab include a variety of local phenomena, such as peptic ulcer disease, diverticulitis, bowel obstruction, chemotherapy-induced colitis, prior bowel irradiation or surgery and bowel ischemia [28]. Additionally, high-dose corticosteroid use in neuro-oncology patients is itself a predisposing factor [29]. Consequently, it is not surprising that the use of bevacizumab in recurrent GBM carries at least a 2% risk of perforation [9,10,30]. Bevacizumab-associated perforation is a severe complication in cancer patients, carrying a 22% mortality rate [31]; this is undoubtedly true in the setting of GBM [30].

BEVACIZUMAB AND POSTERIOR REVERSIBLE ENCEPHALOPATHY SYNDROME (PRES)

PRES (also known as reversible posterior leukoencephalopathy syndrome or RPLS) is a distinctive but rare clinicoradiological entity characterized by headache, confusion, cortical visual loss and seizures in combination with vasogenic edema predominantly of the posterior cerebral white matter seen best with magnetic resonance imaging (MRI) [32,33].

Agents targeting VEGF and its receptor have been associated with PRES [34]. Single case reports of PRES in patients receiving systemic treatment with bevacizumab have been published [35-38]. The mechanism is uncertain:

VEGF inhibition may lead to endothelial cell disruption that ultimately increases vascular permeability of the blood-brain barrier; alternatively, bevacizumab-induced hypertension might also contribute to its development [35-37]. Management includes treatment of hypertension, headaches and seizures along with discontinuation of bevacizumab. It is important early in the clinical course to differentiate this syndrome from acute cerebral ischemia or thromboembolic phenomena, which are also associated with this agent, in order to prevent neurological complications.

BEVACIZUMAB TOXICITIES UNIQUE TO GLIOMAS

Bevacizumab's uncommon but serious effects on wound healing occasionally manifest as craniotomy site wound dehiscence [39.40]. This was a rare complication pre-bevacizumab, even with repeat craniotomy following scalp irradiation. This complication is seen despite withholding bevacizumab for at least four weeks following craniotomy, and it raises potential concerns for the two large randomized trials of bevacizumab for newly diagnosed glioblastomas that recently launched.

Finally, some data suggest that bevacizumab may sometimes alter the pattern of failure of GBM, resulting in a higher percentage of remote and/or multifocal progression [41]. We have seen several cases of optic neuropathy with bevacizumab utilized for GBM; whether this represents microscopic remote tumor failure or a previously unreported bevacizumab toxic effect remains uncertain [42].

Table 1: Selected Bevacizumab-Related Adverse Events in GBM

	Friedman H et al.	**Kreisl et al.**
Hypertension	35.7 (all grades)	12.5 (Grade I & II)
Intracranial hemorrhage	2.4	-
Venous thromboembolism	3.6	10.4
Arterial thromboembolism	4.8	2.1
Proteinuria	4.8	2.1
GI perforation	2.5	2.1
Wound healing complication	6.0	-
RPLS	-	-
Convulsion	6.0	
Neutropenia	1.2	
Lymphopenia	2.4	

REFERENCES

[1]   Folkman J. Role of angiogenesis in tumor growth and metastasis. Semin Oncol. 2002 Dec;29(6 Suppl 16):15-8.

[2]   Folkman J. Tumor angiogenesis: therapeutic implications. N Engl J Med. 1971 Nov 18;285(21):1182-6.

[3]   Gerber HP, Ferrara N. Pharmacology and pharmacodynamics of bevacizumab as monotherapy or in combination with cytotoxic therapy in preclinical studies. Cancer Res. 2005 Feb 1;65(3):671-80.

[4]   Wang Y, Fei D, Vanderlaan M, Song A. Biological activity of bevacizumab, a humanized anti-VEGF antibody in vitro. Angiogenesis. 2004;7(4):335-45.

[5]   Zondor SD, Medina PJ. Bevacizumab: an angiogenesis inhibitor with efficacy in colorectal and other malignancies. Ann Pharmacother. 2004 Jul-Aug;38(7-8):1258-64.

[6]   Jain RK. Antiangiogenic therapy for cancer: current and emerging concepts. Oncology (Williston Park). 2005 Apr;19(4 Suppl 3):7-16.

[7]   Jain RK. Normalizing tumor vasculature with anti-angiogenic therapy: a new paradigm for combination therapy. Nat Med. 2001 Sep;7(9):987-9.

[8]   Vredenburgh JJ, Desjardins A, Herndon JE, 2nd, *et al.* Phase II trial of bevacizumab and irinotecan in recurrent malignant glioma. Clin Cancer Res. 2007 Feb 15;13(4):1253-9.

[9]   Kreisl TN, Kim L, Moore K, *et al.* Phase II trial of single-agent bevacizumab followed by bevacizumab plus irinotecan at tumor progression in recurrent glioblastoma. J Clin Oncol. 2009 Feb 10;27(5):740-5.

[10]   Friedman HS, Prados MD, Wen PY, *et al.* Bevacizumab Alone and in Combination With Irinotecan in Recurrent Glioblastoma. J Clin Oncol. 2009 Aug 31.

[11]   Yang JC, Haworth L, Sherry RM, *et al.* A randomized trial of bevacizumab, an anti-vascular endothelial growth factor antibody, for metastatic renal cancer. N Engl J Med. 2003 Jul 31;349(5):427-34.

[12]   Hurwitz H, Fehrenbacher L, Novotny W, *et al.* Bevacizumab plus irinotecan, fluorouracil, and leucovorin for metastatic colorectal cancer. N Engl J Med. 2004 Jun 3;350(23):2335-42.

[13]   Veronese ML, Mosenkis A, Flaherty KT, *et al.* Mechanisms of hypertension associated with BAY 43-9006. J Clin Oncol. 2006 Mar 20;24(9):1363-9.

[14]   Kreisl TN, Kim L, Moore K, *et al.* Phase II Trial of Single-Agent Bevacizumab Followed by Bevacizumab Plus Irinotecan at Tumor Progression in Recurrent Glioblastoma. J Clin Oncol. 2008 December 29, 2008:JCO.2008.16.3055.

[15]   Pande A, Lombardo J, Spangenthal E, *et al.* Hypertension secondary to anti-angiogenic therapy: experience with bevacizumab. Anticancer Res. 2007 Sep-Oct;27(5B):3465-70.

[16]   Hood JD, Meininger CJ, Ziche M, *et al.* VEGF upregulates ecNOS message, protein, and NO production in human endothelial cells. Am J Physiol. 1998 Mar;274(3 Pt 2):H1054-8.

[17]   Shen BQ, Lee DY, Zioncheck TF. Vascular endothelial growth factor governs endothelial nitric-oxide synthase expression via a KDR/Flk-1 receptor and a protein kinase C signaling pathway. J Biol Chem. 1999 Nov 12;274(46):33057-63.

[18]   Zou AP, Cowley AW, Jr. Role of nitric oxide in the control of renal function and salt sensitivity. Curr Hypertens Rep. 1999 Apr-May;1(2):178-86.

[19]   Frangie C, Lefaucheur C, Medioni J, J*et al.* Renal thrombotic microangiopathy caused by anti-VEGF-antibody treatment for metastatic renal-cell carcinoma. Lancet Oncol. 2007 Feb;8(2):177-8.

[20]   Zhu X, Wu S, Dahut WL, *et al.* Risks of proteinuria and hypertension with bevacizumab, an antibody against vascular endothelial growth factor: systematic review and meta-analysis. Am J Kidney Dis. 2007 Feb;49(2):186-93.

[21]   Levine RJ, Lam C, Qian C, *et al.* Soluble endoglin and other circulating antiangiogenic factors in preeclampsia. N Engl J Med. 2006 Sep 7;355(10):992-1005.

[22]   Kabbinavar FF, Schulz J, McCleod M, *et al.* Addition of bevacizumab to bolus fluorouracil and leucovorin in first-line metastatic colorectal cancer: results of a randomized phase II trial. J Clin Oncol. 2005 Jun 1;23(16):3697-705.

[23]   Elice F, Jacoub J, Rickles FR, *et al.* Hemostatic complications of angiogenesis inhibitors in cancer patients. Am J Hematol. 2008 Nov;83(11):862-70.

[24]   Nalluri SR, Chu D, Keresztes R, *et al.* Risk of venous thromboembolism with the angiogenesis inhibitor bevacizumab in cancer patients: a meta-analysis. JAMA. 2008 Nov 19;300(19):2277-85.

[25]   Marras LC, Geerts WH, Perry JR. The risk of venous thromboembolism is increased throughout the course of malignant glioma: an evidence-based review. Cancer. 2000 Aug 1;89(3):640-6.

[26]   Scappaticci FA, Skillings JR, Holden SN, *et al.* Arterial thromboembolic events in patients with metastatic carcinoma treated with chemotherapy and bevacizumab. J Natl Cancer Inst. 2007 Aug 15;99(16):1232-9.

[27]   Nghiemphu PL, Green RM, Pope WB, *et al.* Safety of anticoagulation use and bevacizumab in patients with glioma. Neuro Oncol. 2008 Jun;10(3):355-60.

[28]   Heinzerling JH, Huerta S. Bowel perforation from bevacizumab for the treatment of metastatic colon cancer: incidence, etiology, and management. Curr Surg. 2006 Sep-Oct;63(5):334-7.

[29]   Fadul CE, Lemann W, Thaler HT, *et al.* Perforation of the gastrointestinal tract in patients receiving steroids for neurologic disease. Neurology. 1988;38(3):348.

[30]   Norden AD, Drappatz J, Ciampa AS, *et al.* Colon perforation during antiangiogenic therapy for malignant glioma. Neuro Oncol. 2009 Feb;11(1):92-5.

[31]   Hapani S, Chu D, Wu S. Risk of gastrointestinal perforation in patients with cancer treated with bevacizumab: a meta-analysis. Lancet Oncol. 2009 Jun;10(6):559-68.

[32]   Hinchey J, Chaves C, Appignani B, *et al.* A reversible posterior leukoencephalopathy syndrome. N Engl J Med. 1996 Feb 22;334(8):494-500.

[33]   Stott VL, Hurrell MA, Anderson TJ. Reversible posterior leukoencephalopathy syndrome: a misnomer reviewed. Intern Med J. 2005 Feb;35(2):83-90.

[34]   Vaughn C, Zhang L, Schiff D. Reversible posterior leukoencephalopathy syndrome in cancer. Curr Oncol Rep. 2008 Jan;10(1):86-91.

[35]   Glusker P, Recht L, Lane B. Reversible posterior leukoencephalopathy syndrome and bevacizumab. N Engl J Med. 2006 Mar 2;354(9):980-2; discussion -2.

[36]   Ozcan C, Wong SJ, Hari P. Reversible posterior leukoencephalopathy syndrome and bevacizumab. N Engl J Med. 2006 Mar 2;354(9):980-2; discussion -2.

[37] Allen JA, Adlakha A, Bergethon PR. Reversible posterior leukoencephalopathy syndrome after bevacizumab/FOLFIRI regimen for metastatic colon cancer. Arch Neurol. 2006 Oct;63(10):1475-8.

[38] Peter S, Hausmann N, Schuster A, *et al.* Reversible posterior leukoencephalopathy syndrome and intravenous bevacizumab. Clin Experiment Ophthalmol. 2008 Jan-Feb;36(1):94-6.

[39] Chamberlain MC. Bevacizumab Plus Irinotecan in Recurrent Glioblastoma. J Clin Oncol. 2008 February 20, 2008;26(6):1012-3.

[40] Lai A, Filka E, McGibbon B, *et al.* Phase II pilot study of bevacizumab in combination with temozolomide and regional radiation therapy for up-front treatment of patients with newly diagnosed glioblastoma multiforme: interim analysis of safety and tolerability. Int J Radiat Oncol Biol Phys. 2008 Aug 1;71(5):1372-80.

[41] Norden AD, Young GS, Setayesh K, *et al.* Bevacizumab for recurrent malignant gliomas: efficacy, toxicity, and patterns of recurrence. Neurology. 2008 Mar 4;70(10):779-87.

[42] Sherman JH, Aregawi DG, Lai A, *et al.* Optic neuropathy in patients with glioblastoma receiving bevacizumab. Neurology (in press)

CHAPTER 10

Is Bevacizumab Administration Safe When Combined with Therapeutic Anticoagulation in Patients with High-grade Glioma?

Lisa R. Rogers[*]

University Hospitals, Case Western Reserve Medical Center, 11100 Euclid Avenue, Hanna House 517, Cleveland, Ohio 44106

Abstract: High-grade gliomas are associated with a small risk of spontaneous intratumoral hemorrhage. A significant percentage of patients with high-grade glioma develop a deep venous thrombosis or pulmonary embolus, requiring anticoagulation. Because bevacizumab administration can be complicated by hemorrhage at the site of tumor or at other sites, a clinical concern for increasing the risk of intracranial hemorrhage arises when treating high-grade glioma patients who have a deep venous thrombosis or pulmonary embolus with therapeutic anticoagulation and concurrent bevacizumab. Evidence to date does not indicate that there is an increased risk of intracranial hemorrhage when bevacizumab is combined with anticoagulation in this setting.

INTRODUCTION

Bevacizumab is approved by the Food and Drug Administration to treat relapsed glioblastoma (GBM), based upon its efficacy in Phase II trials. It is commonly administered to patients with relapsed or progressive GBM or other high-grade gliomas (HGGs). In that setting, the agent may be administered alone or in combination with other systemic antineoplastic agents. Cancer patients, including those with HGGs, are prone to the development of deep venous thrombosis (DVT) and pulmonary embolus (PE) because of coagulation disorders associated with the tumor, patient immobility, and possibly the added thrombotic effects of antineoplastic therapy. Specific to HGG, one prospective study of 77 newly-diagnosed HGG patients who were treated with adjuvant radiation and chemotherapy identified a 20.8% and 31.7% risk of DVT at 12 and 24 months, respectively. Four study patients (5%) developed a PE. In this study, histology of GBM and the presence of limb paresis were significantly associated with the occurrence of DVT [1].

Although the precise frequency has not been quantified, a small rate of spontaneous intracranial hemorrhage (ICH) is observed in patients with HGG in clinical practice. Despite this occurrence, the use of anticoagulation to treat DVT/PE in this patient population is commonly performed and does not appear to increase the risk of ICH [2]. Anticoagulation is preferred to venal caval filters by many clinicians because filters do not reliably prevent PE and because they can be complicated by *in situ* thrombosis.

Hemorrhages, including fatal hemorrhages, at the site of the primary tumor have been reported in a variety of systemic cancers treated with bevacizumab [3, 4]. Because significant thrombocytopenia was not present in the patients with bleeding episodes, the bleeding was attributed to bevacizumab. Rare instances of ICH are reported with the use of bevacizumab in patients with HGG. Because of the small risk of spontaneous ICH in patients with HGG and a possible risk of ICH associated with bevacizumab, a practical consideration is whether the administration of bevacizumab in combination with therapeutic anticoagulation to treat DVT/PE will increase the risk of ICH in HGG patients.

METHODS

Table **1** shows eight studies reporting the administration of bevacizumab alone or in combination with cytotoxic chemotherapy or with molecularly-targeted agents, for relapsed or progressive HGG. The articles are listed in order of the number of study subjects. Tumor histologies include GBM, anaplastic astrocytoma, and oligodendroglioma.

*Address correspondence to Lisa R. Rogers:** University Hospitals, Case Western Reserve Medical Center, 11100 Euclid Avenue, Hanna House 517, Cleveland, Ohio 44106; Tel: 216.844.3717, Fax: 216.844.3014, Email: Lisa.Rogers@uhhospitals.org

Thomas C. Chen (Ed)

Five of the studies were retrospective. The dosage of bevacizumab and schedule was typically 10 mg/kg (rarely 5mg/kg) administered every 2 weeks. Table **1** shows the number of patients with ICH and the number that were symptomatic. In some cases, the ICH associated with bevacizumab led to discontinuation of bevacizumab [6-10]. In two of these reviews [6, 11], the study specifically details relapsed or progressive HGG patients who were treated with anticoagulation (fractionated or unfractionated heparin and/or warfarin) to treat DVT/PE during the time that bevacizumab was given. In combining the data from these two studies, there is no demonstrable evidence of an increased risk of ICH compared with other studies of bevacizumab without anticoagulation in this patient population, in particular regarding symptomatic ICH. In addition, the report by Nghiempu *et al.* [6] included a separate assessment of ICH associated with bevacizumab without anticoagulation in seven HGG patients, each of whom was symptomatic.

Table 1: Frequency of ICH in Patients with Recurrent or Progressive HGG Treated with Bevacizumab.

Author	N	Number of ICH	Symptomatic	Anticoagulation Treatment
Friedman	167	5	1	2
Norden [5]	55	2	0	NS
Vredenburgh	35	1	0	NS
Taillibert	25	6	1	NS
Chamberlain	25	2	0	NS
Dsejardins	24	1	1	NS
Nghiemphu	21	3	1	21
Rogers	18	1	0	18

HGG high-grade gliomas
ICH intracranial hemorrhage
NS not stated

Limitations of the published studies include the small number of patients per study and the retrospective nature of most of the reviews. Another limitation is that the frequency of small bleeds identified on imaging is not known; Nghiempu *et al.* [6] reported two cases with petechial hemorrhages, but a systematic review of brain images for petechial hemorrhage was not performed in any study. Petechial hemorrhages are a common finding in patients who have undergone surgery for HGG and, therefore, the significance of this finding is not certain.

A review of the published literature does not identify an increased risk of ICH when bevacizumab is administered concurrently with anticoagulation in patients with relapsed or progressive HGG. However, the limitations of these studies suggest that caution be used when administering this combination and that careful observation for neurological decline attributed to ICH be exercised. In addition, careful monitoring of the prothrombin time/international normalized ratio (PT/INR) in patients treated with warfarin should be performed.

Because of the demonstrated effectiveness of bevacizumab when used in relapsed or progressive HGG patients, current treatment trials seek to determine the benefit of adding bevacizumab to standard therapy of external beam radiation therapy with concomitant and adjuvant temozolomide in newly-diagnosed GBM. The risk of ICH in this setting has not been determined, although a preliminary report of this treatment schedule in ten patients [13] did not report ICH. This finding needs to be confirmed in larger studies utilizing a prospective, randomized controlled design, such as the ongoing Radiation Therapy Oncology Group 0825 study.

References

[1]   Brandes AA, Scelzi E, Salmistraro G, *et al.* Incidence of risk of thromboembolism during treatment high-grade gliomas: a prospective study. Eur J Cancer 1997;33(10):1592-6.

[2]   Ruff RL, Posner JB. Incidence and treatment of peripheral venous thrombosis in patients with glioma. Ann Neurol 1983 Mar;13(3):334-6.

[3]   Sandler A, Gray R, Perry MC, *et al.* Paclitaxel-carboplatin alone or with bevacizumab for non-small-cell lung cancer. N Eng J Med 2006;355(24):2542-50.

[4]   Johnson DH, Fehrenbacher L, Novotny WF, *et al.* Randomized phase II trial comparing bevacizumab plus carboplatin and paclitaxel with carboplatin and paclitaxel alone in previously untreated locally advanced or metastatic non-small-cell lung cancer. J Clin Oncol 2004;22(11):2184-91.

[5]   Norden AD, Young GS, Setayesh K, *et al.* Bevacizumab for recurrent malignant gliomas: efficacy, toxicity, and patterns of recurrence. Neurology 2008;70(10):779-87.

[6]   Nghiemphu P, Green RM, Pope WB, *et al.* Safety of anticoagulation use and bevacizumab in patients with glioma. Neuro Oncol 2008;10(3):355-60.

[7]   Taillibert S, Vincent LA, Granger B, *et al.* Bevacizumab and irinotecan for recurrent oligodendroglial tumors. Neurology 2009;72(18):1601-6.

[8]   Chamberlain MC, Johnston S. Salvage chemotherapy with bevacizumab for recurrent alkylator-refractory anaplastic astrocytoma. J Neurooncol 2009 Feb;91(3):359-67.

[9]   Desjardins A, Reardon DA, Herndon JE II, *et al.* Bevacizumab plus irinotecan in recurrent WHO grade 3 malignant gliomas. Clin Cancer Res 2008 14(21):7068-73.

[10]   Vredenburgh JJ, Desjardins A, Herndon JE II, *et al.* Bevacizumab plus irinotecan in recurrent glioblastoma multiform. J Clin Oncol 2007;25(30):4722-9.

[11]   Rogers LR, Malkin MG, Bertoni S, *et al.* The safety of therapeutic anticoagulation for DVT/PE and the risk of recurrent DVT/PE in glioma patients receiving bevacizumab-based therapy: the Central Neuro-oncology (CNOG) experience. Neurology 2009.

[12]   Friedman HS, Prados MD, Wen PY, *et al.* Bevacizumab alone and in combination with irinotecan in recurrent glioblastoma. J Clin Oncol 2009;27(28):4733-40.

[13]   Lai R, Filka E, McGibbon B, *et al.* Phase II pilot study of bevacizumab in combination with temozolomide and regional radiation therapy for upfront treatment of patients with newly diagnosed glioblastoma multiforme: interim analysis of safety and tolerability. Int J Radiation Oncology Biol Phys 2008;71(5):1372-80.

CHAPTER 11

Bevacizumab in the Treatment of Glioblastoma: Is there an Optimal Dose or Schedule?

L. Kamsheh, P. Kumthekar and J.J. Raizer[*]

Department of Neurology, Northwestern University, Feinberg School of Medicine

Abstract: Gliomas, particularly those that are malignant, are rapidly fatal often within 2 years despite the use of surgery followed by radiation therapy with concomitant and then maintenance therapy. Angiogenesis is an important aspect of malignant glioma biology that is reviewed. As such it has become a target for therapy, via the ligand (VEGF) or its receptor (VEGFR). There are several trails, prospective and retrospective, that had shown the benefits of bevacizumab therapy alone or in combination with chemotherapy, often CPT-11. We review the scientific basis for targeting this aspect of tumor biology and the prospective data that exists to date. Still many questions remain as to the optimal schedule but also whether there is an added benefit with the addition of chemotherapy.

INTRODUCTION AND BACKGROUND

Gliomas are the most common brain tumor in adults with glioblastoma (GBM) accounting for about 50%. Glioblastoma can be primary or secondary (develop from a lower grade glioma) tumors. Standard management of newly diagnosed GBM includes maximal surgical resection, radiation therapy with concomitant temozolomide followed by maintenance temozolomide [1], despite this approach recurrences almost always occur and survivals are on the order of 15 months. Recently, bevacizumab was FDA approved for recurrent GBM.

Angiogenesis is the process by which new blood vessels sprout from pre-existing vessels through endothelial cell proliferation and migration. In embryonic and early postnatal development, VEGF is essential to embryonic vasculogenesis and angiogenesis. It has an important role in surfactant production, inducing colony formation in bone marrow, it is a potent vascular permeability factor, and has the ability to promote vascular endothelial cells. A single allele mutation of the VEGF gene leads to embryonic death, hence this process is needed for normal development [2]. Angiogenesis is responsible for processes such as wound healing, menstruation, and fetal-placental vascular network [3]. The VEGF family consists of 6 isoforms, A-E and placental growth factor. VEGFA is the prototypic subtype and the main ligand involved in angiogenesis [3].

Glioblastoma is a highly vascular tumor dependent on robust angiogenesis which is mediated via vascular endothelial growth factor (VEGF) and its receptors. Several other pro-angiogenic factors including the angiopoiten family, epidermal growth factor, fibroblast growth factor, tumor growth factor alpha and beta, platelet derived growth factor, and inflammatory cytokines such as Il-8 are also associated with this process.[4] This allows tumor growth and progression past what would be allowed with normal host vasculature.[5] The expression of VEGF and its receptors correlates with astrocytic tumor grade [5]. Vascular endothelial growth factor functions to promote new blood vessels, renders vessels hyperpermeable, stimulates endothelial cells to divide and migrate, protects endothelial cells from apoptosis, and alters endothelial cell gene expression. VEGF acts on tyrosine kinase receptors VEGFR-1 (Flt-1) and 2 (KDR); both upregulated in GBM.[3] VEGFR-2 is the major mediator of endothelial cell mitogenesis, angiogenesis and microvascular permeability. It induces endothelial growth and proliferation by binding to VEGFR-2 which leads to the activation of the Raf-Mek-Erk pathways.[2] VEGF is also known to be a chemo-attractant for monocytes and macrophages which leads to a heightened inflammatory response and vasogenic edema on MRI [4].

VEGF gene expression is regulated by oxygen tension (induces VEGF mRNA), low pH, inflammatory cytokines (Il-8),

*Address correspondence to Jeffrey Raizer:** Northwestern University, Feinberg School of Medicine, Robert H. Lurie Comprehensive Cancer Center, Director, Medical Neuro-Oncology, 710 N. Lake Shore Drive, Abbott Hall, Room 1123, Chicago, IL 60611, Tel: 312-503-4724, Fax: 312-908-5073, Email: Jraizer@nmff.org

and other growth factors [2,6]. The process is as follows: Glioma cells initially accumulate around native vessels, a process known as cooption. This causes mechanical disruption of endothelial cells and basement membrane. These coopted vessels then overexpress Ang-2, another pro-angiogenic factor, causing a destabilization of the blood vessels and decreased pericyte coverage. This allows proliferation of tumor cells around the other existing vessels. With continued proliferation, the blood vessels eventually involute leading to hypoxia and necrosis of surrounding tumor cells. It is this response that causes increased expression of HIF-1α and VEGF release. This facilitates induction of angiogenesis and further growth of tumor [7]. HIF-1α, central to VEGF expression, function and release, is a transcription factor that is upregulated in the setting of hypoxia [2]. Under normal conditions, HIF-1α is inhibited through hydroxylation and ubiquination by Von Hippel Lindau (VHL) protein [5]. HIF-1α activates several genes in gliomas including those responsible for pH regulation, apoptosis, cell proliferation and survival, and extracellular matrix. HIF-1α also promotes tumor expansion and angiogenesis by stimulating bone marrow derived cells (BMDC)s with pro-angiogenic properties. Some of these include pericyte progenitor cells, endothelial progenitor cells, and CD45+cells.[8] Studies have shown that HIF-1α deficient tumor cells have surrounding blood vessels that are more reflective of host vasculature. However, even without this potent stimulator of VEGF, these tumor cells will in fact adapt by coopting host vessels to travel and invade further into brain parenchyma [9]. This illustrates the complexity of angiogenesis and the ability of tumor cells to adapt to the host environment, a phenomenon recently recognized in patients responding to bevacizumab where a gliomatosis pattern, often in the absence of contrast enhancement, is seen while on treatment [10, 11].

Disruption of the VEGF cycle can occur with either VEGF ligand or VEGF receptor based antagonists. Recent clinical evidence has specifically supported the role of the growth factor ligand-based antagonist bevacizumab in the treatment of HGG, the highlights of which are reviewed below along with direction for future research.

REVIEW OF RELEVANT DATA

Most available data, from prospective or retrospective trials, shows efficacy of bevacizumab in the treatment HGG; its use is primarily in the setting of concomitant chemotherapy, mostly with CPT-11 (irinotecan) (Table 1). We will review the prospective clinical trials and highlight some of the issues that remain to be sorted out. Initial data suggesting activity of bevacizumab was by Starke-Vance.[12] This led to a prospective trial by the group at Duke [13]. Vredenburgh *et al.* treated 35 patients with recurrent GBM with bevacizumab (10 mg/kg)/irinotecan and found a response rate of 57%, with a PFS-6, median time to progression (TTP) and OS of 46%, 6 and 10.5 months respectively [13]. Kreisl *et al.* used single agent bevacizumab (10 mg/kg) every 2 weeks in 48 patients with recurrent GBM with a response rate of 35% by Macdonald criteria [14]. The PFS-6 was 29% with a median TTP of 4 months. The 6-month survival and overall survival was 57% and 7.75 months. In a phase II study comparing bevacizumab with or without irinotecan (the only randomized trial--non-comparator); the response rates were 28.2% for single agent bevacizumab and 37.8% for combination therapy with irinotecan. The PFS-6 was 42.6% and 50.3% with a median OS of 9.2 and 8.7 months; median TTP was 4.2 and 5.6 months [15]. The data from the later two trials led to single agent bevacizumab being FDA approved on May 5, 2009. The only other prospective trial has been presented in abstract form using bevacizumab 15 mg/kg every 3 weeks [16]. The PFS-6. Median TTP and OS were 25%, 2.8 months and 6.5 months, respectively [in press].

Importantly, several aspects of bevacizumab have come to pass. First, the approval of bevacizumab was based on high response rates, not PFS-6 or OS, not previously seen in the treatment of GBM. Second, the available data suggests that little, except toxicity and cost, is gained by adding irinotecan to bevacizumab. Third, for patients who fail bevacizumab, survival is short on the order of 6-10 weeks [10, 14, 17, 18]. Fourth, what has become a difficult issue is the ability to assess response and failure due to the permeability changes affecting contrast enhancement on MRI scans of responders and the progressive FLAIR changes that can lead to a gliomatosis pattern, neither of these issues have previously been seen. The phenomenon on gliomatosis may be explained by cooption of normal vessels [4].

Therapeutically, several issues also remain. The optimal schedule remains unknown with a few publications using different doses or schedules (Table 1). Bevacizumab has activity at lower doses of 5 mg/kg given every 2 weeks but also 15 mg/kg given every 3 weeks [16, 18, 19]. No randomized trials exist comparing doses but in two trials of an every 2-week schedule in combination with CPT-11, a subset of patients were treated on a 3-week schedule with no difference in outcome [13, 20]. Furthermore a 3-week schedule appears to have outcomes similar to a 2-week schedule of bevacizumab [14, 16]. We know there is little added benefit of CPT-11 but that agent alone has poor activity, so adding it to bevacizumab should have little added benefit as has been shown. However, other agents exist that might be better when added to bevacizumab or ultimately the activity could remain the same irrespective of adding agents; this will need to be sorted out through clinical trials but to date other chemotherapeutic agents add little to bevacizumab if used in place of CPT-11 [10, 18]. Finally, for patients who fail bevacizumab, a rapid decline can be seen if discontinuing the agent due to rebound cerebral edema, so continuing this agent has some degree of merit, but changing chemotherapies does not [10, 17]. One reason for lack of efficacy of added chemotherapy agents may be due to the vascular normalization and decreased drug penetration [4].

Table 1: Review of Bevacizumab data.

Author	Bev Dose/Schedule	Chemo	PFS-6 %	PFS (m)	OS (m)
Vredenburgh *et al.* [13]	10 mg/kg/q 2 wks	Yes	46	6	10.5
	15 mg/kg q 3 wks	Yes			
Kreisl *et al.*[14]	10 mg/kg/q 2 wks	No	29	NR	7.75
Friedman *et al.*[15]	10 mg/kg/q 2 wks	No	43	5.6	9.7
	10 mg/kg/q 2 wks	Yes	50	4.3	8.9
Gilbert *et al.* [26]	10 mg/kg/q 2 wks	Yes	37	NR	NR
Nghiemphu *et al.* [18]	5 mg/kg/q 2 wks	Yes	41	4.25	9
Chamberlain[27]	10 mg/kg/q 2 wks	No	42	1	8.5
Narayana *et al.*[11]	10 mg/kg/q 2 wks	Yes	44	5	9
Zuniga *et al.* [28]	10 mg/kg/q 2 wks	Yes	63.7	7.6	11.5
			78.6	13.4	NR
Norden *et al.*[10]	10 mg/kg/q 2 wks	Yes	42	NR	9 m (all)
			32	NR	
Quant *et al.*[17]	10 mg/kg/q 2 wks	Yes	33 (all)	4.5	NR
Kang *et al.* [25]	10 mg/kg/q 2 wks	Yes	17	3.8	7.1
	10 mg/kg/q 2 wks		75	9.5	12.6
Desjardins *et al.* [20]	10 mg/kg/q 2 wks	Yes	55 (all)	7.5	16.25
	15 mg/kg q 3 wks		62-AO/52-AA	12.5-AO/7-AA	
Bokstein *et al.*[19]	5 mg/kg/q 2 wks	Yes	25	4.2	7
Taillibert *et al.*[29]	10 mg/kg/q 2 wks	Yes	42	4.6	NR
Chamberlain[30]	10 mg/kg/q 2 wks	No	60	7	9
Chamberlain[31]	10 mg/kg/q 2 wks	No	68	6.75	8.5
Raizer *et al.* {In preparation}	GBM-50	No	25	2.7	6.4
	AG-11		31 (all)	3.3 (all)	7.1 (all)

The anti edema effects of bevacizumab are not trivial as many patients have been able to drastically reduce or stop their steroids once on bevacizumab treatment [14, 15, 18]. This has raised the question of whether the PFS and OS survival seen with bevaciumab is related to anti-edema effects, anti-tumor effects or both. It has been shown with Cedirinab that this agents acts to increase survival by decreasing edema and not by an anti-tumor mechanism [21]. However, the authors have shown that the effects of steroids are not as effective and when treating patients, steroids alone are not enough to increase survival to any significant length.

It would be helpful to predict which patients might benefit from bevacizumab therapy. Two papers from UCLA have shown that ADC (apparent diffusion coefficient) histogram by MRI and FLT-PET scan were predictive of 6 months progression free survival and overall survival, respectively when patients were treated with bevacizumab and CPT-11 [22, 23]. Beyond radiological markers, biomarkers may become the next tool in determining treatment response. VEGF expression in tumors has been shown to correlate with age and outcome[18] and response [24].

Further studies are needed to establish a predictors of response and then validate them prospectively, these studies show that the future method may lie in both radiologic and biomarker methods.

One of the feared complications in treating HGG with bevacizumab is intracranial hemorrhage. This has not been an issue in patients treated on trials. Importantly, the addition of anticoagulation in patients who develop a thrombotic complication is also not an issue [18], nor is treating patients with stable blood products on MRI [25]. It is not known if alterations in dose or schedule change the risk of thrombotic evens but one author had reported a decreases incidence in patients on 5 mg/kg [19].

CONCLUSION

In the case of HGG, where prognosis is poor and patients are often faced with only months to live, the benefits of bevacizumab are real but many questions remain to be answered, most specifically the optimal dose and schedule.

REFERENCES

[1]   Stupp R, Mason WP, van den Bent MJ, *et al.* Radiotherapy plus concomitant and adjuvant temozolomide for glioblastoma. N Engl J Med 2005 352: 987-996.

[2]   Ferrara N, Gerber HP, LeCouter J: The biology of VEGF and its receptors. Nat Med 2003 9: 669-676.

[3]   Chamberlain MC, Raizer J. Antiangiogenic therapy for high-grade gliomas. CNS Neurol Disord Drug Targets 2009 8: 184-194.

[4]   Jain RK, di Tomaso E, Duda DG, *et al.* Angiogenesis in brain tumours. Nat Rev Neurosci 2007 8: 610-622.

[5]   Fischer I, Gagner JP, Law M, *et al.* Angiogenesis in gliomas: biology and molecular pathophysiology. Brain Pathol 2005 15: 297-310.

[6]   Kerbel RS: Tumor angiogenesis. N Engl J Med 2008 358: 2039-2049.

[7]   Holash J, Maisonpierre PC, Compton D, *et al.* Vessel cooption, regression, and growth in tumors mediated by angiopoietins and VEGF. Science 1999 284: 1994-1998.

[8]   Bergers G, Hanahan D. Modes of resistance to anti-angiogenic therapy. Nat Rev Cancer 2008 8: 592-603.

[9]   Du R, Lu KV, Petritsch C, *et al.* HIF1alpha induces the recruitment of bone marrow-derived vascular modulatory cells to regulate tumor angiogenesis and invasion. Cancer Cell 2008 13: 206-220.

[10]   Norden AD, Young GS, Setayesh K, *et al.* Bevacizumab for recurrent malignant gliomas: efficacy, toxicity, and patterns of recurrence. Neurology 2008 70: 779-787.

[11]   Narayana A, Kelly P, Golfinos J, *et al.* Antiangiogenic therapy using bevacizumab in recurrent high-grade glioma: impact on local control and patient survival. J Neurosurg 2009 110: 173-180.

[12]   Stark Vance V. Bevacizumab and CPT-11 in the treatment of relpased malignant glioma. World Federation of Neuro-Oncology Second Quadrennial Meeting, Edinburgh Scotland, 2005

[13]   Vredenburgh JJ, Desjardins A, Herndon JE, *et al.* Bevacizumab plus irinotecan in recurrent glioblastoma multiforme. J Clin Oncol 2007 25: 4722-4729.

[14]   Kreisl TN, Kim L, Moore K, *et al.* Phase II trial of single-agent bevacizumab followed by bevacizumab plus irinotecan at tumor progression in recurrent glioblastoma. J Clin Oncol 2009 27: 740-745.

[15]   Friedman HS, Prados MD, Wen PY, *et al.* Bevacizumab Alone and in Combination With Irinotecan in Recurrent Glioblastoma. J Clin Oncol 2009 [Epub]

[16]   Raizer JJ GS, Rice L, Muro K, *et al.* Phase II trial of single-agent bevacizumab given every 3 weeks for recurrent malignant gliomas. J Clin Oncol 2009 27:15s (abstract 2004)

[17]   Quant EC, Norden AD, Drappatz J, *et al.* Role of a second chemotherapy in recurrent malignant glioma patients who progress on bevacizumab. Neuro Oncol 2009 [Epub]

[18]   Nghiemphu PL, Liu W, Lee Y, *et al.* Bevacizumab and chemotherapy for recurrent glioblastoma: a single-institution experience. Neurology 2009 72: 1217-1222.

[19]   Bokstein F, Shpigel S, Blumenthal DT. Treatment with bevacizumab and irinotecan for recurrent high-grade glial tumors. Cancer 2008 112: 2267-2273.

[20]   Desjardins A, Reardon DA, Herndon JE, 2nd, *et al.* Bevacizumab plus irinotecan in recurrent WHO grade 3 malignant gliomas. Clin Cancer Res 2008 14: 7068-7073.

[21]   Kamoun WS, Ley CD, Farrar CT, *et al.* Edema control by cediranib, a vascular endothelial growth factor receptor-targeted kinase inhibitor, prolongs survival despite persistent brain tumor growth in mice. J Clin Oncol 2009 27: 2542-2552.

[22] Chen W, Delaloye S, Silverman DH, *et al.* Predicting treatment response of malignant gliomas to bevacizumab and irinotecan by imaging proliferation with [18F] fluorothymidine positron emission tomography: a pilot study. J Clin Oncol 2007 25: 4714-4721.

[23] Pope WB, Kim HJ, Huo J, *et al.* Recurrent glioblastoma multiforme: ADC histogram analysis predicts response to bevacizumab treatment. Radiology 2009 252: 182-189.

[24] Sathornsumetee S, Cao Y, Marcello JE, *et al.* Tumor angiogenic and hypoxic profiles predict radiographic response and survival in malignant astrocytoma patients treated with bevacizumab and irinotecan. J Clin Oncol 2008 26: 271-278.

[25] Kang TY, Jin T, Elinzano H, *et al.*Irinotecan and bevacizumab in progressive primary brain tumors, an evaluation of efficacy and safety. J Neurooncol 2008 89: 113-118.

[26] Gilbert MR WM, Aldape K, Lassman A, *et al.* A phase II study of bevacizumab with irinotecan in recurrent glioblastoma (GBM). J Clin Oncol 2009 27:15s (abstract 2011)

[27] Chamberlain MC, Johnston SK. Salvage therapy with single agent bevacizumab for recurrent glioblastoma. J Neurooncol 2009 [Epub]

[28] Zuniga RM, Torcuator R, Jain R, *et al.* Efficacy, safety and patterns of response and recurrence in patients with recurrent high-grade gliomas treated with bevacizumab plus irinotecan. J Neurooncol 2009 91: 329-336.

[29] Taillibert S, Vincent LA, Granger B, *et al.*Bevacizumab and irinotecan for recurrent oligodendroglial tumors. Neurology 2009 72: 1601-1606.

[30] Chamberlain MC, Johnston S. Salvage chemotherapy with bevacizumab for recurrent alkylator-refractory anaplastic astrocytoma. J Neurooncol 2009 91: 359-367.

[31] Chamberlain MC, Johnston S. Bevacizumab for recurrent alkylator-refractory anaplastic oligodendroglioma. Cancer 2009 115: 1734-1743

CHAPTER 12

Assessing Radiographic Response in Glioblastoma Following Avastin Treatment

Whitney B. Pope*

David Geffen School of Medicine, Department of Radiology, University of California, Los Angeles

Abstract: Avastin is thought to normalize tumor vasculature and restore the blood brain barrier, resulting in less enhancement and peritumoral edema. Conventional measurements of tumor response such as the Macdonald criteria are based on the dimensions of enhancing tumor. Converting enhancing to non-enhancing tumor could therefore be considered treatment response, even in the absence of change in tumor size. But it is unknown if reduction in enhancement, by itself, correlates with patient outcome measures such as progression free and overall survival. In general change in tumor size is thought to be a more accurate biomarker of response, underscoring the importance of assessing faintly-enhancing or non-enhancing tumor burden in patients following Avastin therapy. Unfortunately non-enhancing tumor can be difficult to distinguish from other causes of increased T2 signal intensity, including peritumoral edema and radiation-induced gliosis, which are common among glioblastoma patients. This difficulty has led to efforts to find alternative ways to measure non-enhancing tumor, as well as to characterize additional biomarkers for tumor response that correlate with outcome measures and add value to standard MRI. One area of active research is the use of physiologic imaging, which has the potential to detect drug effects before change in tumor size is evident.

INTRODUCTION

Radiographic Response – Conventional Measures

MRI has traditionally been used to provide anatomic data, which in the oncology setting typically consists of tumor size measurements. Changes in enhancing tumor size are the basis for standard biomarkers including the Macdonald criteria for glioma response and progression [1]. Since the vast majority of glioblastoma (GBM) avidly enhance, this method has worked well in the past for monitoring treatment effect. However, with the widespread adoption of bevacizumab (Avastin) as salvage chemotherapy for patients with GBM, limitations of the Macdonald have become more salient. These limitations are related to the effect of Avastin on the blood-brain-barrier (BBB). Typically GBM have extensive abnormal vasculature in which the BBB is significantly more permeable than that of normal brain [2]. As a result, contrast material, typically a gadolinium based agent, is able to leak out of the blood vessels and into the adjacent tumor tissue, resulting in T1 shortening, and thus increase signal (enhancement) on T1-weighted images. The target of Avastin, vascular endothelial growth factor (VEGF), is an active permeability agent, 50 times more potent than histamine [3]. VEGF also induces angiogenesis, leading to the formation of abnormally tortuous and leaky blood vessels [4]. Inhibiting VEGF has several important consequences. One is a reduction in vasculature permeability that can occur within hours of treatment. Another is the progressive pruning over several days of abnormal tumor vasculature [5-8]. Both of these effects act to diminish the leak of gadolinium into the tumor interstitium, reducing contrast enhancement. In malignant gliomas treated with Avastin, reduction in the intensity of contrast enhancement occurs in the majority of tumors, and can be appreciable within days of treatment [9-12] Assessing tumor response based on contrast-enhancing regions therefore becomes problematic, as it can lead to an overestimation of the impact on tumor size. Tumor progression is also more challenging to identify following Avastin therapy because it can take the form of increasing T2-weighted/FLAIR signal change without new enhancement [13, 14]. This progression of non-enhancing tumor can be difficult to differentiate from treatment-related gliosis. Additionally, non-enhancing tumor is often less well-defined than enhancing tumor, making accurate size measurements difficult [15]. Increase in non-enhancing tumor, by itself, does not meet the Macdonald criteria for progressive disease.

In addition to the Macdonald criteria, the World Health Organization [WHO], and the Response Evaluation Criteria

*Address correspondence to Whitney B. Pope:** David Geffen School of Medicine, Department of Radiology, University of California, Los Angeles; Tel: 310.267.9783, Fax: 310.825.2776, Email: WPope@mednet.ucla.edu

Thomas C. Chen (Ed)

in Solid Tumors [RECIST] define overall response and progression-free survival in clinical trials [16, 17]. These are traditionally the only imaging biomarkers that are accepted by the US Food and Drug Administration as surrogate endpoints of clinical outcome after chemotherapy and radiotherapy for phase III trials [18]. Debate about the magnitude of change that is clinically meaningful continues. WHO and RECIST criteria require approximately 65% reduction in total tumor volume for partial response and 40-73% increase in volume for progressive disease [19]. The magnitude of these changes is greater than the 95% confidence interval for repeatability on modern scanners, which are about ≤10-20% by volume [20-22]. Therefore, investigators have questioned whether current criteria for partial response and progressive disease should be less stringent to detect small but significant changes in tumor size.

There also has been debate as to whether one-dimensional, two-dimensional or volumetric measurements are the most effective approach. For example, volumetric change has predicted overall survival in patients with recurrent high-grade glioma, and recurrence-free survival in patients with locally advanced breast cancer who had neoadjuvant chemotherapy [23, 24]. WHO or RECIST measurements did not predict outcome in either study. For both pediatric and adult gliomas, detection of response has been equivalent for 1 dimensional (1D), 2D and 3D measurements, but variable when these measurements are used to define time to progression [25, 26]. Shah *et al* [27] showed that 1D, 2D and enhancing volume were equivalent for predicting overall survival, but that 3D measurements were less predictive. Volumetric measurements are accurate, potentially more so than lower dimension methods and agreement among observers is usually within 10% variation [20, 28, 29]. However volumetric data analysis needs accurate tumor delineation on multiple image slices, and tends to be more time-consuming and complex compared with measurements of size change calculated in one or two dimensions on a single image. With improving software and standardization alleviating some of these drawbacks, it is likely that volumetric methods will become more routinely adopted.

Pitfalls in Detecting Radiographic Response to Bevacizumab Treatment Reduction in Enhancement – Is that True Tumor Response?

Controversy has arisen over how to characterize the impact of Avastin treatment on GBM. Some have suggested that Avastin acts as a "super-steroid", leading to a profound reduction in edema and enhancement that results in an impressive radiographic change, but is not reflective of a true tumor response. Similar to Avastin, corticosteroids have been shown to reduce edema and thus mass effect, as well as diminish enhancement [30]. The steroid effect is often maximal at approximately 2 weeks with 30% of patients having a 25% or more reduction in enhancing tumor volume and 50% having 25% or more reduction in edema. This raises the question of whether Avastin is analogous to steroid treatment and that its anti-permeability effect is being confused with a cytotoxic or cytostatic tumor response.

The potential impact of Avastin on radiation necrosis is another important consideration in interpreting radiographic changes after therapy. Radiation necrosis is often avidly enhancing and associated with edema. Furthermore, radiation necrosis may have mass effect and undergo progressive enlargement on serial imaging, all of which make it difficult to distinguish with certainty from viable tumor. The physiology underlying the imaging appearance of necrosis, whether from tumor or radiation, may have common features. For instance, analogous to tumoral necrosis, areas of radiation induced necrosis are associated with leaky blood vessel and increased VEGF levels [31]. Response to Avastin also is similar. Just as Avastin can rapidly improve the radiographic appearance of necrotic tumor, it also has a substantial impact on the morphology of radiation necrosis, by reducing edema and enhancement [32, 33]. This response can be sustained, of clinical benefit, and result in reduced steroid requirements [32]. Thus it has been suggested that some of the responses seen in Avastin-treated patients may actually be due to palliation of radiation necrosis that has been mistaken for true tumor response [32].

A variety of MR techniques have recently been promulgated to help differentiate tumor recurrence from radiation necrosis including MR spectroscopy, MR perfusion and MR diffusion, but the proven clinical utility of these techniques remains elusive [34-36]. The application of metabolic imaging, such as FDG-PET, has also been challenging for several reasons. For instance it has been shown that uptake of FDG may not be well coupled to glucose uptake in tumors. Furthermore radiation can change metabolic activity in normal brain as well as in tumors in unpredictable ways. Thus it has been advocated that any increase in metabolic activity over adjacent normal brain, or increased metabolic activity in areas that enhance on MRI, should be interpreted as tumor recurrence. Absolute uptake values and uptake values normalized against contralateral brain are less helpful. Newer PET tracers may improve the ability to distinguish recurrent tumor from radiation necrosis [discussed below; 37].

Whether related to tumor or radiation necrosis, the anti-permeability effect of Avastin often has a dramatic impact on edema and enhancement. In patients with GBM, complete resolution of edema is not uncommon (Fig. **1**), and this can occur within weeks of treatment, if not before [9].

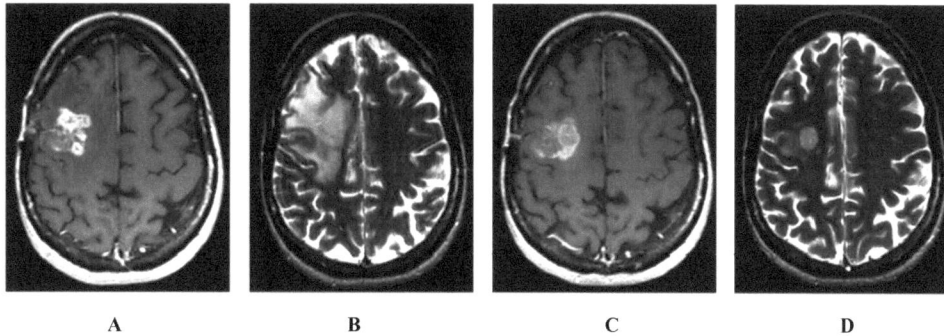

A   **B**   **C**   **D**

Figure 1: Patient with recurrent GBM before (A, B) and after (C, D) treatment with Avastin. Note the slight reduction in enhancement intensity between then pre- and post-treatment T1 contrast enhanced images (A and C, respectively). There is complete resolution of edema as shown on the corresponding T2-weighted images (B and D). Adapted from Pope *et al.*, MRI in patients with high-grade gliomas treated with bevacizumab and chemotherapy. Neurology. 2006 Apr 25;66(8):1258-60. http://www.neurology.org/ Copyright © 2001 by AAN Enterprises, Inc.

In animal studies, substantial change in vascular permeability is detectable within 24 hours of Avastin treatment [5,38,39]. Changes in vascular permeability may be partially or wholly independent of tumor response, as edema and enhancement can be significantly reduced in patients whose tumors are stable in size. Steroid requirements for patients are often diminished following Avastin therapy, presumably due to diminished edema [40]. Inhibition of edema persists, even at tumor progression [13,41]. Decreased edema and reduction in side effects from higher steroid doses are two potential benefits of keeping patients on Avastin therapy, even following tumor progression. This is supported by preclinical data in which asymptomatic tumors were larger in Avastin-treated rats compared to controls, suggesting that suppression of edema has clinical benefit even in the face of disease progression [42]. The anti-permeability effect of Avastin is not limited to primary CNS malignancies, as a similar effect on edema and enhancement is also seen in brain metastases from a variety of tumors [43-45].

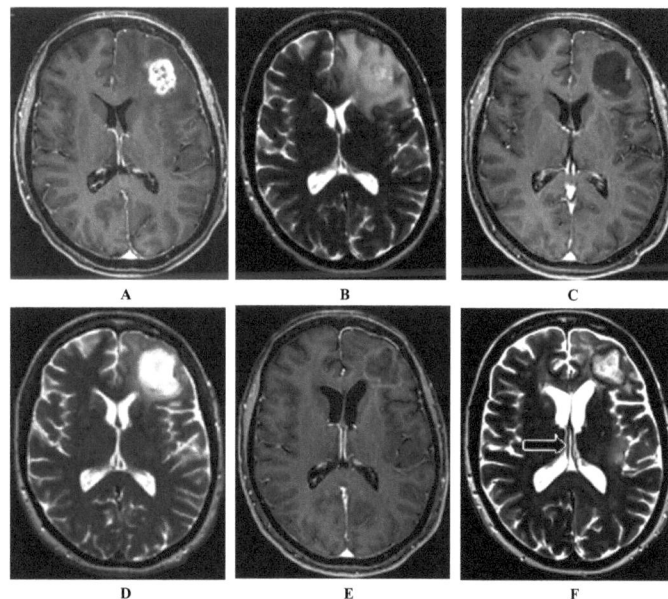

A   **B**   **C**

D   **E**   **F**

Figure 2: Patient with recurrent GBM at baseline (A, B), 6-week post-Avastin treatment (C, D) and 12-weeks post-Avasin treatment (E, F). The first column is T1 post-contrast images. The second column is T2-weighted images. On first follow-up

(C,D), there is reduction in edema and enhancement, but tumor size appears little changed. On second follow-up, there is clearly reduction in tumor size, but a new area of non-enhancing tumor has developed in the posterior insular region (F, arrow).

The interpretation of the anti-permeability effect of Avastin remains controversial, as some argue it may lack prognostic significance. Certainly this is true in some patients in which significant reductions in edema and enhancement are followed by rapid tumor growth. However, the occasional patient without any reduction in edema and enhancement following initiation of Avastin therapy may be at high risk for early treatment failure. Thus there may be a negative predictive value in these cases, although this hypothesis has yet to be formally tested. An example of the difficulties in interpreting tumor response to Avastin is illustrated in Fig. **2**. This patient with recurrent GBM was treated with Avastin and on first follow-up (approximately 6 weeks after initiation of therapy) showed near complete resolution of tumor-associated contrast enhancement. However, T2-weighted images suggested that the tumor was little changed in size. Should this be considered a response? By Macdonald criteria the answer is yes, because this methodology is based on enhancing tumor alone. Others would argue that as tumor size is unchanged, this is merely an anti-permeability effect of Avastin, and should not be considered tumor response. Ultimately the answer depends on how these changes are able to stratify patient response according to outcome measures such as overall survival, which is currently not well characterized.

Additional follow-up was acquired for the patient described above. At approximately 12 weeks after initiation of therapy, the initial tumor showed clear evidence of size reduction, but also a new area of involvement in the posterior insular region. This second region of tumor was non-enhancing. Progressive tumor that is non- or faintly enhancing is common following Avastin therapy. Additional examples are shown in Fig. **3**. Thus the case in Fig. **2** illustrates several key features of Avastin treated tumor: there is often a rapid and dramatic reduction in tumor enhancement and edema, with or without change in tumor size; Tumor size reduction may become evident only upon additional follow-up, taking several months to reach a nadir in responders [13]; Non-enhancing or faintly enhancing tumor progression is common, whereas new areas of highly necrotic tumor, typical of GBM at initial presentation, are not; And lastly, tumor progression is often accompanied by little concomitant increase in edema as the ratio of edema to tumor is significantly lower in progressive tumor following Avastin therapy compared to that at initial presentation.

The observation that there is progressive reduction in tumor size occurring after initial post-treatment follow-up provides evidence that Avastin does, in fact, shrink GBM. A time course of months for reduction in tumor size is in contrast to the much more rapidly occurring anti-permeability effect. A cytotoxic effect of Avastin is supported by preclinical studies. For instance in a mouse model of glioma, Avastin treatment resulted in substantially increased apoptosis, which could account for reduction in tumor size [46]. Other CNS tumors show size diminishment following Avastin therapy. Volume changes in vestibular schwannomas after Avastin therapy are easily characterized as these tumors are typically surrounded by CSF in and around the porus acousticus [47]. Avastin also appears to shrink breast cancer brain metastases [44]. Thus one potential way to discriminate the anti-permeability effect of Avastin from the anti-tumor effect (or effect on tumor size) would be to re-image patients treated with Avastin a few days after initiation of therapy and use this as the baseline for additional follow-up.

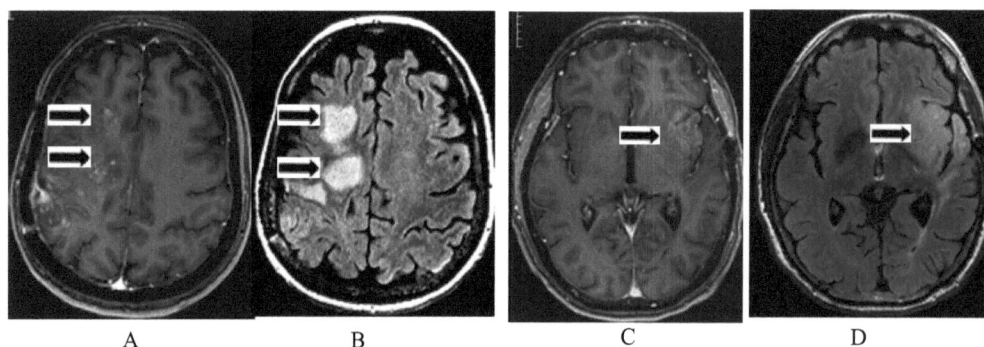

A   B   C   D

Figure 3: Patients with recurrent GBM following Avastin treatment demonstrating faint and speckled enhancement (A, C). Corresponding FLAIR images are shown in (B, D). Each row contains images from a single patient. Note that tumor can be well (B) or poorly (D) defined on FLAIR images, which may portray the extent of tumor better than post-contrast images (A, C).

Another interesting observation illustrated in Fig. **2** is that Avastin can have varying effects on tumor, even within the same patient. Specifically it appears that non-enhancing or solidly enhancing tumor is less affected by Avastin therapy than necrotic tumor [9,14]. A possible explanation is that necrosis induces VEGF expression as an adaptive response by tumors to low oxygen levels. Thus necrotic regions may have more VEGF-dependent growth and viability compared to non-necrotic areas.

Interpretation of Diffusion Abnormality

We and others have also noted that some patients with recurrent GBM develop areas of persistent restricted diffusion following Avastin treatment. An example is show in Fig. **4**. Diffusion signal abnormality has previously been described in GBM patients following tumor resection, potentially related to devascularization or direct operative tissue trauma from retraction or other causes [48]. However, such diffusion change usually resolves within 90 days, whereas the diffusion abnormality we have noticed is not temporally associated with surgery, and persists for many months, if not indefinitely. Another possible explanation is that this abnormality is related to tumor recurrence which is characterized by high cell density and low edema, resulting in diminished diffusion. Alternately this could represent some form of non-ischemia cytotoxic change, given the observation that this finding can persist, stable in size, for many months. More research including histopathologic correlation will be necessary to determine the underlying mechanism.

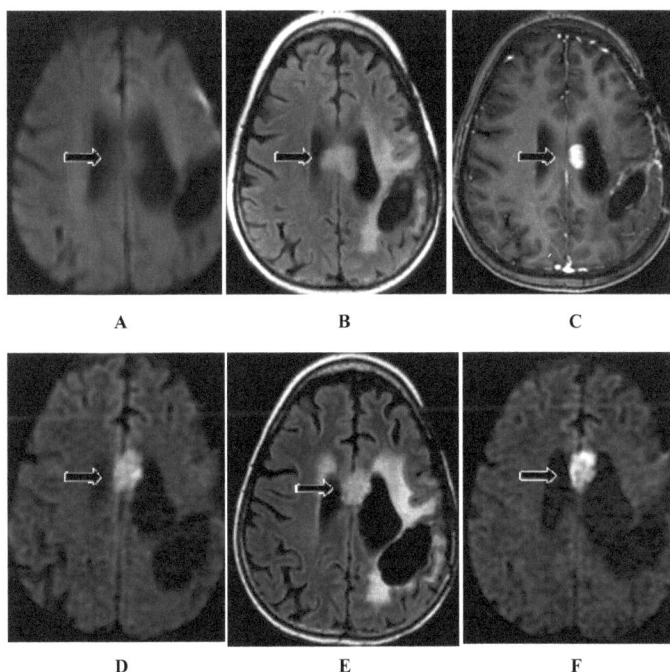

Figure 4: Patient with GBM who developed persistent diffusion signal abnormality. Baseline diffusion (A), FLAIR (B) and post-contrast T1-weighted images (C) show a focus of enhancement and high FLAIR signal in the corpus callosum (arrow). The corresponding region showed no diffusion signal abnormality (A). After 5 months, high diffusion signal (D) developed in the previously seen region of enhancement and FLAIR signal change. This diffusion signal abnormality persisted unchanged for 21 months (E) and the FLAIR signal abnormality also was stable (F).

Detecting Non-Enhancing Tumor

Due to reduction in enhancement, detection of non-contrast enhancing tumor is critical for the accurate evaluation of patients treated with Avastin. Many groups have used the amount of FLAIR signal change as a surrogate for non-enhancing tumor [14,49]. However, this method is suboptimal as gliosis and edema secondary to treatment effect, in particular radiation, also result in high FLAIR signal that may progress over time [50]. Yet, as shown in Fig. **3**, tumor and tumor margins can be more apparent on FLAIR images compared to post-contrast sequences. Various MR techniques to identify recurrent tumor from post-treatment change have been advanced as discussed above. Metabolic imaging with PET and SPECT also has been investigated [51]. Although an in-depth analysis of these techniques is beyond the scope of this discussion, none of these methods have been widely adopted, suggesting significant limitations in their applicability remain. At UCLA we favor FDOPA-PET scans. FDOPA is an amino acid analog which has low background activity in the brain and does not depend on BBB breakdown for tumor uptake [37]. An example of the potential utility of FDOPA-PET is shown in Fig. **5**, in which a small focus of non-enhancing tumor developed at a resection cavity margin. Without FDOPA-PET, it would be very difficult to differentiate this tumor focus from post-treatment gliosis. Amino acid tracers that do not rely on BBB breakdown may be helpful in detecting small amounts of non-enhancing tumor in patients with recurrence following Avastin therapy, but sensitivity and specificity in this setting have yet to be adequately characterized. The impending commercial availability of MR-PET will likely speed the adoption of such newer PET tracers. In the meantime, close analysis of standard MRI scans may be able to distinguish non-enhancing tumor from other causes of increased T2-weighted/FLAIR signal change with fairly high inter-observer reliability [52]. In general, non-enhancing tumor is composed of intermediate T2-weighted signal intensity that is brighter than cortex, but not nearly as bright as CSF (Fig. **6**). Additionally, non-enhancing tumor should give rise to mass effect that is combined with architectural distortion such as blurring of the interface between the white matter and either the cortex or deep nuclei.

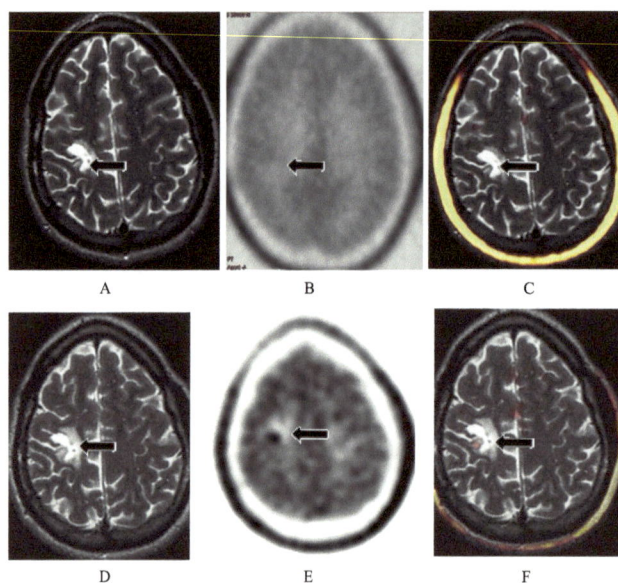

Figure 5: Patient with mixed grade II glioma. Baseline post-resection scan (A-C) shows a nodular focus (arrow) protruding into the right posterior frontal lobe resection cavity. The nodule is associated with increased T2-weighted signal (A), but there is no corresponding metabolic activity on the FDOPA-PET scan (B). T2-weighted images fused with the PET scan (C) show only background activity but no signal in the nodule (arrow). Follow-up images several months later show little change in the appearance on T2-weighted scans (D), and no enhancement (not shown), but there is now a focus of activity associated with this nodule (E, FDOPA-PET and F, fused image). Additional surgery confirmed the presence of recurrent tumor.

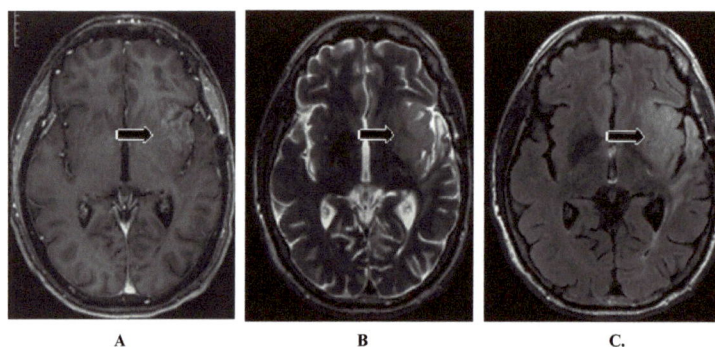

Figure 6: Patient with recurrent GBM following Avastin treatment. Post-contrast images (A) show faint and non-enhancing tumor in the left insular region (arrow). T2-weighted images (B) demonstrates intermediate T2-weighted signal intensity associated with blurring of the gray-white interface in the insula and with mass effect, indicating tumor. Note how the overlying

temporal lobe shows much higher T2-weighted signal confined to the white matter, consistent with edema and or gliosis. The differentiation of non-enhancing tumor from edema/gliosis is more difficult on FLAIR images (C).

Measures of Radiographic Response: Potential New Biomarkers MR Perfusion

The use of perfusion imaging as a biomarker for tumor response in the setting of anti-angiogenic therapy has generated significant interest. Partly this is because changes in tumor perfusion appear to occur soon after therapy initiation with several anti-angiogenic drugs, potentially preceding change in tumor size. And it has been suggested that biomarkers of angiogenesis would greatly facilitate the clinical development of antiangiogenic therapies. Currently there are no validated biomarkers of angiogenesis or antiangiogenesis that are available for routine clinical use.

There are several common methods of perfusion imaging of brain tumors including dynamic susceptibility contrast (DSC), and dynamic contrast enhanced (DCE). DSC imaging can be used to generate maps of relative cerebral (or tumor) blood volume (CBV), cerebral blood flow (CBF) and mean transit time (MTT). In general CBV is the most useful parameter for the evaluation of brain tumors as CBV correlates with blood vessel density within tissues, and is abnormally elevated in tumors, due to increased and irregular neovasculature [53].

DCE can be used to measure K-trans which is a constant for the rate of contrast material going from the vasculature into the extracellular space in the tissue. K-trans is dependent on the surface area of the capillaries (more surface area allows greater flow of contrast) as well as the leakiness of the blood vessels. K-trans can be used as a surrogate for vascular permeability in brain tumor patients [54].

Increased CBV is associated with shortened survival and has been shown to predict transformation of low grade tumors into malignant gliomas [55,56]. CBV has been correlated with vessel tortuosity in GBM, and with histological and angiographic vascularity [57,58]. Maximum CBV has been shown to be an independent prognostic biomarker for survival in patients with malignant astrocytoma [59]. Early changes in CBV and vascular permeability in tumors after radiation treatment have been correlated with better outcomes in some studies [60, 61]. However, others have found that perfusion changes were not predictive of progression in GBM, whereas the amount of enhancing tumor with corresponding T2-weighted signal change was predictive [62].

For malignant glioma patients treated with Cilengitide, an angiogenesis inhibitor, decreased CBV and CBF correlate with a clinical response [63]. Similar findings for other anti-angiogenic therapies including vandetanib, and cediranib have been reported [64,65]. Sorensen *et al* demonstrated that changes in perfusion imaging acquired one day after initiation of anti-angiogenic therapy could stratify outcomes [65]. By combining K-trans and changes in microvessel volume with measurements of circulating collagen IV levels, they were able to obtain a "vascular normalization index", which was closely associated with overall and progression free survival following cediranib treatment.

Avastin treatment has been shown to alter perfusion parameters in a variety of tumors. For instance perfusion in breast adenocarcinoma is significantly reduced following Avastin combination therapy [66]. For hepatocellular carcinoma, Avastin therapy results in decreased CBV, CBF, permeability surface area product and increased MTT. However, only change in MTT correlates with clinical outcome [67]. In a neuroblastoma xenograft model, a single dose of Avastin resulted in reduction of microvessel density by more than 70% within 7 days of treatment as well as a decrease in vessel permeability [68]. In pre-clinical glioma models reduction in CBV and vascular permeability is apparent 24 hours after treatment [39,42,69]. Interestingly, although steroids, like Avastin, reduce tumor permeability, they do not seem to have a significant impact on CBV or CBF, as least in patients with GBM [70, 71]. For glioblastoma, Avastin treatment can reduce tumor vascular permeability within 24 hours, and results in reduced microvessel density by histopathology [72,73].

Although it has been shown that anti-angiogenic drugs, including Avastin, can have a rapid impact on perfusion parameters, there is, as of yet, no data demonstrating that changes in perfusion in response to Avastin therapy can predict outcome in patients with GBM. In fact, some evidence indicates that changes in perfusion parameters do not correlate with either 6 month progression free or overall survival [12]. Most tumors seem to undergo change in perfusion parameters shortly after Avastin treatment. However, a substantially lower percentage of patients treated with Avastin have a good clinical response. Therefore, although change in perfusion might be necessary for eventual response, many non-responders also will show diminished perfusion. This may significantly lower the signal to noise ratio of this metric, and potentially limiting its clinical application.

MR Diffusion and ADC Histogram Analysis

Another physiologic MRI sequence under investigation in evaluating gliomas is diffusion weighted imaging (DWI). DWI measures the amount of motion of water molecules within tissue. Values from DWI scans are expressed as the apparent diffusion coefficient (ADC), and have been shown to be highly reproducible in multi-center trials [74]. Lower ADC values correspond to lower (more restricted) diffusion. Several physiologic properties of tumors may impact ADC measurements [reviewed in 54]. Water molecules are more restricted in their movement within cells than in the extra-cellular space. Since necrosis results in degradation of cellular integrity, necrosis is thought to increase ADC. Similarly, since edema increases interstitial water, edema also acts to increase ADC. Conversely, increased cell density results in diminished diffusion. DWI has been used to assess treatment effect of radiation and chemotherapies on malignant glioma [75,76]. It has also been suggested that diffusion values may correlate with malignancy and survival, potentially due to correlations with cell density, which can be reflective of cell proliferation rates and hence tumor malignancy [77].

Because tumors may show heterogeneous changes in ADC following therapy, the use of a voxel-by-voxel approach to assess impact on diffusion has been advocated [75]. Changes in ADC at the voxel level are measured to ensure that potentially offsetting regions of increasing and decreasing ADC will not cancel each other out, as would be the case if one considered the overall mean tumor ADC. This analysis has been termed a functional diffusion map (fDM). It has been reported that there is a positive correlation between increased diffusion measured 3-weeks after therapy, and 1-year survival in patients with malignant glioma. The prognostic value was similar to that obtained from radiographic response at 10 weeks. The rationale for this association is that effective chemotherapy and radiation induces cell death, tumoral edema, while inhibiting cell division (and thus increased cell density). These changes are then reflected in larger regions of increasing ADC values in responders compared to non-responders. None of the patients in this study were treated with Avastin, however, which raises some concerns. Specifically, Avastin inhibits edema resulting in decreased ADC thereby counteracting the signal being detected by fDM [5,78]. Since Avastin is becoming standard therapy for patients with GBM, this may substantially limit the utility the current fDM approach.

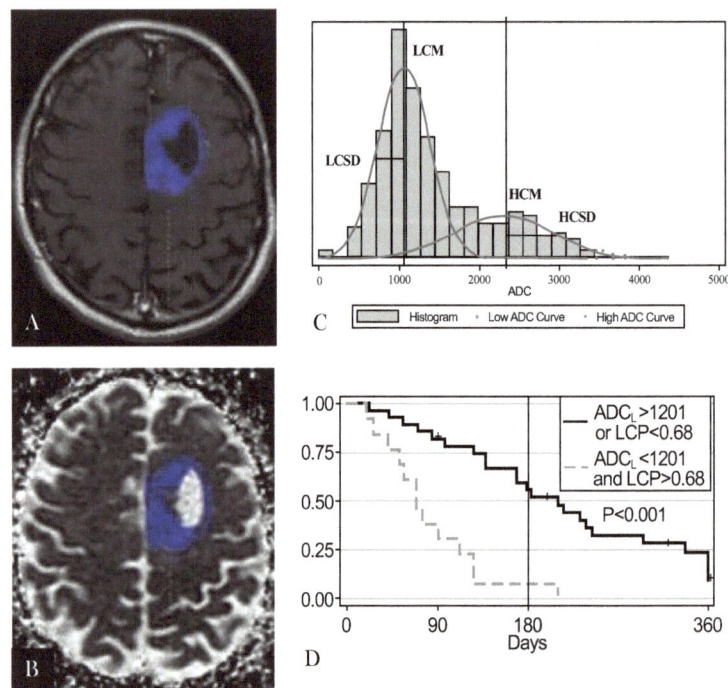

Figure 7: Patient with recurrent GBM following prior to Avastin treatment. Post-contrast images (A) show enhancing tumor which is then mapped to the corresponding ADC image (B) for ADC histogram generation (C). Several ADC classifiers are

generated including the lower and higher curve mean and standard deviation (LCM, HCM, LCSD, HCSD respectively). Combining the mean of the lower histogram curve with the proportion of values under the lower curve as a proportion of the total (LCP), results in the ability to stratify progression-free survival by the Kaplan-Meier method (D). Reprinted with permission from Pope *et al.*,"Recurrent glioblastoma multiforme: ADC histogram analysis predicts response to bevacizumab treatment." Radiology. 2009 Jul;252(1):182-9. Copyright © 2009 by RSNA

Some work indicates that the concentration of VEGF is predictive of response to Avastin treatment and survival [79,80]. GBM with regions of non-enhancing tumor, which typically have lower ADC values, express lower VEGF levels, and have a better prognosis than GBM lacking areas of non-enhancing tumor [81]. VEGF is concentrated in regions of pseudopallisading necrosis, a prominent pathologic feature of GBM, and high levels of necrosis are associated with worse outcomes [82]. Since ADC values are affected by cell density, necrosis, and edema, it is possible that ADC can be used as a non-invasive surrogate for VEGF expression, and thus susceptibility to Avastin therapy. Recently we published a report assessing the ability of ADC histogram analysis as a predictive biomarker of response to Avastin in patients with recurrent GBM [78]. Enhancing tumor portions were segmented and mapped to ADC images for histogram generation. We found that tumors with low ADC values prior to initiation of Avastin therapy were more likely to progress by 6 months, compared to those with higher ADC values. This ADC histogram analysis was more than 70% accurate at predicting 6-month progression free survival, and was superior to the Macdonald criteria at first follow-up (Fig. **7**). ADC values were not predictive of median survival in a non-Avastin treated cohort. If confirmed in a larger study (currently ongoing), this would be the first MRI-based predictive biomarker for Avastin response in GBM.

Radiotracers

One other class of potential biomarkers that should be mentioned are radiotracers used in combination with PET scans. Typical PET scans are performed after the injection of the glucose analogue 2-deoxy-2-[18F]fluoro-d-glucose (FDG). Unfortunately FDG has high background uptake in the cortex and basal ganglia due to active metabolism in these areas. Recently, additional PET tracers have been investigated. 18F-fluorothymidine (FLT) is a non-invasive biomarker of cell proliferation that has been shown to correlate with the proliferation index Ki-67 in gliomas [83]. Patients with reduction in FLT uptake at 6 weeks post treatment initiation survive three times longer than those that do not [84]. Thus FLT shows promise for being able to predict which patients will respond to bevacizumab treatment at a relatively early time point. Several amino acid based tracers also are available and appear to label tumor well. The best-studied is methyl-^{11}C-l-methionine (^{11}C-methionine), which is limited by its 20 minute half-life [85,86]. ^{18}F-labeled amino acid analogs with longer half-lives such as *O*-(2-[^{18}F]fluoroethyl)-l-tyrosine (FET) and ^{18}F-FDOPA have also been used to image brain tumors [87,88]. ^{18}F-FDOPA and ^{11}C-methionine have similar tumor uptake [85], and the diagnostic accuracy of ^{18}F-FDOPA appears to be superior to that of ^{18}F-FDG in evaluating both low and high grade gliomas [88]. Radiotracers specific for angiogenesis also are being developed, based on molecules that are preferentially expressed by new blood vessels. Radiolabeled ligands for these angiogenic molecules, including cyclic RGD peptides (which bind angiogenesis-associated forms of integrin) and prostate specific membrane antigen antibodies, are in use in animal and phase I human studies. [89]. Lastly bevacizumab itself has been radiolabeled and shown clinically to label liver metastasis from colorectal cancer [90]. Potentially this tracer could help determine which gliomas are susceptible to bevacizumab therapy.

Recurrence Following Bevacizumab Treatment: More Aggressive?

Several groups have suggested that tumor progression following bevacizumab therapy tends to be more infiltrative, often approaching a "gliomatosis cerebri" pattern (Fig. **8**), and may be even more difficult to treat [14,49,91,92]. This is supported by animal studies in which progressive tumor in a rat glioblastoma model appeared to co-opt the host vasculature resulting in increased infiltration of distant areas [46,93]. Similar patterns have been described in preclinical models of metastatic disease treated with VEGF pathway inhibitors [94].

Distant recurrence in GBM following current standard therapy (radiation and temozolomide) has been estimated at 20% [95]. In a recent study of 32 patients with GBM treated with a COX-II inhibitor (a presumed anti-angiogenic agent), an astounding 63% of patients had tumor recurrence > 3 cm from the primary site [96]. In a study of 61 patients with malignant glioma treated with bevacizumab and irinotecan or carboplatin, 30% had diffuse relapse [92]. In another study of malignant gliomas treated with bevacizumab and irinotecan, 23 of 38 patients (60%) had distant relapse [14].

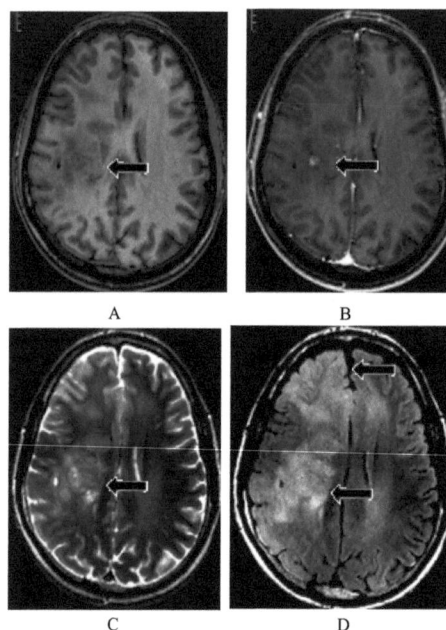

Figure 8: Patient with recurrent GBM following Avastin treatment. Pre and post-contrast images (A and B respectively) show a single small focus of enhancement (B, arrow). T2-weighted (C) and FLAIR images (D) show extensive infiltration of tumor in the right cerebrum (arrows), with some likely extension into the left cerebral hemisphere as well. There is relatively little mass effect, as is also seen with primary gliomatosis.

These results must be interpreted with some caution, however. Firstly, there is a wide range in reported distal relapse rates (20-60%), and the lower end of this range is not substantially higher than that for non-Avastin treated patients. Secondly, what constitutes distal disease is not well defined, particularly regarding non-enhancing tumor. Thirdly, these reports combine grade III and grade IV tumors, which may respond differently to Avastin treatment. Fourthly, increase in diffuse/distant disease is attributed to Avastin, when the patients were treated with Avastin plus chemotherapy. Fifthly, there was no control group in which the impact of important clinical factors such as age could be assessed, as well as the establishment of rates of diffuse disease in non-Avastin treated patients. Lastly there was no control for time to progression. The natural history of GBM is widely infiltrative, contributing to its high relapse rate. It might be that drugs which extend patient survival allow infiltrating tumor cells to migrate farther from the original tumor site, without underlying change in tumor biology. Studies in which rates of distant recurrence are assessed for GBM only, before and following Avastin monotherapy, should provide additional insight into this phenomenon.

Side Effects

One of the reported side effects of Avastin therapy that is diagnosed by imaging is posterior reversible encephalopathy syndrome (PRES) [97,98]. PRES is typically associated with hypertension (particularly in pregnancy) and immunosuppressive drugs, and thought to involve failure of autoregulatory CNS vascular mechanisms. PRES typically results in vasogenic edema of the posterior cerebrum, but can have a much larger distribution of affected areas, and also may result in infarction, with or without hemorrhage [99]. In the cases of PRES associated with Avastin, the patients made complete clinical recovery as is commonly the case.

CONCLUSION

It remains a challenge to select the best biomarker for treatment response for malignant gliomas, particularly given the limits of assessing non-enhancing tumor in patients treated with Avastin. Recently there has been a broadening of focus from strictly anatomic measurements to characterizing the utility of MRI techniques that quantify changes in tumor physiology. One resultant advantage is the potential to detect drug susceptibility or resistance prior to tumor size change. This could allow earlier treatment decisions saving patients from side-effects of ineffective therapies and allowing them to try alternative treatments sooner. However, in part because these physiologic imaging techniques have undergone rapid evolution, their utility remains clinically unproven and they are not currently incorporated into patient management decisions in a standardized way. Despite initial enthusiasm for perfusion imaging to assess response to Avastin, no perfusion-based imaging biomarkers for this therapy have been identified. To date only ADC histogram analysis has been shown to be predictive of response to Avastin therapy in patients with GBM. However, perfusion imaging combined with blood markers has been of value to predict response to another anti-angiogenic drug, suggesting that perfusion imaging may yet prove of clinical utility in monitoring or predicting Avastin treatment response. With the development of therapies that target specific biochemical pathways such as angiogenesis which impact tumor physiology in potentially predictable ways, the validation of physiologic biomarkers is becoming more critical.

REFERENCES

[1]   Macdonald DR, Cascino TL, Schold SC, Jr., Cairncross JG. Response criteria for phase II studies of supratentorial malignant glioma. J Clin Oncol 1990 8:1277–1280.

[2]   Rees JH, Smirniotopoulos JG, Jones RV, Wong K. Glioblastoma multiforme: radiologic-pathologic correlation. RadioGraphics 1996 16:1413-1438.

[3]   Hicklin DJ, Ellis LM. Role of the vascular endothelial growth factor pathway in tumor growth and angiogenesis. J Clin Oncol 2005 23:1011-1027.

[4]   Fischer I, Gagner JP, Law M, *et al.* Angiogenesis in gliomas: biology and molecular pathophysiology. Brain Pathology 2005 15:297-310.

[5]   Jordan BF, Runquist M, Raghunand N, *et al.* Dynamic contrast-enhanced and diffusion MRI show rapid and dramatic changes in tumor microenvironment in response to inhibition of HIF-1alpha using PX-478. Neoplasia 2005 7:475-485.

[6]   Jain RK. Normalizing tumor vasculature with anti-angiogenic therapy: a new paradigm for combination therapy. Nat Med 2001 7:987–989.

[7]   Jain RK. Normalization of tumor vasculature: an emerging concept in antiangiogenic therapy. Science 2005 307:58–62.

[8]   Yuan F, Chen Y, Dellian M, *et al.* Time-dependent vascular regression and permeability changes in established human tumor xenografts induced by an anti-vascular endothelial growth factor/vascular permeability factor antibody. Proc Natl Acad Sci U S A 1996 93:14765–14770

[9]   Pope WB, Lai A, Nghiemphu P, *et al.* MR Imaging in Patients with High Grade Gliomas Treated with Bevacizumab and Chemotherapy. Neurol 2006 66:1258-1260.

[10]   Vredenburgh JJ, Desjardins A, Herndon JE, *et al.* Phase II trial of bevacizumab and irinotecan in recurrent malignant glioma. Clin Cancer Res 2007 13:1253-1259.

[11]   Vredenburgh JJ, Desjardins A, Herndon JE 2nd, *et al.* Bevacizumab plus irinotecan in recurrent glioblastoma multiforme. J Clin Oncol 2007 Oct 20;25(30):4722-4729.

[12]   Desjardins A, Reardon DA, Herndon JE 2nd, *et al.* Bevacizumab plus irinotecan in recurrent WHO grade 3 malignant gliomas. Clin Cancer Res 2008 Nov 1;14(21):7068-7073.

[13]   Ananthnarayan S, Bahng J, Roring J, *et al.* Time course of imaging changes of GBM during extended bevacizumab treatment. J Neurooncol 2008 Jul;88(3):339-347. Epub 2008 Apr 4.

[14]   Norden AD, Young GS, Setayesh K, *et al.* Bevacizumab for recurrent malignant gliomas: efficacy, toxicity, and patterns of recurrence. Neurology 2008 Mar 4;70(10):779-787.

[15]   Hayward RM, Patronas N, Baker EH, *et al.* Inter-observer variability in the measurement of diffuse intrinsic pontine gliomas. Journal Neurooncol 2008 90(1):57-61.

[16]   Miller, AB, Hoogstraten, B, Staquet, M, Winkler, A. Reporting results of cancer treatment. Cancer 1981 47:207-214.

[17]   Therasse, P, Arbuck, SG, Eisenhauer, EA, *et al.* New guidelines to evaluate the response to treatment in solid tumors. European Organization for Research and Treatment of cancer, National Cancer Institute of the United States, National Cancer Institute of Canada. J. Natl. Cancer Inst. 2000 92:205-216.

[18]   US Food and Drug Administration, Guidance for industry: clinical trial endpoints for the approval of cancer drugs and biologics. 2007 http://www.fda.gov/cder/guidance/7478fnl.pdf.

[19]   Padhani AR, Ollivier L. The RECIST (Response Evaluation Criteria in Solid Tumors) criteria: implications for diagnostic radiologists. Br J Radiol 2001 74: 983–986.

[20]   Poussaint TY, Jaramillo D, Chang Y, *et al.* Interobserver reproducibility of volumetric MR imaging measurements of plexiform neurofibromas. AJR Am J Roentgenol 2003 Feb;180(2):419-423.

[21]   Reeves AP, Chan AB, Yankelevitz DF, *et al.* On measuring the change in size of pulmonary nodules. IEEE Trans Med Imaging 2006 25:435–450.

[22]   Kostis WJ, Yankelevitz DF, Reeves AP, *et al.* Small pulmonary nodules: reproducibility of three-dimensional volumetric measurement and estimation of time to follow-up CT. Radiology 2004 231:446–452.

[23]   Dempsey MF, Condon BR, Hadley DM. Measurement of tumor "size" in recurrent malignant glioma: 1D, 2D, or 3D? AJNR Am J Neuroradiol 2005 26: 770–776.

[24]   Partridge SC, Gibbs JE, Lu Y *et al.* MRI measurements of breast tumor volume predict response to neoadjuvant chemotherapy and recurrence-free survival. AJR 2005 184:1774–1781.

[25]   Warren KE, Patronas N, Aikin AA, *et al.* Comparison of one-, two-, and three-dimensional measurements of childhood brain tumors. J Natl Cancer Inst 2001 Sep 19;93(18):1401-1405.

[26]   Galanis E, Buckner JC, Maurer MJ, *et al.* Validation of neuroradiologic response assessment in gliomas: measurement by RECIST, two-dimensional, computer-assisted tumor area, and computer-assisted tumor volume methods. Neuro Oncol 2006 Apr;8(2):156-165. Epub 2006 Mar 2.

[27]   Shah GD, Kesari S, Xu R, *et al.* Comparison of linear and volumetric criteria in assessing tumor response in adult high-grade gliomas. Neuro Oncol 2006 Jan;8(1):38-46.

[28]   Sorensen AG, Patel S, Harmath C, *et al.* Comparison of diameter and perimeter methods for tumor volume calculation. J Clin Oncol 2001 Jan 15;19(2):551-557.

[29]   Sorensen AG, Batchelor TT, Wen PY, *et al.* Response criteria for glioma. Nat Clin Pract Oncol 2008 Nov;5(11):634-644. Epub 2008 Aug 19.

[30]   Watling CJ, Lee DH, Macdonald DR, *et al.* Corticosteroid-induced magnetic resonance imaging changes in patients with recurrent malignant glioma. J Clin Oncol 1994 Sep;12(9):1886-1889.

[31]   Kim JH, Chung YG, Kim CY, *et al.* Upregulation of VEGF and FGF2 in normal rat brain after experimental intraoperative radiation therapy. J Korean Med Sci 2004 Dec;19(6):879-886

[32]   Gonzalez J, Kumar AJ, Conrad CA, *et al.* Effect of bevacizumab on radiation necrosis of the brain. Int J Radiat Oncol Biol Phys 2007 Feb 1;67(2):323-326.

[33]   Torcuator R, Zuniga R, Mohan YS, *et al.* Initial experience with bevacizumab treatment for biopsy confirmed cerebral radiation necrosis. J Neurooncol 2009 Aug;94(1):63-68. Epub 2009 Feb 3.

[34]   Peca C, Pacelli R, Elefante A, *et al.* Early clinical and neuroradiological worsening after radiotherapy and concomitant temozolomide in patients with glioblastoma: tumour progression or radionecrosis? Clin Neurol Neurosurg 2009 May;111(4):331-334. Epub 2008 Dec 30

[35]   Cha S, Knopp EA, Johnson G, *et al.* Intracranial mass lesions: dynamic contrast-enhanced susceptibility-weighted echo-planar perfusion MR imaging. Radiology 2002 Apr;223(1):11-29.

[36]   Hein PA, Eskey CJ, Dunn JF, *et al.* Diffusion-weighted imaging in the follow-up of treated high-grade gliomas: tumor recurrence versus radiation injury. AJNR Am J Neuroradiol 2004 Feb;25(2):201-209.

[37]   Chen W. Clinical applications of PET in brain tumors. J Nucl Med. 2007 Sep;48(9):1468-1481. Epub 2007 Aug 17.

[38]   Raatschen HJ, Simon GH, Fu Y, *et al.* Vascular permeability during antiangiogenesis treatment: MR imaging assay results as biomarker for subsequent tumor growth in rats. Radiology 2008 May;247(2):391-399. Epub 2008 Mar 27.

[39]   Varallyay CG, Muldoon LL, Gahramanov S, *et al.* Dynamic MRI using iron oxide nanoparticles to assess early vascular effects of antiangiogenic versus corticosteroid treatment in a glioma model. J Cereb Blood Flow Metab 2009 Apr;29(4):853-860. Epub 2009 Jan 14.

[40]   Cloughesy T, Prados M, Wen P, *et al.* A phase II, randomized, noncomparative clinical trial of bevacizumab alone or in combination with irinotecan prolongs six-month PFS in recurrent, treatment-refractory glioblastoma. Late-breaking abstract. Twelfth Annual Meeting of the Society of Neuro-Oncology (SNO), 2007.

[41]   Chi AS, Sorensen AG, Jain RK, *et al.* Angiogenesis as a therapeutic target in malignant gliomas. Oncologist 2009 Jun;14(6):621-636. Epub 2009 Jun 1.

[42]   Jahnke K, Muldoon LL, Varallyay CG, *et al.* Bevacizumab and carboplatin increase survival and asymptomatic tumor volume in a glioma model. Neuro Oncol 2009 Apr;11(2):142-150. Epub 2008 Sep 4.

[43]   Karimi S, Lis E, Gilani S, *et al.* Nonenhancing Brain Metastases. J Neuroimaging 2009 May 20. [Epub ahead of print].

[44]   Labidi SI, Bachelot T, Ray-Coquard I, *et al.* Bevacizumab and paclitaxel for breast cancer patients with central nervous system metastases: a case series. Clin Breast Cancer 2009 May;9(2):118-121.

[45]   Mathews MS, Linskey ME, Hasso AN, *et al.* The effect of bevacizumab (Avastin) on neuroimaging of brain metastases. Surg Neurol 2008 Dec;70(6):649-652; discussion 653. Epub 2008 Feb 8.

[46]   Rubenstein JL, Kim J, Ozawa T, *et al.* Anti-VEGF antibody treatment of glioblastoma prolongs survival but results in increased vascular cooption. Neoplasia 2000 Jul-Aug;2(4):306-314.

[47]   Plotkin SR, Stemmer-Rachamimov AO, Barker FG 2nd, *et al.* Hearing improvement after bevacizumab in patients with neurofibromatosis type 2. N Engl J Med 2009 Jul 23;361(4):358-367. Epub 2009 Jul 8.

[48]   Smith JS, Cha S, Mayo MC, *et al.* Serial diffusion-weighted magnetic resonance imaging in cases of glioma: distinguishing tumor recurrence from postresection injury. J Neurosurg 2005 Sep;103(3):428-438.

[49]   Zuniga RM, Torcuator R, Jain R, *et al.* Efficacy, safety and patterns of response and recurrence in patients with recurrent high-grade gliomas treated with bevacizumab plus irinotecan. J Neurooncol 2009 Feb;91(3):329-336. Epub 2008 Oct 25.

[50]   Kumar AJ, Leeds NE, Fuller GN, *et al.* Malignant gliomas: MR imaging spectrum of radiation therapy- and chemotherapy-induced necrosis of the brain after treatment. Radiology 2000 Nov;217(2):377-384.

[51]   Siepmann DB, Siegel A, Lewis PJ. Tl-201 SPECT and F-18 FDG PET for assessment of glioma recurrence versus radiation necrosis. Clin Nucl Med 2005 Mar;30(3):199-200.

[52]   Pope WB, Sayre J, Perlina A, Villablanca JP, Mischel PS, Cloughesy TF. MR imaging correlates of survival in patients with high-grade gliomas. AJNR Am J Neuroradiol 2005 Nov-Dec;26(10):2466-2474.

[53]   Aronen HJ, Perkiö J. Dynamic susceptibility contrast MRI of gliomas. Neuroimaging Clin N Am 2002 Nov;12(4):501-523.

[54]   Provenzale JM, Mukundan S, Barboriak DP. Diffusion-weighted and perfusion MR imaging for brain tumor characterization and assessment of treatment response. Radiology 2006 Jun;239(3):632-649.

[55]   Saraswathy S, Crawford FW, Lamborn KR, *et al.* Evaluation of MR markers that predict survival in patients with newly diagnosed GBM prior to adjuvant therapy. J Neurooncol 2009 Jan;91(1):69-81. Epub 2008 Sep 23.

[56]   Danchaivijitr N, Waldman AD, Tozer DJ, *et al.* Low-grade gliomas: do changes in rCBV measurements at longitudinal perfusion-weighted MR imaging predict malignant transformation? Radiology 2008 Apr;247(1):170-178.

[57]   Parikh AH, Smith JK, Ewend MG, *et al.* Correlation of MR perfusion imaging and vessel tortuosity parameters in assessment of intracranial neoplasms. Technol Cancer Res Treat 2004 Dec;3(6):585-590.

[58]   Sugahara T, Korogi Y, Kochi M, *et al.* Correlation of MR imaging-determined cerebral blood volume maps with histologic and angiographic determination of vascularity of gliomas. AJR Am J Roentgenol 1998 Dec;171(6):1479-1486.

[59]   Hirai T, Murakami R, Nakamura H, *et al.* Prognostic value of perfusion MR imaging of high-grade astrocytomas: long-term follow-up study. AJNR Am J Neuroradiol 2008 Sep;29(8):1505-1510. Epub 2008 Jun 12.

[60]   Cao Y, Tsien CI, Nagesh V, *et al.* Survival prediction in high-grade gliomas by MRI perfusion before and during early stage of RT [corrected] Int J Radiat Oncol Biol Phys 2006 Mar 1;64(3):876-885. Epub 2005 Nov 18. Erratum in: Int J Radiat Oncol Biol Phys 2006 Jul 1;65(3):960.

[61]   Cao Y, Sundgren PC, Tsien CI, *et al.* Physiologic and metabolic magnetic resonance imaging in gliomas. J Clin Oncol 2006 Mar 10;24(8):1228-1235.

[62]   Leimgruber A, Ostermann S, Yeon EJ, *et al.* Perfusion and diffusion MRI of glioblastoma progression in a four-year prospective temozolomide clinical trial. Int J Radiat Oncol Biol Phys 2006 Mar 1;64(3):869-875. Epub 2005 Oct 13.

[63]   Akella NS, Twieg DB, Mikkelsen T, *et al.* Assessment of brain tumor angiogenesis inhibitors using perfusion magnetic resonance imaging: quality and analysis results of a phase I trial. J Magn Reson Imaging 2004 Dec;20(6):913-922.

[64]   Claes A, Gambarota G, Hamans B, *et al.* Magnetic resonance imaging-based detection of glial brain tumors in mice after antiangiogenic treatment. Int J Cancer 2008 May 1;122(9):1981-1986.

[65]   Sorensen AG, Batchelor TT, Zhang WT, *et al.* A "vascular normalization index" as potential mechanistic biomarker to predict survival after a single dose of cediranib in recurrent glioblastoma patients. Cancer Res 2009 Jul 1;69(13):5296-5300. Epub 2009 Jun 23.

[66]   Baar J, Silverman P, Lyons J, *et al.* A vasculature-targeting regimen of preoperative docetaxel with or without bevacizumab for locally advanced breast cancer: impact on angiogenic biomarkers. Clin Cancer Res 2009 May 15;15(10):3583-3590. Epub 2009 May 5.

[67]   Zhu AX, Holalkere NS, Muzikansky A, Horgan K, Sahani DV. Early antiangiogenic activity of bevacizumab evaluated by computed tomography perfusion scan in patients with advanced hepatocellular carcinoma. Oncologist 2008 Feb;13(2):120-125.

[68]   Dickson PV, Hamner JB, Sims TL, *et al.* Bevacizumab-induced transient remodeling of the vasculature in neuroblastoma xenografts results in improved delivery and efficacy of systemically administered chemotherapy. Clin Cancer Res. 2007 Jul 1;13(13):3942-3950.

[69]   Preda A, Novikov V, Moglich M, *et al.* MRI monitoring of Avastin antiangiogenesis therapy using B22956/1, a new blood pool contrast agent, in an experimental model of human cancer. J Magn Reson Imaging 2004 Nov;20(5):865-873.

[70]   Armitage PA, Schwindack C, Bastin ME, *et al.* Quantitative assessment of intracranial tumor response to dexamethasone using diffusion, perfusion and permeability magnetic resonance imaging. Magn Reson Imaging 2007 Apr;25(3):303-310. Epub 2006 Nov 13.

[71] Bastin ME, Carpenter TK, Armitage PA, *et al*. Effects of dexamethasone on cerebral perfusion and water diffusion in patients with high-grade glioma. AJNR Am J Neuroradiol 2006 Feb;27(2):402-408.

[72] Barboriak D, DesJardins A, Rich J, *et al*. Treatment of Recurrent Glioblastoma Multiforme with Bevacizimab and Irinotecan Leads to Rapid Decreases in Tumor Plasma Volume and Ktrans. Abstract SST09-05. Radiological Society of North America Annual Meeting 2007.

[73] Fischer I, Cunliffe CH, Bollo RJ, *et al*. High-grade glioma before and after treatment with radiation and Avastin: initial observations. Neuro Oncol 2008 Oct;10(5):700-708. Epub 2008 Aug 12.

[74] Koh DM, Blackledge M, Collins DJ, *et al*. Reproducibility and changes in the apparent diffusion coefficients of solid tumours treated with combretastatin A4 phosphate and bevacizumab in a two-centre phase I clinical trial. Eur Radiol 2009 Jun 23. [Epub ahead of print]

[75] Hamstra DA, Galbán CJ, Meyer CR, *et al*. Functional diffusion map as an early imaging biomarker for high-grade glioma: correlation with conventional radiologic response and overall survival. J Clin Oncol 2008 Jul 10;26(20):3387-3394. Epub 2008 Jun 9.

[76] Mardor Y, Pfeffer R, Spiegelmann R, *et al*. Early detection of response to radiation therapy in patients with brain malignancies using conventional and high bvalue diffusion-weighted magnetic resonance imaging. J Clin Oncol 2003; 21: 1094-1100.

[77] Oh J, Henry RG, Pirzkall A, *et al*. Survival analysis in patients with glioblastoma multiforme: predictive value of choline-to-N-acetylaspartate index, apparent diffusion coefficient, and relative cerebral blood volume. J Magn Reson Imaging 2004 May;19(5):546-554.

[78] Pope WB, Kim HJ, Huo J, *et al*. Recurrent glioblastoma multiforme: ADC histogram analysis predicts response to bevacizumab treatment. Radiology 2009 Jul;252(1):182-189.

[79] Flynn JR, Wang L, Gillespie DL, *et al*. Hypoxia-regulated protein expression, patient characteristics, and preoperative imaging as predictors of survival in adults with glioblastoma multiforme. Cancer 2008 Sep 1;113(5):1032-1042.

[80] Sathornsumetee S, Cao Y, Marcello JE, *et al*. Tumor angiogenic and hypoxic profiles predict radiographic response and survival in malignant astrocytoma patients treated with bevacizumab and irinotecan. J Clin Oncol 2008 Jan 10;26(2):271-278.

[81] Pope WB, Chen JH, Dong J, *et al*. Relationship between gene expression and enhancement in glioblastoma multiforme: exploratory DNA microarray analysis. Radiology 2008 Oct;249(1):268-277.

[82] Pierallini A, Bonamini M, Pantano P, *et al*. Radiological assessment of necrosis in glioblastoma: variability and prognostic value. Neuroradiology 1998 Mar;40(3):150-153.

[83] Chen W, Cloughesy T, Kamdar N, *et al*. Imaging proliferation in brain tumors with 18F-FLT PET: comparison with 18F-FDG. J Nucl Med 2005 Jun;46(6):945-952.

[84] Chen W, Delaloye S, Silverman DH, *et al*. Predicting treatment response of malignant gliomas to bevacizumab and irinotecan by imaging proliferation with [18F] fluorothymidine positron emission tomography: a pilot study. J Clin Oncol 2007 Oct 20;25(30):4714-4721.

[85] Becherer A, Karanikas G, Szabó M, *et al*. Brain tumour imaging with PET: a comparison between [18F]fluorodopa and [11C]methionine. Eur J Nucl Med Mol Imaging 2003 Nov;30(11):1561-1567. Epub 2003 Jul 23.

[86] Pötzi C, Becherer A, Marosi C, *et al*. [11C] methionine and [18F] fluorodeoxyglucose PET in the follow-up of glioblastoma multiforme. J Neurooncol 2007 Sep;84(3):305-314. Epub 2007 May 11.

[87] Laverman P, Boerman OC, Corstens FH, *et al*. Fluorinated amino acids for tumour imaging with positron emission tomography. Eur J Nucl Med Mol Imaging 2002 May;29(5):681-690. Epub 2002 Jan 11. Review. Erratum in: Eur J Nucl Med Mol Imaging 2002 Jun;29(6):834.

[88] Chen W, Silverman DH, Delaloye S, *et al*. 18F-FDOPA PET imaging of brain tumors: comparison study with 18F-FDG PET and evaluation of diagnostic accuracy. J Nucl Med 2006 Jun;47(6):904-911.

[89] Stollman TH, Ruers TJ, Oyen WJ, *et al*. New targeted probes for radioimaging of angiogenesis. Methods 2009 Jun;48(2):188-192. Epub 2009 Mar 24.

[90] Scheer MG, Stollman TH, Boerman OC, *et al*. Imaging liver metastases of colorectal cancer patients with radiolabelled bevacizumab: Lack of correlation with VEGF-A expression. Eur J Cancer 2008 Sep;44(13):1835-1840. Epub 2008 Jul 14.

[91] Waldman AD, Jackson A, Price SJ, *et al*. Quantitative imaging biomarkers in neuro-oncology. Nat Rev Clin Oncol 2009 Aug;6(8):445-454. Epub 2009 Jun 23.

[92] Narayana A, Kelly P, Golfinos J, *et al*. Antiangiogenic therapy using bevacizumab in recurrent high-grade glioma: impact on local control and patient survival. J Neurosurg 2009 Jan;110(1):173-180.

[93] Lamszus K, Kunkel P, Westphal M. Invasion as limitation to anti-angiogenic glioma therapy. Acta Neurochir Suppl 2003;88:169–177.

[94]   Leenders WP, Küsters B, Verrijp K, *et al.* Antiangiogenic therapy of cerebral melanoma metastases results in sustained tumor progression via vessel co-option. Clin Cancer Res 2004 Sep 15;10(18 Pt 1):6222-6230.

[95]   Wick W, Stupp R, Beule AC, *et al.* A novel tool to analyze MRI recurrence patterns in glioblastoma. Neuro Oncol 2008 Dec;10(6):1019-1024. Epub 2008 Jul 31.

[96]   Tuettenberg J, Grobholz R, Seiz M, *et al.* Recurrence pattern in glioblastoma multiforme patients treated with anti-angiogenic chemotherapy. J Cancer Res Clin Oncol 2009 Sep;135(9):1239-1244. Epub 2009 Mar 10.

[97]   Glusker P, Recht L, Lane B. Reversible posterior leukoencephalopathy syndrome and bevacizumab. N Engl J Med 2006 Mar 2;354(9):980-982.

[98]   Allen JA, Adlakha A, Bergethon PR. Reversible posterior leukoencephalopathy syndrome after bevacizumab/FOLFIRI regimen for metastatic colon cancer. Arch Neurol 2006 Oct;63(10):1475-1478.

[99]   Bartynski WS, Boardman JF. Distinct imaging patterns and lesion distribution in posterior reversible encephalopathy syndrome. AJNR Am J Neuroradiol 2007 Aug;28(7):1320-1327.

CHAPTER 13

The Radiographic Interpretation of Response to Avastin in Glioblastoma Multiforme

Nicholas Butowski* and Susan Chang

Department of Neuro-Oncology, Brain Tumor Research Center, University of California, San Francisco, San Francisco, California, 400 Parnassus Avenue, A808, San Francisco, California 94143-0350

Abstract: Avastin generates a decrease in vascular permeability in GBM which is marked by a decrease in cerebral edema and a decrease in contrast enhancement as seen on magnetic resonance imaging. These effects on the tumor vasculature may be mistakenly referred to as tumor responses because the historical method of measuring tumor response is based on tumor size assessed by contrast enhancement. This may explain why the few prospective phase II trials and several retrospective studies of Avastin in GBM report high radiographic response rates (30-60%) but modest improvements in progression-free survival and overall survival. Improved radiographic criteria for detecting disease progression in this context are needed and should be used in larger, randomized clinical trials which determine the magnitude of the survival benefit from Avastin.

INTRODUCTION

Glioblastoma mutiforme (GBM) is difficult to treat and associated with a high degree of morbidity and mortality. Standard treatment consists of cytoreductive surgery followed by radiation therapy in combination with temozolomide chemotherapy followed by adjuvant temozolomide which leads to a median survival of 14.6 months [1]. Key prognostic factors that influence outcome include functional performance status, age, and extent of surgical resection. Based on several meta-analyses, other types of adjuvant chemotherapy, mainly nitrosoureas, seem to add some survival benefit but the gain is modest [2-4]. Efforts are ongoing to develop more novel, effective agents or combinations of agents that may improve overall survival or prolong time to progression.

Such efforts led to the use of Avastin, a humanized monoclonal antibody against vascular endothelial growth factor (VEGF). The main hypothesis supporting the use of Avastin in GBM is that by eliminating poorly perfused and erratic tumor vasculature, perfusion is comparatively normalized leading to improved tissue oxygenation and drug delivery when used with concurrent cytotoxic chemotherapy [5,6]. This 'normalized' vasculature may lead to decreased extravasation of imaging contrast into interstitial spaces and consequently to a decrease in enhancement seen on MRI [7, 8].

Studies to date using Avastin in GBM recently resulted in the approval of Avastin as a single agent for the treatment of recurrent GBM following prior therapy. However, it is important to note that Avastin's effectiveness in GBM is based solely on an improvement in objective radiographic response rate (ORR) rather than data demonstrating an improvement in disease-related symptoms or increased survival. Per the '*Avastin Prescribing Information*' released by Genentech, Inc. in May 2009, the efficacy and safety of Avastin in GBM is based on 2 studies: the first was an open-label, multicenter, randomized, non-comparative study of patients with previously treated GBM. Patients received Avastin alone or Avastin plus irinotecan every 2 weeks until disease progression. All patients received prior radiotherapy and temozolomide. Of the 85 patients randomized to the Avastin arm, the median age was 54 years, 81% were in first relapse, Karnofsky performance status (KPS) was 90–100 for 45%. The efficacy of Avastin was demonstrated using MRI radiographic response assessment criteria and by stable or decreasing corticosteroid use, which occurred in 25.9% of the patients. Median duration of response was 4.2 months. The second study was a single-arm, single institution trial with 56 patients with GBM. All patients had disease progression after receiving temozolomide and radiation therapy. Patients received Avastin every 2 weeks until disease progression. The median age was 54 and 68% had a KPS of 90–100. The efficacy of Avastin was supported by an objective response rate of

*Address correspondence to Nicholas Butowski:** Department of Neuro-Oncology, Brain Tumor Research Center, University of California, San Francisco, San Francisco, California, 400 Parnassus Avenue, A808, San Francisco, California 94143-0350; Tel: 415-353-7500; Fax: 415-353-2187; Email: butowski@neurosurg.ucsf.edu

19.6% using the same response criteria as in the first study. Median duration of response was 3.9 months. These data were compared to the single digit radiographic response rates of several previous GBM studies and considered to be a vast improvement [9-11].

Yet before Avastin's approval there existed substantial challenges in the radiologic evaluation of ORR during brain tumor clinical trials and its use as a surrogate for survival benefit [7]. Imaging measurement approaches, response criteria, selection of lesions for measurement, technical imaging factors, intervals between tumor measurements and response confirmation, and validity of imaging as a measure of efficacy are all continuing topics of debate in the neuro-oncology community [7,8]. This debate now involves the added challenge of using antiangiogenic agents, such as Avastin, that may change the appearance of a tumor on an imaging study in a manner that indicates radiographic response but does not translate into considerable overall survival benefit. In this context, added questions to the debate over interpretation of ORR have arisen; these include whether radiographic response is a valid endpoint in Avastin studies and a valid surrogate measure for improved overall survival and whether it should it be the sole or primary endpoint? Some non-Avastin based, retrospective studies of patients with progressive high-grade gliomas demonstrate a positive correlation between radiographic response and progression free survival, but not overall survival [9,12]. Therefore, prior data, to some extent, support the validity of radiographic response as a predictor of progression free survival but its use as a surrogate of overall survival is in question. Of course, the definition of what is a true radiographic response --in general and in the context of an antiangiogenic agent-- remains up for debate. We'll explore this issue below first in general and then with specific regard to Avastin.

GENERAL RADIOGRAPHIC RESPONSE IN CANCER AND GBM

In systemic cancers, one dimensional tumor measurements have become the standard criteria to determine radiographic response [13]. The Response Evaluation Criteria in Solid Tumors (RECIST) instituted the use of one dimensional measurements in 2000. Several retrospective studies compared the RECIST criteria, with two- and three-dimensional measurements and volumetric measurements in GBM. These studies suggest that there is good concordance between the different methods in determining radiographic response in patients with both newly-diagnosed and recurrent GBM. However, studies prospectively validating the RECIST criteria in gliomas have not been performed.

Table 1: The Macdonald Criteria:

Complete Response:

1) Complete disappearance of all enhancing measurable and non-measurable disease sustained for at least 4 weeks.
     2) No new lesions.
     3) No steroids.
     4) Stable or improved clinically.

Partial Response:

1) $>$ 50% decrease compared to baseline in the sum of products of perpendicular diameters of all measurable enhancing lesions sustained for at least 4 weeks.
     2) No new lesions.
     3) Stable or reduced steroid dose
     4) Stable or improved clinically.

Stable Stable Disease:
1) Does not qualify for complete response, partial response, or progression.   2) Stable clinically.
Tumor Progression:

1) $>$ 25% increase in sum of the products of perpendicular diameters of enhancing lesions
     2) Any new lesion
     3) Clinical deterioration

Instead, the most commonly used criteria, termed the Macdonald Criteria (Table **1**), for assessing radiographic response to therapy in GBM is based on guidelines written in 1990 by Macdonald *et al* [14]. These guidelines are based on two-dimensional tumor measurements from computed tomography (CT) or magnetic resonance imaging (MRI) of the contrast enhancing portion of the tumor, in conjunction with clinical assessment and corticosteroid dose --meaning that a significant increase in a contrast enhancing lesion is used as an indicator of tumor progression or a decrease in enhancement is seen as a tumor response to treatment.

Contrast enhancement on a CT or MRI though is a non-specific process which reveals the passage of contrast across a disrupted blood-tumor barrier, across an area of tumor with abnormal vascular architecture, or across an area of disrupted integrity of the blood brain barrier. Thus, decreased enhancement can be promoted by a number of things other than a tumor's response to therapy including changes in corticosteroid doses, chemotherapy agents, and different radiological techniques. Increased enhancement can be produced by treatment-related inflammation, seizure activity, post-surgical changes, ischemia, radiation effects, and tumor growth.

Taking the above into consideration, there are evident limitations to the Macdonald criteria [7, 8, 15]. First and foremost among these limitations is that they only address the contrast-enhancing component of a GBM as seen on CT or MRI. Other confines include the difficulty in measuring irregularly shaped tumors, the lack of guidance for the assessment of multi-focal tumors, the difficulty in measuring enhancing lesions in the wall of cystic or surgical cavities as the cyst/cavity itself may be included in the tumor, and the inter-observer variability amongst those physicians interpreting the scans. These limitations also include evaluating pseudoprogression or the transient increase in tumor enhancement seen in 20-30% of patients with GBMs on their post-radiation MRI which is difficult to differentiate from genuine tumor progression [7, 8, 15]. In addition, a transient increase in enhancement that can be difficult to distinguish from recurrent disease can also occur following several additional therapies like chemotherapy wafers, therapies delivered by convection enhanced delivery, regional immunotherapies, and radiosurgery.

RADIOGRAPHIC RESPONSE IN AVASTIN TRIALS

Despite the above concerns about the Macdonald criteria, the majority of clinical trials and retrospective studies examining the use of Avastin in GBM used radiographic response as a primary endpoint and based it on the Macdonald criteria (see Table **2** for examples of a number of studies published in 2008 and 2009). Some of these studies slightly modified the Macdonald criteria but most did not and modifications were still centered on enhancing disease [16, 17]. Even studies analyzing the ability to predict treatment response of GBM to Avastin with fluorothymidine Positron Emission Tomography did so in a manner in which the MRI comparison was based only on the MacDonald criteria [18]. Utilizing the Macdonald criteria, nearly all of these Avastin studies in GBM demonstrated a significantly improved radiographic tumor response than previously reported data; they also reported reduced edema and to some extent reduced necrotic areas [19,30]. A few studies did comment on atypical, nonenhancing imaging patterns of GBM recurrence but most did not [16, 31].

Table 2: Recent Avastin studies in GBM and their endpoints

CLINICAL TRIAL	LEAD AUTHOR	PRIMARY ENDPOINTS
Phase II Trial of Bevacizumab and Irinotecan in Recurrent Malignant Glioma	Vrendenburgh *et al.* 2007	1) Radiographic response (Macdonald criteria) 2) PFS 3) 6m PFS
Bezacizumab Plus Irinotecan in Recurrent GBM	Vrendenburgh et al 2007	1) Radiographic Response (Macdonald criteria) 2) 6m PFS
Bevacizumab for recurrent malignant gliomas *retrospective study	Norden *et al.* 2008	1) radiographic response determined by Macdonald criteria 2) Volumetric MRI
Treatment With Bevacizumab and Irinotecan for Recurrent High-Grade Glial Tumors	Bokstein et al 2008	1) Radiographic Response (Macdonald criteria) 2) 6m PFS
Salvage Therapy With Single Agent Bevacizumab For Recurrent Glioblastoma *retrospective study	Chamberlain et al 2009	1) 6m PFS 2) radiographic response determined by Macdonald criteria
Bevacizumab plus irinotecan in the treatment patients with progressive recurrent malignant brain tumors. *retrospective study	Skovgaard et al 2009	1) 6m PFS 2) radiographic response determined by Macdonald criteria

Safety and Efficacy of Bevacizumab with Hypofractionated Stereotactic Irradiation for Recurrent Malignant Gliomas	Gutin *et al.* 2009	1) 6m PFS 2) radiographic response determined by Macdonald criteria
Phase II trial of single-agent bevacizumab followed by bevacizumab plus irinotecan at tumor progression in recurrent glioblastoma	Kreisl et al 2009	1) 6m PFS 2) radiographic response determined by Macdonald criteria
Bevacizumab and chemotherapy for recurrent glioblastoma: a single-institution experience. *retrospective study	Nghiemphu *et al.* 2009	1) PFS 2) OS
An exploratory survival analysis of anti-angiogenic therapy for recurrent malignant glioma. *retrospective	Norden *et al.* 2009	1) PFS 2) OS
Bevacizumab plus irinotecan in the treatment patients with progressive recurrent malignant brain tumours *retrospective	Poulsen *et al.* 2009	1) 6m PFS 2) radiographic response determined by Macdonald criteria 3) OS
Role of a second chemotherapy in recurrent malignant glioma patients who progress on bevacizumab *retrospective	Quant *et al.* 2009	1) 6m PFS 2) median PFS 3) radiographic response determined by Macdonald criteria
Efficacy, safety and patterns of response and recurrence in patients with recurrent high *retrospective	Zuniga *et al.* 2009	1) 6m PFS 2) radiographic response determined by Macdonald criteria
A Phase II, Randomized, Non-comparative Clinical Trial of Bevacizumab Alone or in Combination with CPT-11 Prolongs 6-Month Progression-free Survival in Recurrent, Treatment-Refractory Glioblastoma	Cloughesy *et al.*	1) 6m PFS 2) radiographic response determined by Macdonald criteria

OS= overall survival; PFS =progression free survival.

In this background and in addition to the continued concern over the limitations of the Macdonald criteria in connecting changes in enhancement with changes in tumor growth, now arises the added challenge of how such changes in enhancement are made more difficult to evaluate appropriately when considering the introduction of therapies, such as Avastin, that affect the permeability of tumor vasculature [32]. Antiangiogenic agents may produce decreased enhancement shortly after the initiation of therapy or long after its start indicating several possible biological mechanisms for such varied findings [23, 33]. Also, in all likelihood these "responses" are due in part to normalization of abnormally permeable tumor blood vessels and not to an antitumor effect [6-8, 16]. As a result, radiographic responses in studies with Avastin should be interpreted with prudence that accounts for the apparent inconsistency between the high response rates produced in recurrent GBM and the modest survival benefit that has been reported [16, 31, 34]. In fact, a recent study examined this issue when patients treated at a single institution on phase II clinical trials of Avastin and cediranib were compared to 18 patients treated on clinical trials of cytotoxic chemotherapies [28]. In univariate and multivariate analyses, antiangiogenic treatment group was a significant predictor of progression-free but not overall survival. These results suggest that anti-angiogenic therapy may fail to prolong overall survival in patients with recurrent malignant glioma and that progression free survival data for the antiangiogenic treatment group may be unduly influenced by inappropriate interpretation of imaging. If this conclusion proves correct, progression-free survival may be a less desirable endpoint for trials of anti-angiogenic therapies in patients with brain tumors.

Other recent studies do indicate a modest survival benefit from using Avastin in recurrent GBM but highlight another concern: a more invasive and possible multifocal recurrence pattern seen on imaging in those patients with GBMs that become resistant to Avastin [17, 31, 35, 36]. This invasive and perhaps multifocal pattern is in contradistinction to the more typical enhancing, edematous GBM recurrence pattern which generally also shows considerable mass effect. In this vein, there appears to be increasing acknowledgment that a number of patients with GBM treated with Avastin develop tumor recurrence characterized by an increase in the non-enhancing component depicted on T2-weighted/ fluid attenuated inversion recovery (FLAIR) sequences which may be solitary or multifocal [16, 37]. This pattern of recurrence may be due to the fact that anti-VEGF therapy increases the ability of tumor cells to co-opt existing normal blood vessels which results in an invasive non-enhancing tumor. This mechanism may be particularly important when VEGF-mediated angiogenesis is blocked in patients with GBM and may influence the response or lack thereof to additional therapy [35, 37].

Determination of the extent of this non-enhancing component of the tumor can be difficult on MRI as peritumoral edema and treatment related change may also appear as T2/FLAIR abnormality. Since the Macdonald Criteria do not account for the non-enhancing component of the tumor these areas of tumor progression may go unevaluated. A recent study by Norden et al examined this issue but was unable to demonstrate a significant difference in the pattern of recurrence between Avastin-treated and control patients --although there was a trend toward more diffuse or distant recurrences in the Avastin group, particularly among subjects who achieved a radiographic response. The study was limited by small numbers of patients and its inability to differentiate abnormal FLAIR in the Avastin treated group, which was presumably reflective of infiltrating tumor, from abnormal FLAIR hyperintensity in the control group which was likely reflective of a combination of infiltrating tumor and peritumoral edema. The authors suggested that the trend toward diffuse recurrence by Avastin therapy represented a combination of increased suppression of local enhancing tumor recurrence with decreased suppression of nonenhancing, infiltrative tumor progression. Certainly, if this were to be proven true in future studies then correlation with tumor genotypes may identify a molecular substrate that explains this observation and may help guide therapy. Preliminary studies along these lines have been done but on small numbers of patients [38].

Other retrospective studies have attempted to better understand the imaging response to Avastin as well. A recent study demonstrated that higher tumor expression levels of VEGF were associated with radiographic response and that expression of other markers of angiogenesis and hypoxia, such as carbonic anhydrase 9, were associated with poorer survival outcome.[39] However, the duration of the response and the patterns of recurrence were not discussed. Another retrospective study of 15 patients with recurrent GBM who responded to Avastin regimen treatment, and had extended follow-up revealed that the relative reduction of edema and necrosis was sustained even in patients who developed tumor progression indicating a more invasive phenotypic recurrence versus the more expected necrotic and edematous recurrence pattern [23]. A further retrospective study demonstrated 60% (23/38) of patients with high grade glioma treated with Avastin demonstrated a 'distant' (defined as at least one new focus of enhancement observed outside of 2-cm limit around the index lesion) pattern of recurrence on post contrast studies, with or without evidence of local progression [17]. A "diffuse" (defined by areas of recurrence seen on FLAIR that were not concordant with increased areas of enhancement) was seen in 18% (7/38) of patients who progressed while on treatment with Avastin. Based on this information the study suggested that FLAIR MRI sequences may more accurately reflect the infiltrating tumor burden because some patients whose tumors recur while on Avastin demonstrate a lack of concordance between areas of increased enhancement and areas of hyperintensity on FLAIR sequences. Such studies support the conclusion that the morphology of recurrent GBM following Avastin regimen therapy is distinct from that on other chemotherapy and requires different imaging criteria to properly assess radiographic response and progression.

THE FUTURE

Inadequate radiographic response criteria may be overestimating the true clinical benefits of Avastin in studies completed to date. Published proposals that account for such difficulties with radiographic response suggest that clinical studies report both radiographic and clinical response rates and use volumetric rather than cross-sectional area to measure lesion size [8]. Other studies suggested that techniques such as apparent diffusion coefficient (ADC) histogram analysis, diffusion weighted imaging, or dynamic perfusion MRI measurements can assist in stratifying progression-free survival in patients with recurrent GBM prior to Avastin treatment [17, 40, 41].

These suggestions and the increased awareness that contrast enhancement is nonspecific and not always a surrogate of tumor response together with the need to assess the non-enhancing component of GBM, inspired the recent creation of The Response Assessment in Neuro-Oncology (RANO) Working Group [15]. This group is charged with the development of new standardized response criteria for clinical trials for patients with brain tumors which accounts for both the known challenges of radiographic assessment of GBM and the emerging challenges associated with antiangiogenic agents like Avastin. Unlike the Macdonald criteria which do not take into account progressive non-enhancing disease, the new response criteria will regard enlarging areas of non-enhancing tumor as evidence of tumor progression. However, the group cautions that the quantification of the increase in T2/FLAIR signal must be differentiated from other causes of increased T2/FLAIR signal including radiation effects, decreased corticosteroid dosing, demyelination, ischemic injury, infection, seizures, and post-operative changes. The RANO also advises that changes in T2/FLAIR signal that raises the possibility of infiltrating tumor include mass effect, infiltration of the cortical ribbon, and location outside of the radiation field.

Future, if not current, trials will likely combine therapies which inhibit angiogenesis with those which prevent invasion. Thus, in addition to the RANO group criteria it may also be wise to include, as a primary endpoint, the duration of response and the overall survival as a more accurate indicator of a true antitumor effect. It is also very important to incorporate novel imaging techniques such as perfusion and permeability imaging and diffusion imaging into clinical trials of these combination agents to develop better ways of measuring biologic effects. Such additional imaging techniques may help answer the critical questions which remain about how antiangiogenic agents work and how to combine them with other therapies. Work is also left to be completed in understanding the progress relating to the identification of potential biomarkers for anti-VEGF-agent efficacy in humans [42]. Lastly, an ongoing area of interesting research involves examining whether MRI based classifications of GBM may help predict tumor recurrence patterns of patients on Avastin or other novel agents [43, 44].

REFERENCES

[1]   Stupp R. Radiotherapy plus concomitant and adjuvant temozolomide for glioblastoma. N Engl J Med 2005; 352(10): 987-96.

[2]   Fine H.A. Meta-analysis of radiation therapy with and without adjuvant chemotherapy for malignant gliomas in adults. Cancer 1993; 71(8): 2585-97.

[3]   Stenning, S.P., L.S. Freedman, N.M. Bleehen. An overview of published results from randomized studies of nitrosoureas in primary high grade malignant glioma. Br J Cancer 1987; 56(1): 89-90.

[4]   Stewart, L.A. Chemotherapy in adult high-grade glioma: a systematic review and meta-analysis of individual patient data from 12 randomised trials. Lancet 2002; 359(9311): 1011-8.

[5]   Gerstner, E.R. Antiangiogenic agents for the treatment of glioblastoma. Expert Opin Investig Drugs 2007; 16(12): 1895-908.

[6]   Jain, R.K. Angiogenesis in brain tumours. Nat Rev Neurosci, 2007. 8(8): 610-22.

[7]   Henson, J.W., S. Ulmer, G.J. Harris. Brain tumor imaging in clinical trials. AJNR Am J Neuroradiol 2008; 29(3): 419-24.

[8]   Sorensen, A.G., et al., Response criteria for glioma. Nat Clin Pract Oncol 2008; 5(11): 634-44.

[9]   Ballman, K.V. The relationship between six-month progression-free survival and 12-month overall survival end points for phase II trials in patients with glioblastoma multiforme. Neuro Oncol 2007; 9(1): 29-38.

[10]   Lamborn, K.R. Progression-free survival: an important end point in evaluating therapy for recurrent high-grade gliomas. Neuro Oncol 2008; 10(2): 162-70.

[11]   Wong, E.T. Outcomes and prognostic factors in recurrent glioma patients enrolled onto phase II clinical trials. J Clin Oncol 1999; 17(8): 2572-8.

[12]   Hess, K.R. Response and progression in recurrent malignant glioma. Neuro Oncol 1999; 1(4): 282-8.

[13]   Therasse, P. New guidelines to evaluate the response to treatment in solid tumors. European Organization for Research and Treatment of Cancer, National Cancer Institute of the United States, National Cancer Institute of Canada. J Natl Cancer Inst 2000; 92(3): 205-16.

[14]   Macdonald, D.R. Response criteria for phase II studies of supratentorial malignant glioma. J Clin Oncol 1990; 8(7): 1277-80.

[15]   van den Bent, M.J. End point assessment in gliomas: novel treatments limit usefulness of classical Macdonald's Criteria. J Clin Oncol, 2009. 27(18): 2905-8.

[16]   Norden, A.D. Bevacizumab for recurrent malignant gliomas: efficacy, toxicity, and patterns of recurrence. Neurology 2008; 70(10): 779-87.

[17]   Zuniga, R.M. Efficacy, safety and patterns of response and recurrence in patients with recurrent high-grade gliomas treated with bevacizumab plus irinotecan. J Neurooncol 2009; 91(3): 329-36.

[18]   Chen, W. Predicting treatment response of malignant gliomas to bevacizumab and irinotecan by imaging proliferation with [18F] fluorothymidine positron emission tomography: a pilot study. J Clin Oncol 2007; 25(30): 4714-21.

[19]   Gonzalez, J. Effect of bevacizumab on radiation necrosis of the brain. Int J Radiat Oncol Biol Phys 2007; 67(2): 323-6.

[20]   Vredenburgh, J.J. Phase II trial of bevacizumab and irinotecan in recurrent malignant glioma. Clin Cancer Res 2007; 13(4): 1253-9.

[21]   Vredenburgh, J.J. Bevacizumab plus irinotecan in recurrent glioblastoma multiforme. J Clin Oncol 2007; 25(30): 4722-9.

[22]   Bokstein, F., S. Shpigel, D.T. Blumenthal. Treatment with bevacizumab and irinotecan for recurrent high-grade glial tumors. Cancer 2008; 112(10): 2267-73.

[23]   Ananthnarayan, S. Time course of imaging changes of GBM during extended bevacizumab treatment. J Neurooncol 2008; 88(3): 339-47.

[24]   Chamberlain, M.C., S.K. Johnston. Salvage therapy with single agent bevacizumab for recurrent glioblastoma. J Neurooncol 2009.

[25]   Gutin, P.H. Safety and Efficacy of Bevacizumab with Hypofractionated Stereotactic Irradiation for Recurrent Malignant Gliomas. Int J Radiat Oncol Biol Phys 2009.

[26]   Kreisl, T.N. Phase II trial of single-agent bevacizumab followed by bevacizumab plus irinotecan at tumor progression in recurrent glioblastoma. J Clin Oncol 2009; 27(5): 740-5.

[27]   Nghiemphu, P.L. Bevacizumab and chemotherapy for recurrent glioblastoma: a single-institution experience. Neurology 2009; 72(14): 1217-22.

[28]   Norden, A.D. An exploratory survival analysis of anti-angiogenic therapy for recurrent malignant glioma. J Neurooncol 2009; 92(2): 149-55.

[29]   Poulsen, H.S. Bevacizumab plus irinotecan in the treatment patients with progressive recurrent malignant brain tumours. Acta Oncol 2009; 48(1): 52-8.

[30]   Quant, E.C. Role of a second chemotherapy in recurrent malignant glioma patients who progress on bevacizumab. Neuro Oncol 2009.

[31]   Narayana, A. Antiangiogenic therapy using bevacizumab in recurrent high-grade glioma: impact on local control and patient survival. J Neurosurg 2009; 110(1): 173-80.

[32]   Fischer, I. High-grade glioma before and after treatment with radiation and Avastin: initial observations. Neuro Oncol 2008; 10(5): 700-8.

[33]   Pope, W.B. MRI in patients with high-grade gliomas treated with bevacizumab and chemotherapy. Neurology 2006; 66(8): 1258-60.

[34]   de Groot, J.F., W.K. Yung. Bevacizumab and irinotecan in the treatment of recurrent malignant gliomas. Cancer J 2008; 14(5): 279-85.

[35]   Bergers, G., D. Hanahan. Modes of resistance to anti-angiogenic therapy. Nat Rev Cancer 2008; 8(8): 592-603.

[36]   Miletic, H. Anti-VEGF therapies for malignant glioma: treatment effects and escape mechanisms. Expert Opin Ther Targets 2009; 13(4): 455-68.

[37]   Chi, A., A.D. Norden, P.Y. Wen. Inhibition of angiogenesis and invasion in malignant gliomas. Expert Rev Anticancer Ther 2007; 7(11): 1537-60.

[38]   Zhang, W. Antiangiogenic therapy with bevacizumab in recurrent malignant gliomas: analysis of the response and core pathway aberrations. Chin Med J (Engl) 2009; 122(11): 1250-4.

[39]   Sathornsumetee, S. Tumor angiogenic and hypoxic profiles predict radiographic response and survival in malignant astrocytoma patients treated with bevacizumab and irinotecan. J Clin Oncol 2008; 26(2): 271-8.

[40]   Pope, W.B. Recurrent glioblastoma multiforme: ADC histogram analysis predicts response to bevacizumab treatment. Radiology 2009; 252(1): 182-9.

[41]   Varallyay, C.G. Dynamic MRI using iron oxide nanoparticles to assess early vascular effects of antiangiogenic versus corticosteroid treatment in a glioma model. J Cereb Blood Flow Metab 2009; 29(4): 853-60.

[42]   Jain, R.K. Lessons from phase III clinical trials on anti-VEGF therapy for cancer. Nat Clin Pract Oncol 2006; 3(1): 24-40.

[43]   Lim, D.A. Relationship of glioblastoma multiforme to neural stem cell regions predicts invasive and multifocal tumor phenotype. Neuro Oncol 2007; 9(4): 424-9.

[44]   Saraswathy, S. Evaluation of MR markers that predict survival in patients with newly diagnosed GBM prior to adjuvant therapy. J Neurooncol 2009; 91(1): 69-81.

CHAPTER 14

Imaging Responses of Bevacizumab

R Thind, Y.S Mohan and T Mikkelsen*

Hermelin Brain Tumor Center, Henry Ford Hospital

Abstract: Although, the recent use of bevacizumab has resulted in significant imaging responses, it appears that the impact on overall survival may be more limited, likely illustrating the fact that imaging responses may not correlate well with overall survival. given that vascular endothelial growth factor (VEGF) the ligand to which bevacizumab binds is responsible for a significant component of the permeability of the blood-brain-barrier (BBB), it will be important to distinguish effects on the BBB from true anti-tumor effects. This paper will illustrate the patterns of responses seen typically on post-Gd and FLAIR MRI. We also illustrate several patterns of tumor progression seen in patients treated with long-term bevacizumab in order to illustrate the range of novel imaging changes being seen in this clinical setting. The addition of bevacizumab to the clinical armamentarium for the treatment of glioblastoma has enhanced clinical outcomes, but it has come with the need to understand the range of imaging effects for this novel targeted therapy.

INTRODUCTION

Glioblastoma multiforme (GBM) is the most aggressive and infiltrative of primary brain tumors, characterized by diffuse parenchymal infiltration and prominent angiogenesis. The overall prognosis of patients with glioblastoma remains poor with a median survival rate of 14.6 months. Key prognostic factors that influence outcome include tumor histology, patient age, their functional performance status, and extent of surgical resection. Standard treatment for patients with GBM includes maximal safe resection, focal fractionated radiation with concurrent temozolomide, an oral alkylating chemotherapeutic agent, followed by 6-12 cycles of adjuvant temozolomide [1].

PATHOPHYSIOLOGY

Angiogenesis in GBM involves complex paracrine interactions between glioma cells, stromal cells and endothelial cells. As tumor growth outstrips its own blood supply, hypoxia and necrosis develop triggering an "angiogenic switch", which leads to the secretion of proangiogenic growth factors and new blood vessel formation [2]. These blood vessels are histologically abnormal and have enlarged vessel diameter, gaps in pericyte coverage with increased vessel permeability and thickened basement membranes. The resulting vascular network is functionally inhomogenous with regions of differential perfusion which may cause hypoxia and impair delivery of chemotherapeutic agents to the tumor. Disruption of the normal blood brain barrier leads to vasogenic peritumoral edema, which correlates with poorer survival [3].

Due to the highly vascular nature of GBM, antiangiogenic strategies are a promising approach in the treatment of GBM. Multiple signaling pathways and growth factors implicated in tumor angiogenesis have been elucidated. Vascular endothelial growth factor (VEGF) is a highly expressed proangiogenic molecule in GBM. Oversecretion of VEGF has been linked with a permeable blood brain barrier with leakage of intravascular components into the peritumor space and resulting vasogenic edema. Bevacizumab is a newly developed antiangiogenic drug which acts as a non-selective monoclonal antibody to VEGF [4]. As a monoclonal antibody, it offers the advantages of high specificity, limited cross-reactivity, and a relatively long half life requiring less frequent drug administration. Monoclonal antibodies are expensive to produce and the current formulation of bevacizumab requires intravenous infusion.

Bevacizumab has been shown to reduce tumor burden and peritumoral edema in patients with GBM patients and has applications as adjunctive therapy in other forms of malignancy such as colorectal cancer, non small cell lung cancer and breast cancer.

*Address correspondence to T Mikkelsen: Hermelin Brain Tumor Center, Depts. Neurology & Neurosurgery, E&R3096 Henry Ford Hospital 2799 West Grand Blvd., Detroit, MI 48202; Tel: 313 916-1094 or 8133, Fax: 313 916-9855, E-mail: tmikkel1@hfhs.org

Studies demonstrate improved progression-free and overall survival with bevacizumab [5-7]. Decreased edema improves patient quality of life by reducing corticosteroid dependence and related side effects (Fig. **1a, b, c** and **d**). After national multicenter phase 2 studies with Genentech, bevacizumab was granted accelerated approval for use in recurrent GBM in May 2009.

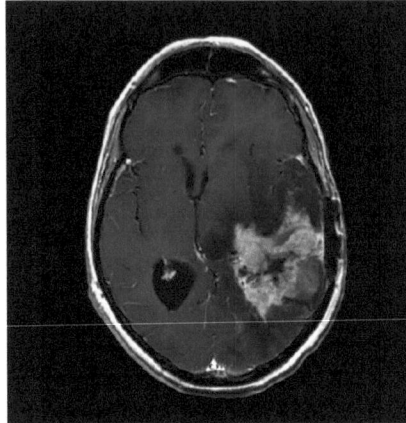

Figure 1a: Gadolinium enhanced MRI showing tumor in the left temporo-parietal lobe with surrounding edema and mass effect causing midline shift.

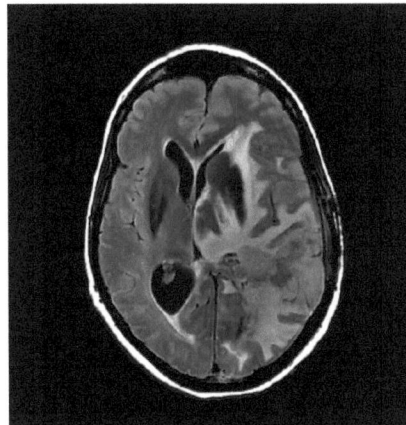

Figure 1b: Corresponding FLAIR image showing significant T2 hyperintensity.

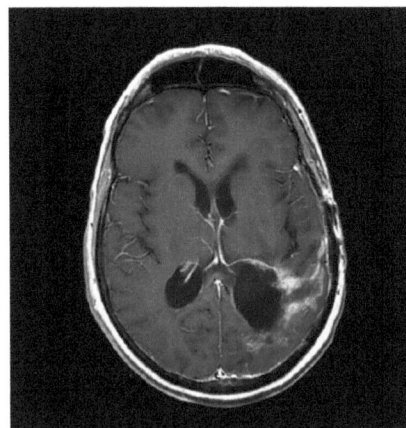

Figure 1c: Gadolinium enhanced MRI showing significant improvement in the contrast enhancing lesion and surrounding edema with resolution of midline shift.

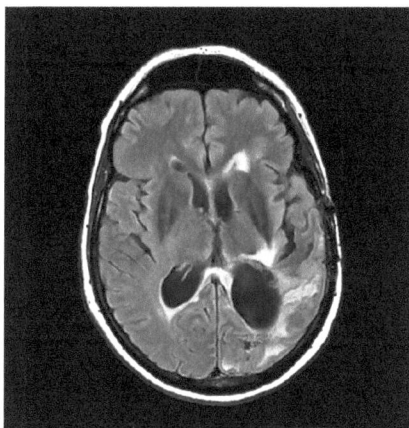

Figure 1d: FLAIR image after 6 weeks of bevacizumab therapy showing improvement in peritumoral edema and mass effect.

Diffuse brainstem glioma carries a poor prognosis with an overall median survival time of 44-74 weeks. Conventional chemotherapy appears to be ineffective and case reports have analyzed the use of bevacizumab in brainstem glioma [8]. With lesions in critical anatomic regions such as the brainstem, the anti-edema effect of anti-VEGF agents may play a significant role in symptom control and overall clinical improvement (Fig. **2a, b, c** and **d**).

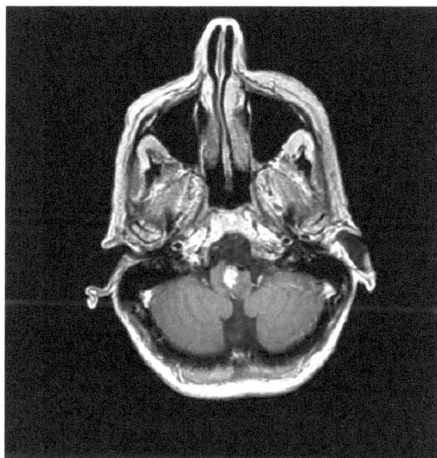

Figure 2a: Gadolinium enhanced MRI showing medullary lesion.

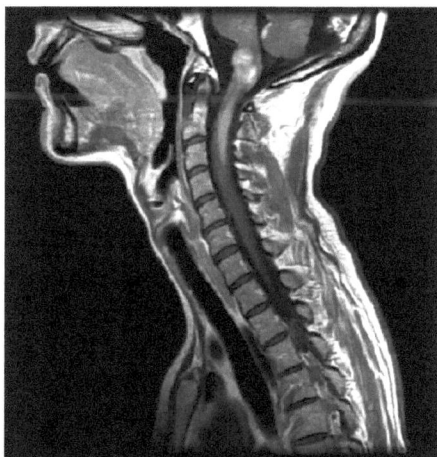

Figure 2b: Gadolinium enhanced spine MRI showing medullocervical lesion.

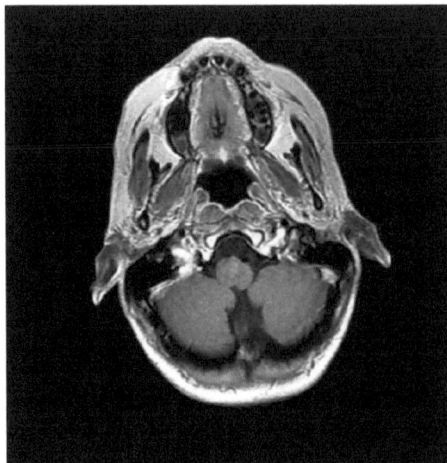

Figure 2c: Near complete response in medullary lesion following 8 weeks of bevacizumab therapy.

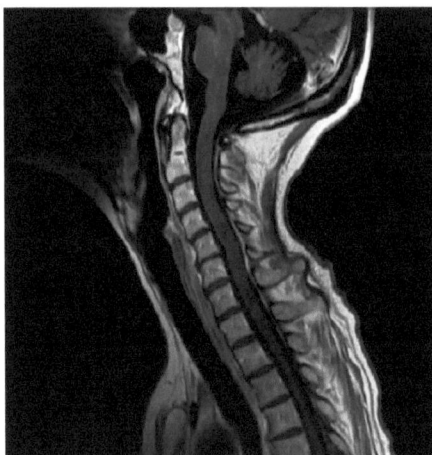

Figure 2d: Saggital view of same patient showing near complete response in the cervical lesion.

Bevacizumab is traditionally used as an adjunct with a chemotherapeutic agent (such as irinotecan) where its role is to promote vascular normalization and inhibit neovasculature formation (Fig. **3a** and **b**). Efficient vascular normalization may enhance cytotoxic chemotherapy delivery and improve oxygen delivery to the tumor.

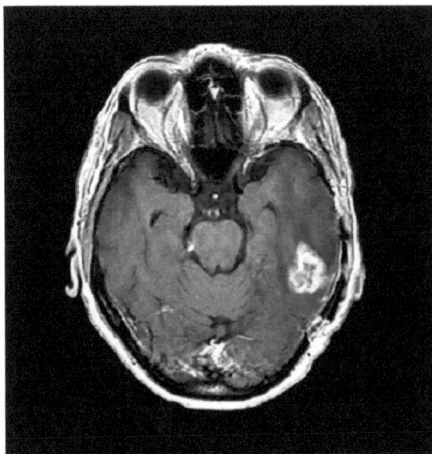

Figure 3a: Post gadolinium MRI showing enhancing lesion in the left temporal lobe.

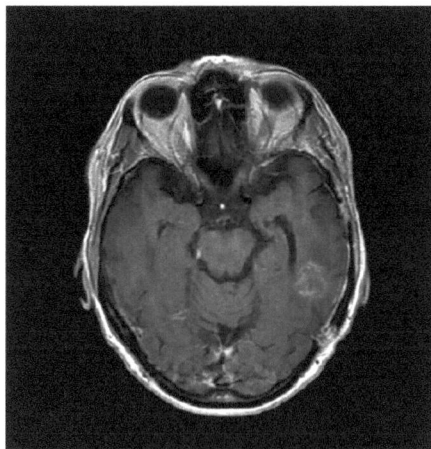

Figure 3b: Post gadolinium MRI after 8 weeks of bevacizumab therapy showing major partial response.

For recurrent GBM, bevacizumab at 10mg/kg administered intravenously every two weeks is a well tolerated regimen. Potential adverse reactions are related to the drug's inhibition of circulating VEGF and include arterial and venous thromboembolic events and hemorrhage ranging from mild to severe has also been reported. It also poses a risk for clinically significant hypertension, proteinuria, and impaired wound healing [9]. Careful monitoring is required to detect and treat these complications.

RADIOGRAPHIC FINDINGS

On pretreatment brain magnetic resonance imaging (MRI), GBM tumors enhance after intravenous injection of contrast because the blood brain barrier of tumor vasculature is dysfunctional and permeable, allowing extravasation of contrast media into the surrounding brain parenchyma. A decrease in enhancement after therapy with bevacizumab and standard cytotoxic chemotherapy agents is typically interpreted as a decrease in tumor burden (Fig. **4a, b, c** and **d**). The MacDonald criteria have traditionally been used to assess radiographic response to treatment and tumor progression [10]. It is based on two-dimensional measurement of the enhancing tumor on computed tomography (CT) or MRI. A 50% decrease in cross sectional area of enhancement on T1 weighted post gadolinium sequences defines tumor response, while a 25-49% decrease in largest area of cross sectional enhancement constitutes a minimal partial response as proposed by Norden *et al* [11]. Cloughesy *et al.* performed a retrospective analysis of the time course of radiographic response to bevacizumab in GBM patients [12]. The investigators observed that maximal reduction in tumor volume in patients with an initial response to bevacizumab treatment may occur as early as 16 days, but took an average of approximately 5 months (Fig **5a** and **b**). All patients had a maximal response within approximately 8 months.

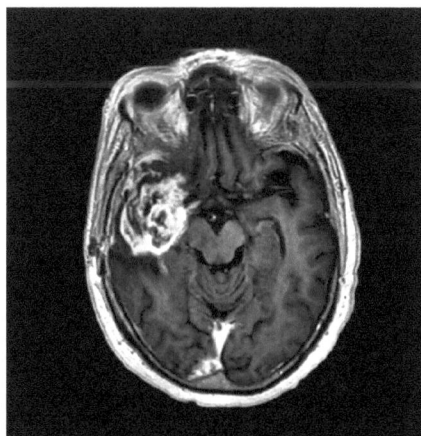

Figure 4a: Gadolinium enhanced MRI showing right temporal lobe lesion.

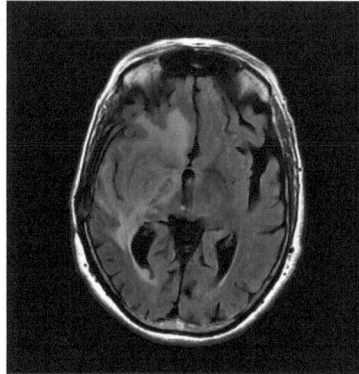

Figure 4b: FLAIR sequence corresponding to the above lesion.

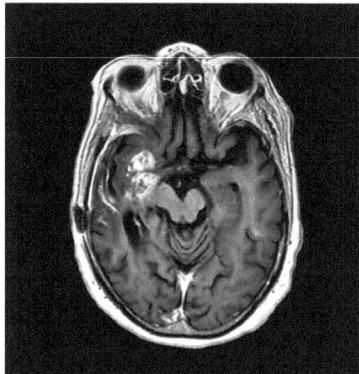

Figure 4c: Following 6 weeks of bevacizumab treatment, major partial response noted.

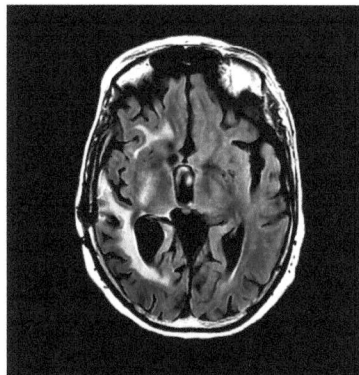

Figure 4d: Significant improvement in the T2 abnormality after 6 weeks of bevacizumab therapy.

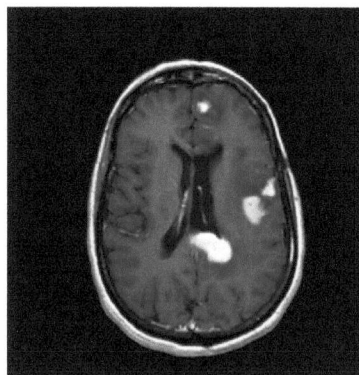

Figure 5a: Gadolinium enhanced MRI showing multifocal contrast enhancing lesions in the left cerebral hemisphere.

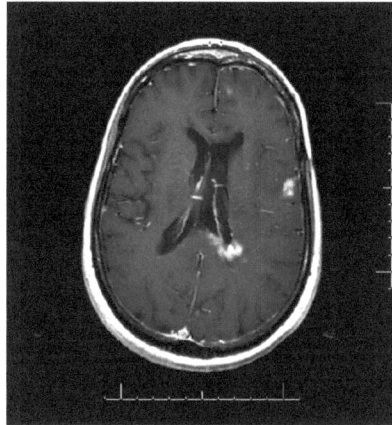

Figure 5b: Following 6 weeks of bevacizumab, gadolinium enhanced MRI showing significant improvement in the multifocal contrast enhancing lesions.

However, in the setting of therapy anti-VEGF therapy the correlation between decreased contrast enhancement and decreased tumor burden is less clear. Neutralization of VEGF stabilizes the blood brain barrier, decreases vascular permeability, and subsequently mitigates gadolinium extravasation into the surrounding brain parenchyma. The anti-permeability effect of bevacizumab is believed to explain the high initial radiographic response rate. Tumor progression on bevacizumab lacks necrosis, but a blanched or smudged pattern of enhancement has been reported (Fig. **6a, b** and **c**).

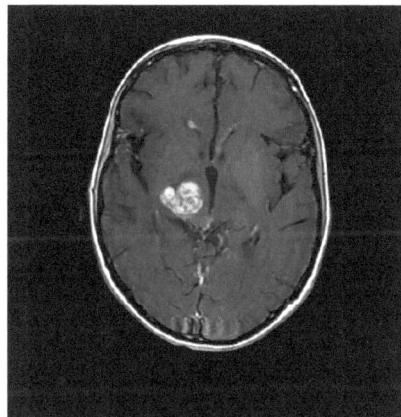

Figure 6a: Gadolinium enhanced MRI showing nodular enhancing lesion in the right thalamic area.

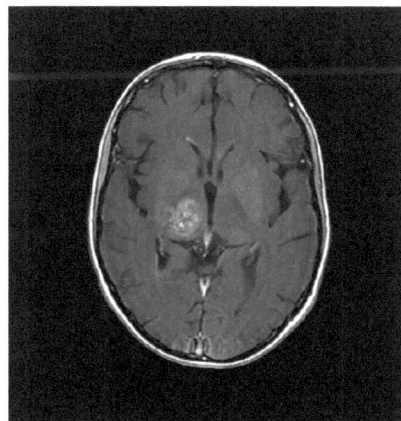

Figure 6b: Gadolinium enhanced MRI showing improvement in the enhancing lesion after 6 weeks of bevacizumab therapy.

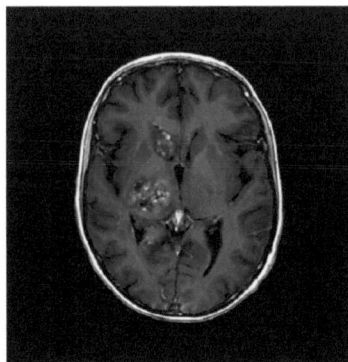

Figure 6c: Progressive disease following 6 months of bevacizumab therapy in the index right thalamic lesion and distally in the right frontal horn with blanching or smudged pattern.

Therefore, tumor growth may not be visible on standard post contrast MRI sequences and the clinical utility of standard MacDonald's criteria of radiographic response following VEGF inhibition is an area of active debate, with some suggesting alternative methods to measure tumor response to anti-VEGF therapies. Contrast enhancement is not specicfic to tumor progression and is also seen in treatment related inflammation and radiation necrosis or "pseudoprogression". Other limitations associated with Macdonald's criteria include difficulty of measuring irregularly shaped lesions, lack of assessment of the non-enhancing component of the tumor, absence of guidelines to assess multi-focal lesions and difficulty in measuring rim enhancing cystic lesions. This could lead to inaccurate assessment of the efficacy of treatment modalities.

It is unclear to what extent if any that anti-VEGF agents cause direct tumor cytotoxicity independent of their vascular effects. Failure to directly alter neoplastic cell biology likely accounts for subsequent progression in the majority of initial responders. Although anti-VEGF therapies have been associated with prolonged progression free survival and overall survival, most glioma patients treated with these drugs eventually relapse. The patients who initially respond but then relapse have likely developed escape mechanisms to bypass VEGF inhibition.

After treatment with bevacizumab, brain MRI imaging shows decreased peritumoral edema and necrotic changes which persist even in patients who develop tumor progression. This radiographic finding suggests that the morphology of recurrent GBM following bevacizumab therapy is distinct from progression after other forms of chemotherapy. Some studies have suggested that blocking VEGF induced angiogenesis may trigger the tumor to draw from native brain blood vessels for adequate nutrition and oxygenation. Tumor spread may occur via direct infiltration into surrounding brain tissue or by cooptation along native brain blood vessels. These blood vessels maintain an impermeable blood brain barrier, therefore perivascular tumor is not detected on contrast enhanced MRI studies. Some have postulated that changes seen on fluid attenuation inversion recovery (FLAIR) sequences or diffusion weighted imaging (DWI) may represent progressive tumor, even in the absence of contrast enhancement (Fig. **7a, b, c** and **d**). Currently, the MacDonald criteria do not include FLAIR or DWI sequences to assess tumor progression hence making it difficult to reliably assess infiltrative tumor burden. New neuroimaging criteria or biomarkers may be needed to assess glioma response in the setting of bevacizumab.

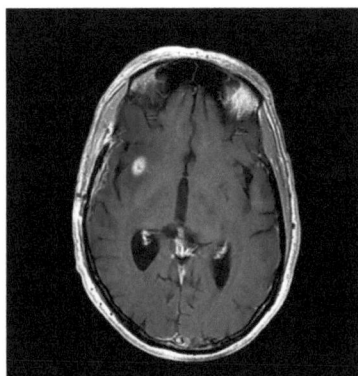

Figure 7a: Post gadolinium MRI showing a nodular enhancing lesion in the right temporal lobe.

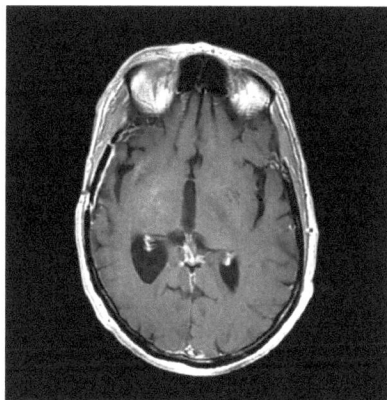

Figure 7b: Following 6 months of bevacizumab therapy, sustained near complete response of the enhancing lesion.

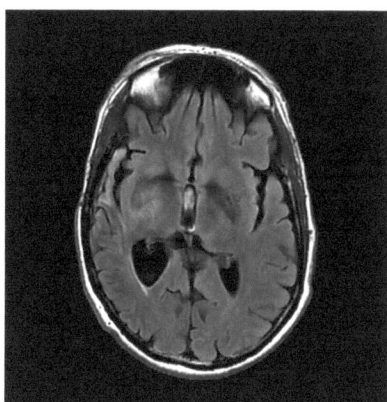

Figure 7c: FLAIR sequence after 6 months of bevacizumab showing minimal T2 hyperintensity.

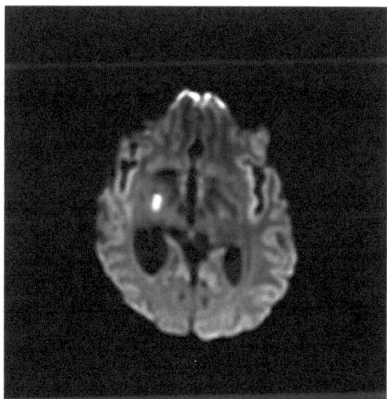

Figure 7d: DWI image after 6 months of bevacizumab therapy after patient presented with new neurological symptoms localizing to the above right internal capsule lesion.

A clinical study on efficacy, safety and patterns of response and recurrence in patients with recurrent high grade gliomas treated by bevacizumab and irinotecan by Mikkelsen *et al.* [13] recognized three patterns of tumor recurrence on bevacizumab. Local recurrence is defined as an increase of at least 25% in the maximal cross-sectional area of enhancement. Distant recurrence is defined as a new focus of contrast enhancement distal to the index lesion. Finally, diffuse recurrence is defined by areas of diffuse infiltrative tumor growth seen on FLAIR sequences not correlating with increased enhancement. The authors have noted that prior to recurrence seen on post gadolinium sequences, one can find increased signal intensity on DWI or worsening hyper intensity on FLAIR sequences, which might suggest high tumor cellularity and early progressive disease, however further clinical trials are needed (Fig. **8a-i**).

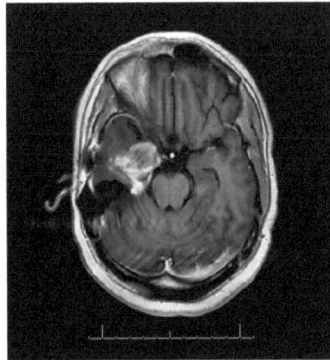

Figure 8a: Post gadolinium MRI showing right temporal contrast enhancing lesion.

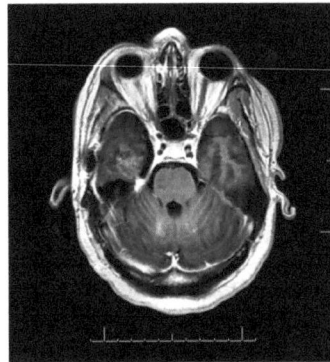

Figure 8b: Following 8 weeks of bevacizumab near complete response of the enhancing lesion noted.

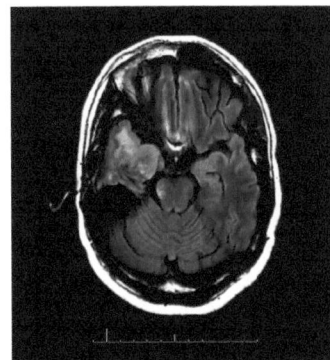

Figure 8c: Minor T2 hyperintensity on FLAIR prior to bevacizumab.

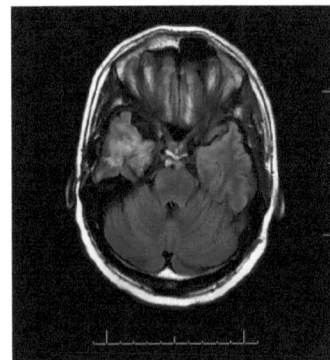

Figure 8d: Persisting T2 abnormality on FLAIR after 8 weeks of bevacizumab.

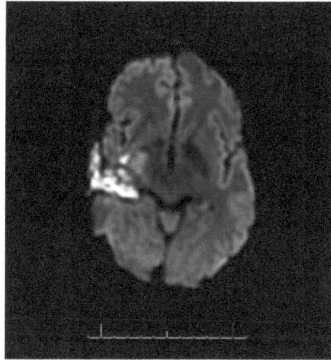

Figure 8e: DWI sequence prior to bevacizumab.

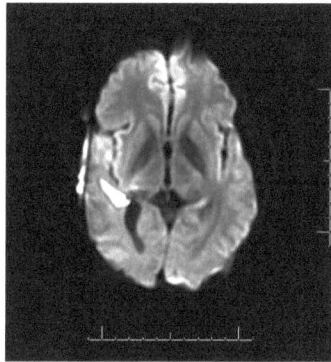

Figure 8f: DWI sequence after 8 weeks of bevacizumab therapy showing improvement in the external capsular lesion.

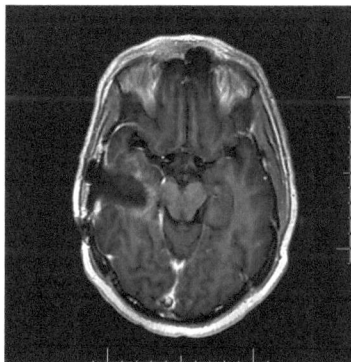

Figure 8g: Post contrast sequence after 4 months of bevacizumab treatment and new symptoms of left sided weakness.

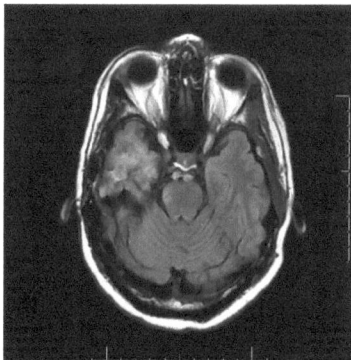

Figure 8h: FLAIR sequence showing stable T2 hyperintensity after 4 months of bevacizumab.

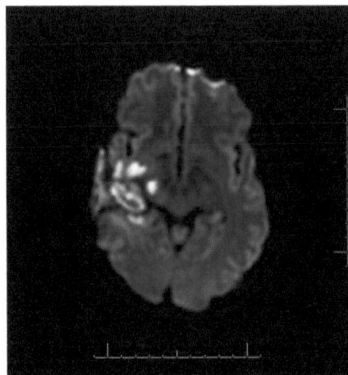

Figure 8i: DWI sequence after 4 months of bevacizumab showing new lesions in the right cerebral peduncle and globus pallidus externa.

It is known that FLAIR or T2 signal abnormality can be a combined result of edema, infiltrative tumor, gliosis or treatment related encephalopathy, hence making it difficult to assess actual tumor size. A recent retrospective review of 20 patients by R. Jain *et al.* [14] used volumetric assessment of the contrast enhancing lesion in addition to the nonenhancing lesion and employed DWI and apparent diffusion coefficient (ADC) to assess imaging response in patients on bevacizumab. DWI can assess tumor cellularity based on water diffusivity within the tumor. DWI and ADC have been used to distinguish normal brain tissue from necrosis, edema and solid enhancing tumor [15-18]. An inverse relationship has been noted between ADC values and tumor cellularity [19]. A progressive decrease in ADC values was found early on [6 weeks to 3 months) in the nonenhancing lesion in patients with progressive disease on bevacizumab, even though the contrast enhancing lesion continued to decrease, suggesting that ADC values can be used as an early tool to measure nonenhancing infiltrative cellular tumor growth.

While contrast extravasation is accepted as a useful radiographic marker for tumor progression, the pattern of response and progression seen on MRI in patients treated with bevacizumab reflects its unique antiangiogenic properties and non enhanced MRI sequences may need to be included in future response and recurrence criteria [20, 21]. Due to the fundamental limitations associated with the currently used Macdonald's criteria, there is an ongoing international effort to develop new standardized response criteria under the auspices of Response Assessment in Neuro-Oncology (RANO) working group. The initial proposal for updated response criteria in the setting of anti-angiogenic therapy by the RANO working group includes significant increase in T2/FLAIR non-enhancing lesion on stable or increasing doses of corticosteroids as well as clear clinical deterioration not attributable to other causes apart from the tumor.

RADIATION NECROSIS

Cerebral radiation necrosis is a recognized potential treatment complication that usually develops in brain tumor patients one to two years after radiation treatment. The primary mechanism of the delayed injury in radiation necrosis is secondary to vascular endothelial injury resulting in endothelial thickening, lymphocytic and macrophagic infiltrates, presence of cytokines, hyalinization, fibrinoid deposition, thrombosis and occlusion. It is a continuous process leading to tissue hypoxia, necrosis, edema, and concomitant release of vascular endothelial growth factor (VEGF), resulting partly in disruption of the blood brain barrier. The damage is usually irreversible and in some cases relentlessly progressive with an overall guarded prognosis. Many therapies have been tried for radiation necrosis without much success including anticoagulants, hyperbaric oxygen and steroids. T.Mikkelsen *et al.* confirmed 100% radiographic response noted by Gonzales *et al.* with bevacizumab treatment for biopsy confirmed cerebral radiation necrosis [22, 23]. The rationale for use of bevacizumab in cerebral radiation necrosis is due to the relative normalization of the blood brain barrier secondary to decreased levels of VEGF.

REFERENCES

[1]　　Stupp R, Mason WP, Van Den Bent MJ *et al.* Radiotherapy plus concomitant and adjuvant temozolomide for glioblastoma. N Engl J Med 2005;352:987-996.

[2]   Elizabeth R Gerstner, A. Gregory Sorensen, Rakesh K Jain *et al.* Anti-vascular endothelial growth factor therapy for malignant glioma. Current Neurology and Neuroscience reports 2009;9:254-26.2

[3]   Pope WB, Sayre J, Perlina A *et al.* MR imaging correlates of survival in patients with high grade gliomas. Am J Neuroradiol 2005;26:2466-2474.

[4]   Duda DJ, Batchelor TT, Willett CG *et al.* VEGF targeted cancer therapy strategies: current progress, hurdles and future prospects. Trends Mol Med 2007;13(6):223-230.

[5]   Teri N Kreisl, Lyndon Kim, Paul Duic *et al.* Phase 2 trial of single agent bevacizumab followed by bevacizumab plus irinotecan at tumor progression in recurrent glioblastoma. Journal of Clinical Oncology 2008;27:740-745.

[6]   P.L. Nghiemphu, W Liu, Y Lee *et al.* Bevacizumab and chemotherapy for recurrent glioblastoma. Neurology 2009;72:1217-1222.

[7]   Vredenburgh JJ, Desjardins A, Herndon JE *et al.* Phase 2 trial of bevacizumab and irinotecan in recurrent malignant glioma. Clin Cancer Res 2007;13:1253-1259.

[8]   Roy Torcuator, Richard Zuniga, Randa Loutfi *et al.* Bevacizumab and irinotecan treatment for progressive diffuse brainsten glioma: case report. J Neuro Oncology 2009;93:409-412.

[9]   Larry W Buie and John M Valgus. Bevacizumab: A treatment option for recurrent glioblastoma multiforme. Annals of pharmacotherapy 2008;42:1486-90.

[10]   Macdonald DR, Cascino TL, Schold SC *et al.* Response criteria for phase 2 studies of malignant glioma. J Clin Oncol 1990;8:1277-80.

[11]   Norden AD, Young GS, Setayesh K *et al.* Bevacizumab for recurrent malignant gliomas: efficacy, toxicity and patterns of recurrence. J Neuro Oncology 2009;91:329-336.

[12]   Suchitra Ananthnarayan, Jennie Bahng, James Roring *et al.* Time course of imaging changes of GBM during extended bevacizumab treatment. J Neuro Oncology 2008;88:339-347.

[13]   R.M. Zuniga, R Torcuator, R Jain *et al.* Efficacy, safety and patterns of response and recurrence in patients with recurrent high grade gliomas treated with bevacizumab plus irinotecan. J Neuro Oncology 2009;91:329-336.

[14]   R. Jain, L Scarpace, S.K. Ellika *et al.* Imaging response criteria for recurrent gliomas treated with bevacizumab: Role of diffusion weighted imaging as an imaging biomarker. in press, J. Neuro Oncology, 2009.

[15]   Le Bihan D, Breton E, Lallemand D *et al.* MR imaging of intravoxel incoherent motions: application to diffusion and perfusion in neurologic disorders. Radiology 1986;161:401-7.

[16]   Tien RD, Felsberg GJ, Friedman H *et al.* MR imaging of high grade cerebral gliomas: value of diffusion weighted echoplanar pulse sequences. AJR Am J Roentgenol 1994;162:671-77.

[17]   Brunberg JA, Chenevert TL, McKeever PE *et al.*MR determination of water diffusion coefficients and diffusion anisotropy: correlation with structural alteration in gliomas of the cerebral hemispheres. AJNR Am J Neuroradiol 1995;16:361-71.

[18]   Noguchi K, Watanabe N, Nagayoshi T *et al.* Role of diffusion weighted echo-planar MRI in distinguishing between brain abscess and tumor: a preliminary report. Neuroradiology 1999;41:171-74.

[19]   Gupta RK, Sinha U, Cloughesy TF *et al.* Inverse correlation between choline magnetic resonance spectroscopy signal intensity and the apparent diffusion coefficient in human glioma. Magn Reson Med 1999;41:2-7.

[20]   Martin J van den Bent, Michael A Vogelbaum, Patrick Y Wen *et al.* End point assessment in gliomas: Novel treatments limit usefulness of classical Macdonald's criteria. J Clin Oncol 2009;27(18): 2905-2908.

[21]   R.K. Jain, D.G. Duda *et al.* Biomarkers of response and resistance to antiangiogenic therapy. Nat Rev Clin Oncol 2009;6(6):327-338.

[22]   Roy Torcuator, Richard Zuniga, Yethadore S Mohan *et al.* Initial experience with bevacizumab treatment for biopsy confirmed cerebral radiation necrosis. J Neuro Oncology 2009;94:63-68.

[23]   Gonzales J, Kumar AJ, Conrad CA *et al.* Effect of bevacizumab on radiation necrosis of the brain. Int J Radiat Oncol Biol Phys 2007;67(2):323-326.

CHAPTER 15

Assessing Radiographic Response to Bevacizumab in Patients with GBM

John W. Henson[1,*] and Bart Keogh[2,3]

[1]Neurology, [2]Neuroradiology, Swedish Neuroscience Institute, and [3]Radia PS, Seattle, WA

Abstract: Abnormal gadolinium enhancement has been the standard characteristic for the measurements of brain tumors in clinical trials, but new therapies that target the vascular components of tumors have highlighted the shortcomings of enhancement as a measurement tool. Inhibitors of vascular endothelial growth factor (VEGF), such as bevacizumab, can produce rapid changes in the degree of contrast enhancement within malignant gliomas and in the extent of surrounding hyperintense T2-weighted signal. These effects, which are consistent with decreasing permeability of tumor capillaries, make it exceedingly difficult to employ conventional measures of tumor size in the setting of clinical trials. This chapter will review these issues and describe approaches to tumor measurement in the era of VEGF inhibitors.

INTRODUCTION

Clinical trials for malignant gliomas have relied heavily on neuroimaging to assess the activity of cytotoxic agents, particularly in Phase II trials. Radiographic response for each patient is assigned according to predetermined criteria, using some measure of the size of a gadolinium enhancing lesion as the key parameter. There have been challenges with imaging and determination of efficacy, however. There are at least four significant issues in this regard.

- Gadolinium enhancement reflects the state of the blood-brain barrier and thus is an indirect measure of a cytotoxic effect on tumor cells.

- There are significant technical issues in the selection and measurement of enhancing lesions in patient with malignant gliomas [1].

- Malignant gliomas have been very resistant to treatment, historically, with a complete response (CR) or partial response (PR) being seen in only 10% of patients in clinical trials for newly diagnosed malignant gliomas [2] and in 1–10% of patients with progressive disease [3, 4]. As a result, many studies have reported the duration of stable disease (SD) as a measure of "response", using either time to progression (TTP) or progression free survival (PFS) [5]. Despite this, there is reasonable evidence to support the fact that, depending on the criteria employed, radiographic response correlates with survival in patients with malignant gliomas.

- The fourth issue concerns the recent introduction of the vascular endothelial growth factor (VEGF) inhibitor bevacizumab (Avastin®) into treatment for glioblastoma multiforme (GBM). As a result of the rapid reduction in lesion enhancement induced by bevacizumab, the interpretation of neuroimaging studies in brain tumor practice and trials has been greatly altered, and these new considerations are the subject of this chapter.

BEVACIZUMAB RELATED NEUROIMAGING CHANGES IN ENHANCING MALIGNANT GLIOMAS

There has been more rapid accrual of clinical experience with the administration of bevacizumab for malignant glioma patients with progressive disease than with any other newly-introduced agent in the history of neuro-oncology. The speed with which bevacizumab has been accepted by neuro-oncologists reflects primarily the profound changes seen on neuroimaging and rapid improvement in edema-related symptoms, and secondarily, the recent suggestion in clinical trials that bevacizumab prolongs PFS in brain tumor patients. The imaging changes can be divided into those associated with an apparent response upon initiating treatment, and features that are seen with disease progression during administration of bevacizumab.

*****Address correspondence to John W. Henson**: Neurology, Swedish Neuroscience Institute, 550 17th Avenue, Suite 500, Seattle, WA 98122; Tel: (206) 320-2300, Fax (206) 320-8282, E-mail: john.henson@swedish.org

Thomas C. Chen (Ed)

<u>Response</u>. At least four imaging changes are associated with an apparent response upon initiating treatment. The fact that these changes are not in seen every patient likely indicates that bevacizumab is not active in every tumor. The reasons for this dichotomous response remain unclear, but likely relate to variations in the role of VEGF in each tumor.

- A rapid decrease in the degree of lesional enhancement with gadolinium contrast.

A profound decrease in the intensity of abnormal contrast enhancement may occur within nodular components of the tumor (Fig. 1). This change can be seen within 24 to 48 hours of receiving the first dose of bevacizumab, and continuing decrease in intensity of enhancement can occur over several weeks[6]. This feature is noted in about 50% of patients with glioblastoma, and it seems to be correlated with older age [7] and the presence of central nonenhancing areas with the mass that likely represent necrosis [6]. Decreased enhancement is thought to relate to normalization of the blood brain barrier in tumor capillaries. Of note, there is evidence that bevacizumab reduces the enhancement (and edema, see below) seen with treatment related changes in brain tissue. Early decrease in enhancement correlates with improved survival [8]. Mixed responses, with necrotic appearing areas showing changes and solidly enhancing areas lacking changes, can be seen [9].

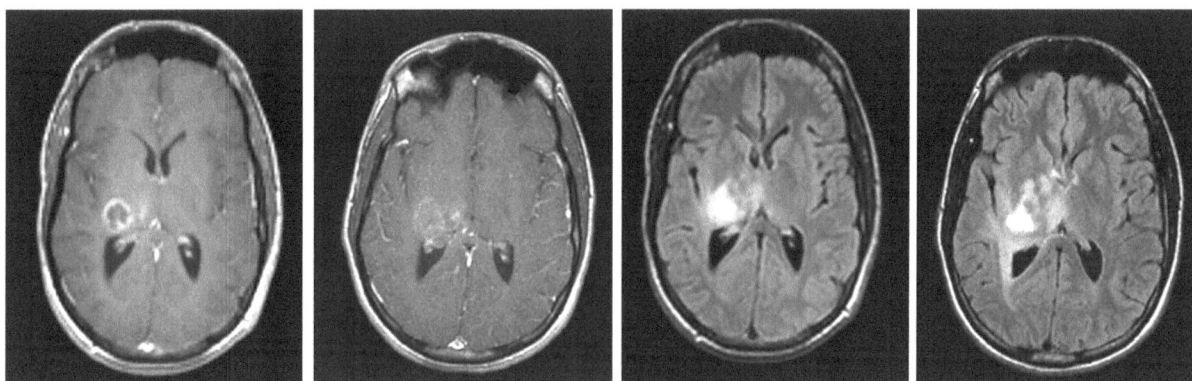

Figure 1: Decrease in contrast enhancement within a right thalamic region GBM on T1-weighted gadolinium-enhanced images before (A) and after (B) treatment with anti-VEGF therapy. Progression in the infiltrating component can be seen on T2/FLAIR images after treatment (before C, and after D).

- Decrease in the extent of vasogenic edema surrounding the lesion.

Vasogenic edema has a characteristic appearance on fast spin echo (FSE) T2-weighted and T2 fluid attenuated inversion recovery (FLAIR) images. It is very hyperintense, approximately equal to the intensity of cerebrospinal fluid (CSF) on FSE T2-weighted images. Edema exhibits finger-like projections into the white matter surrounding the enhancing mass lesion, with relative sparing of the cortex. By comparison, infiltrating tumor is only mildly hyperintense, does not spare cortex, and projections into subcortical white matter are not prominent. A remarkable decrease in the extent of vasogenic edema can be seen within several days of bevacizumab administration in approximately 50% of patients [8]. This may or may not accompany decrease in enhancement, and is thought to another manifestation of blood brain barrier normalization [9].

- Decrease in size of the enhancing mass lesion.

The above-noted features are notable for two reasons. First, reduction in enhancement makes it difficult to accurately follow the size of the lesion. Secondly, the finding makes plausible mechanistic sense since bevacizumab inactivates circulating VEGF, and VEGF is thought to have roles in tumor capillary proliferation, blood brain barrier function, and generation of edema. It is unlikely that bevacizumab has a direct cytotoxic effect on tumor cells. Thus it would seem that clear evidence of tumor shrinkage that is seen in many cases, superimposed on decreases in enhancement and vasogenic edema, is likely due to a secondary effect on the tumor tissue via the vascular effects. Tumor shrinkage usually occurs in concert with decreased enhancement, and is seen in about 20-25% of patients [9].

- Advanced Imaging

Perfusion magnetic resonance imaging allows the measurement of hemodynamic parameters (e.g. cerebral blood flow, cerebral blood volume, mean transit time) by imaging the first pass of a paramagnetic agent (most commonly gadolinium chelates) through the vascular bed. This technique can provide both absolute and relative values, which have been investigated widely, particularly in stroke imaging.

A large body of data supports a correlation between tumor hypervascularity and poor prognosis [10]. Relative cerebral blood volume (rCBV) correlates with vascular proliferation as seen on histopathologic evaluation [11]. These two facts would suggest that rCBV should be an independent predictor of patient clinical course. This has been shown in a series of 69 patients with low grade gliomas at two institutions [12]. rCBV has been shown to correlate with both grade and survival in patients with diffuse astrocytomas, but not oligodendrogliomas [13]. A negative association between rCBV and survival has also been demonstrated retrospectively in 189 patients in a population with both high grade and low grade gliomas [14].

Perfusion parameters have been used to evaluate response to therapy, and limited data indicate that VEGF inhibitors produce rapid and marked decrease in rCBV values that occurs with decreased enhancement (Fig. 2) [15, 16].

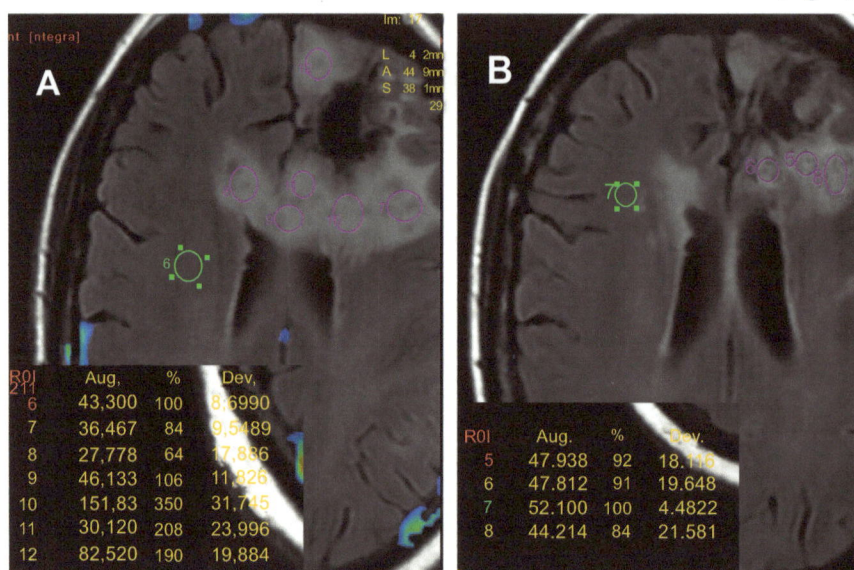

Figure 2: Interval reduction in maximal rCBV values from 3.5 to 1.0 after treatment with bevacizumab. Bevacizumab was initiated after the day 0 (A). Perfusion imaging was performed at 3Tesla (TR 2100 ms, TE 14.1 ms, matrix 128 x 128, gadolinium dose was 0.1 mmol/kg, injection rate 4 cc/sec, flip angle 60 degrees), with rCBV approximated by negative enhancement integral (GE – Advantage Workstation, Functools 6.3.1e). All values are normalized to normal appearing white matter. Pre-loading of contrast was controlled for effects of capillary leak. Substantial interval reduction in both rCBV and T2 signal change was seen at day 47 (B). There was a corresponding decrease in enhancement (not shown).

Published data suggests that not only can advanced imaging predict clinical course, but that these parameters may predict an individual patient's likelihood of responding to bevacizumab therapy.

Evaluation of the degree to which water may freely diffuse within the brain is a commonly used parameter in the evaluation of stroke, and reflects the level of microstructure with the brain - this parameter may be approximated by the apparent diffusion coefficient (ADC). The distribution of apparent diffusion coefficients may predict the response of patients with recurrent glioblastoma to bevacizumab [17].

Flurodeoxyglucose positron emission tomography (FDG-PET) is an indicator of tumor metabolic activity, and has been reported to show little change after administration of bevacizumab [8]. Fluorthymidine PET (FLT-PET) is thought to image cell proliferation and decreases in uptake during bevacizumab therapy have been shown to correlate with survival in patients with progressive GBM [18].

<u>Progression</u>. The features that are seen with disease progression during administration of bevacizumab can be categorized into three groups [19, 20]. The three types of progression are often overlapping.

- New enhancement that is contiguous with the previous enhancing disease, or, in the case of a gross total resection of enhancing tumor, immediately adjacent to the resection cavity.

This pattern presumably reflects the loss of VEGF inhibition. The mechanism by which this form of progression occurs in not yet known, but could relate to development of an escape pathway by which tumor cells develop a new molecular pathway for angiogenesis, or relate to a change in the availability of bevacizumab, such as the development of neutralizing antibodies as is seen with protein-based multiple sclerosis therapies [21].

- New enhancement that is "distant" or not contiguous as described above.

It is common to see new foci of enhancement that are distant from the original areas of enhancing tumor. These foci may be relatively close or quite distant (e.g., opposite cerebral hemisphere) and often arise while the original site of tumor continues to have decreased enhancement. These foci of new enhancement often appear within an area of diffusely infiltrating tumor, as described in the next paragraph, and thus likely represent the development of a mitotically active population of tumor cells that can invoke angiogenesis despite the presence of bevacizumab among a previously infiltrating population.

- Enlarging extent of diffusely infiltrating tumor, as defined by abnormal signal on T2-FLAIR images that does not exhibit features of vasogenic edema.

Diffuse gliomas such as glioblastoma are well known to be highly infiltrative tumors. This feature is responsible for the failure of intensified local therapies, such as more extensive surgery and brachytherapy, to significantly improve survival. A common feature of bevacizumab-treated patients is to see gradual extension of T2-weighted hyperintensity away from the original site of tumor. This imaging finding is known to represent infiltrating tumor cells. A pattern of gliomastosis cerebri often develops (Fig. **3**).

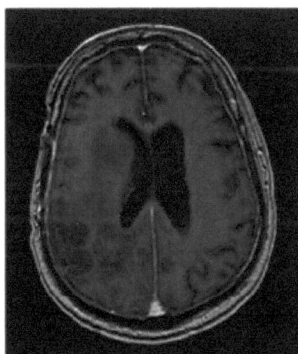

Figure 3: Progression of infiltrating tumor is seen before (A) and after (B) treatment with bevacizumab in T2/FLAIR images. Minimal enhancement is present at the latter time point on postcontrast T1-weighted images (C).

CLINICAL CORRELATES OF BEVACIZUMAB RELATED NEUROIMAGING CHANGES

The remarkable changes seen on magnetic resonance imaging (MRI) are frequently accompanied by a prompt improvement in clinical signs and symptoms. It is common to see improvements in deficits such as hemiparesis within 24 hours of the initial infusion of bevacizumab. This most likely relates to the reduction in vasogenic edema, much as is seen with the administration of a glucocorticoid such as dexamethasone. Clinical experience also indicates that the pattern of diffuse tumor infiltration may be accompanied by deterioration of cognitive function and gait. The effect on seizures is not well understood.

Older patients may exhibit a better response to bevacizumab than do younger patients [7, 8]. Not only is this encouraging news for the elderly patient with glioblastoma, for whom the benefit of previous treatments has been less than with younger patients, but it likely reflects important biological differences, such as the level of VEGF expression in the tumors of older patients [7]. A similar consideration likely applies to the observation that tumors with areas indicative of necrosis are more likely to respond to bevacizumab [6].

CONSIDERATIONS FOR MEASURING RESPONSE IN BEVACIZUMAB-CONTAINING REGIMENS

The changes described on gadolinium-enhanced MRI under "Response", above, are valuable indicators of the activity of bevacizumab on the tumor vasculature, and as such, serve as a plausible biomarker of the agent's function. Early results indicate that a radiographic response to bevacizumab correlates with improved PFS and overall survival. Thus, it might be possible to "personalize" bevacizumab therapy based on the presence of absence of an early response on MRI. Measures that could be employed include presence or absence of response, time to first response, and time to best response. Definitions of response are being developed by the Response Assessment in Neuro-oncology (RANO) study group.

Reduction in degree of enhancement make the standard measures of response based on the size of an enhancing lesion (e.g., Mcdonald measurements of enhancing tumor area) very difficult, if not impossible, to apply. Initially it seemed that the only remaining measure of response would be clinically-based measures such as overall survival or time to clinical progression. Emerging data, however, suggest that TTP or PFS, as based on neuroimaging, may be useful. Given the rapid changes in the appearance of the tumor after initiation of bevacizumab, it would likely be necessary to obtain a baseline MRI study within a week or so after beginning treatment. Using this baseline study, progression would then require a set of criteria for progression, such as a new area of enhancement that exceeds a certain minimal diameter, an area of existing enhancement that enlarges by a certain amount, and increase in the extent of infiltrating tumor by a defined amount. These are challenges currently being taken up by RANO.

Quantification of infiltrating tumor is technically more difficult that the identification of new or enlarging areas of enhancing tumor. This could be performed using a longest diameter approach or using a volumetric approach (Fig. 4). Reliable distinction of infiltrating tumor and edema will be important, and ADC measurements could be helpful in this analysis.

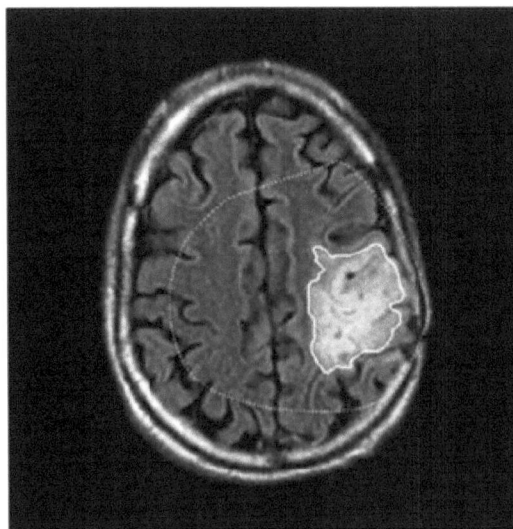

Figure 4: Computer-assisted volumetrics can be used to assess the volume of the infiltrating component of some tumors, as shown in this T2/FLAIR image.

CONCLUSIONS

The introduction of bevacizumab has changed neuroimaging in clinical practice and clinical trials for patients with malignant gliomas, but this complication should be seen as a sign of much-needed progress in finding active agents in the treatment of GBM.

REFERENCES

[1]   Henson JW, Ulmer S, Harris GJ. Brain tumor imaging in clinical trials. AJNR Am J Neuroradiol 2008;29:419-424.

[2]   Galanis E, Buckner JC, Maurer MJ, *et al.* Validation of neuroradiologic response assessment in gliomas: measurement by RECIST, two-dimensional, computer-assisted tumor area, and computer-assisted tumor volume methods. Neuro-oncol 2006;8:156-165.

[3]   Hess KR, Wong ET, Jaeckle KA, *et al.* Response and progression in recurrent malignant glioma. Neuro-oncol 1999;1:282-288.

[4]   Shah GD, Kesari S, Xu R, *et al.* Comparison of linear and volumetric criteria in assessing tumor response in adult high-grade gliomas. Neuro-oncol 2006;8:38-46.

[5]   Batchelor T, Stanley K, Andersen J. Clinical trials in neuro-oncology. Curr Opin Neurol 2001;14:689-694.

[6]   Ananthnarayan S, Bahng J, Roring J, *et al.* Time course of imaging changes of GBM during extended bevacizumab treatment. J Neurooncol 2008;88:339-347.

[7]   Nghiemphu PL, Liu W, Lee Y, *et al.* Bevacizumab and chemotherapy for recurrent glioblastoma: a single-institution experience. Neurology 2009;72:1217-1222.

[8]   Kreisl TN, Kim L, Moore K, *et al.* Phase II trial of single-agent bevacizumab followed by bevacizumab plus irinotecan at tumor progression in recurrent glioblastoma. J Clin Oncol 2009;27:740-745.

[9]   Pope WB, Lai A, Nghiemphu P, Mischel P, Cloughesy TF. MRI in patients with high-grade gliomas treated with bevacizumab and chemotherapy. Neurology 2006;66:1258-1260.

[10]   Chow KL, Gobin YP, Cloughesy T, Sayre JW, Villablanca JP, Vinuela F. Prognostic factors in recurrent glioblastoma multiforme and anaplastic astrocytoma treated with selective intra-arterial chemotherapy. AJNR Am J Neuroradiol 2000;21:471-478.

[11]   Aronen HJ, Gazit IE, Louis DN, *et al.* Cerebral blood volume maps of gliomas: comparison with tumor grade and histologic findings. Radiology 1994;191:41-51.

[12]   Caseiras GB, Chheang S, Babb J, *et al.* Relative cerebral blood volume measurements of low-grade gliomas predict patient outcome in a multi-institution setting. Eur J Radiol 2009. [Epub ahead of print]

[13]   Lev ML, Ozsunar Y, Henson JW, *et al.* Glial Tumor Grading and Outcome Prediction using Dynamic Spin-Echo MR Susceptibility Mapping compared to Conventional Contrast Enhanced MRI: Confounding Effect of Elevated relative Cerebral Blood Volume of Oligodendrogliomas. American Journal of Neuroradiology 2004;25:214-221.

[14]   Law M, Young RJ, Babb JS, *et al.* Gliomas: predicting time to progression or survival with cerebral blood volume measurements at dynamic susceptibility-weighted contrast-enhanced perfusion MR imaging. Radiology 2008;247:490-498.

[15]   Narayana A, Golfinos JG, Fischer I, *et al.* Feasibility of using bevacizumab with radiation therapy and temozolomide in newly diagnosed high-grade glioma. Int J Radiat Oncol Biol Phys 2008;72:383-389.

[16]   Narayana A, Kelly P, Golfinos J, *et al.* Antiangiogenic therapy using bevacizumab in recurrent high-grade glioma: impact on local control and patient survival. J Neurosurg 2009;110:173-180.

[17]   Pope WB, Kim HJ, Huo J, *et al.* Recurrent glioblastoma multiforme: ADC histogram analysis predicts response to bevacizumab treatment. Radiology 2009;252:182-189.

[18]   Chen W, Delaloye S, Silverman DH, *et al.* Predicting treatment response of malignant gliomas to bevacizumab and irinotecan by imaging proliferation with [18F] fluorothymidine positron emission tomography: a pilot study. J Clin Oncol 2007;25:4714-4721.

[19]   Zuniga RM, Torcuator R, Jain R, *et al.* Efficacy, safety and patterns of response and recurrence in patients with recurrent high-grade gliomas treated with bevacizumab plus irinotecan. J Neurooncol 2009;91:329-336.

[20]   Norden AD, Young GS, Setayesh K, *et al.* Bevacizumab for recurrent malignant gliomas: efficacy, toxicity, and patterns of recurrence. Neurology 2008;70:779-787.

[21]   Cohen BA, Oger J, Gagnon A, Giovannoni G. The implications of immunogenicity for protein-based multiple sclerosis therapies. J Neurol Sci 2008;275:7-17.

CHAPTER 16

Neurosurgical Implications of Bevacizumab Therapy of Malignant Gliomas

Manish K. Aghi[1,*] and Mitchel S. Berger[1]

[1]*University of California, San Francisco (UCSF) Department of Neurosurgery*

Abstract: Glioblastomas are histopathologically defined by endothelial proliferation and exhibit a uniquely elevated microvessel density compared to the surrounding normal tissue from which they derive, as compared to other tumor types. Clinical efficacy of the VEGF neutralizing antibody bevacizumab (avastin) in the treatment of other solid tumors led to a pair of phase II clinical trials studying bevacizumab treatment in recurrent human glioblastomas. Encouraging results from these trials led to the accelerated FDA approval of bevacizumab in the treatment of recurrent glioblastomas. However, extended bevacizumab treatment can lead to the development of infiltrative tumor on MRI with limited neurosurgical or chemotherapy options. Future studies will be needed to be able to identify tumors that are on their way to developing this appearance before it happens, in order to effectively use new potent anti-angiogenic agents like bevacizumab in the treatment of glioblastomas or symptomatic radiation necrosis associated with glioblastomas for which bevacizumab treatment may also be effective.

INTRODUCTION

Recognition of the role of vascular endothelial growth factor (VEGF) in developing the rich vascularity of glioblastomas, which contributes to their growth and resistance to radiation and chemotherapy has led to clinical trials of agents targeting VEGF or VEGF receptors 1 and 2 (VEGFR-1 and 2). VEGF has been targeted most frequently using the monoclonal mouse anti-human VEGF neutralizing antibody bevacizumab (avastin), which, when combined with topoisomerase inhibitor irinotecan in a pair of phase II clinical trials, led to a median progression-free survival of 23 weeks in 67 recurrent glioma patients [1,2]. In these two trials, the overall toxicity rate necessitating discontinuation of therapy was 34%, with thromboembolic complications being the most common toxicity [1,2]. There was only one patient (1.5%) with intracranial hemorrhage in these two trials. The rate of thromboembolic complications was 18% in these two trials, even greater than the 12% rate of thromboembolic complications in all types of cancer patients reported in a recent meta-analysis of cancer patients treated with bevacizumab [3], suggesting that VEGF blockade-induced hypercoaguability is particularly elevated in glioblastoma patients. This hypercoaguability in cancer patients undergoing bevacizumab treatment could be explained by pharmacologic inhibition of VEGF inhibiting endothelial regeneration and exposing subendothelial procoagulant phospholipids, but the exact reason it is particularly elevated in glioblastoma patients remains to be determined. A subsequent phase II clinical trial confirmed the benefits of bevacizumab monotherapy for recurrent glioblastomas in 48 patients, with a median overall survival of 31 weeks, with no treatment-associated intracranial hemorrhages and a 12.5% rate of thromboembolic events [4]. The encouraging efficacy of bevacizumab therapy of glioblastomas led to the May 6, 2009 FDA accelerated approval of bevacizumab in the treatment of recurrent glioblastoma, making bevacizumab only the third FDA approved treatment for glioblastoma in the past three decades, following implantable carmustine (BCNU)-containing wafers (gliadel), which were approved in 1996, and temozolomide, which was approved in 2005.

RADIOGRAPHIC PATTERNS AFTER BEVACIZUMAB TREATMENT OF GLIOBLASTOMAS

The phase II clinical trials showed that bevacizumab treatment reduced the amount of enhancing tumor [5], as with most effective chemotherapies. However, even more striking than direct effects on the tumor are the ability of bevacizumab to reduce peritumoral edema and mass effect, as manifested by a reduced dexamethasone requirement [6]. These effects of bevacizumab led, in one of the phase II clinical trials [4] to a 71% radiographic response rate when using the Levin criteria [7], which were developed in 1977 and are based on neurologic exam, but a 35%

*Address for correspondence to Manish K. Aghi: Department of Neurological Surgery, 505 Parnassus Avenue, Rm M779, San Francisco, CA 94143-0112; Tel: 415-353-1172, Fax: 415-353-3907, Email: aghim@neurosurg.ucsf.edu

Thomas C. Chen (Ed)

response rate when using the more commonly used Macdonald criteria [8], which were developed in 1990 and are based on the amount of T1 gadolinium enhancement seen on MRI. Gadolinium enhancement is a direct and proportional measure of tumor mass for discrete intracranial masses, such as brain metastases, making the circumferential decrease in the size of the enhancing mass assessed by the Macdonald criteria a reasonable radiographic response by which to judge therapeutic efficacy when treating these discrete masses. On the other hand, glioblastomas contain asymmetrically infiltrating tumor cells causing variable blood-brain barrier disruption, making spatial measurements of enhancement an inaccurate surrogate marker for total glioblastoma tumor burden at pre-treatment baseline and making such measurements even more inaccurate after VEGF inhibition. The limitations of the Macdonald criteria, particularly in the area of anti-angiogenic treatments like bevacizumab have recently led to the creation of an international Response Assessment in Neuro-oncology (RANO) task force, a team of experts whose goals will be to develop new criteria for glioblastoma progression applicable to today's targeted therapies [9].

Soon after the initial use of bevacizumab in glioblastoma treatment, neuro-oncologists began reporting that prolonged bevacizumab treatment of glioblastomas led to a FLAIR bright non-enhancing infiltrative abnormality [10], as demonstrated in Fig. **1**. The median time to maximal reduction in total tumor volume (enhancing plus non-enhancing) was shown in one study to be 158 days, and when FLAIR bright infiltration occurs it tends to occur shortly thereafter [5]. Biopsies of these FLAIR bright abnormalities have shown that they contain infiltrating glioblastoma cells, as shown in Fig. **2**. Another study showed that 60% of the tumor progressions occurring after bevacizumab treatment were distant progression with maintenance of local tumor control [11], consistent with studies in murine models [12]. These findings suggest that bevacizumab treatment normalizes the blood-brain barrier and exerts a direct antitumoral effect on glioblastoma, but tumor cells that survive bevacizumab treatment can emerge with a propensity for greater perivascular infiltration or greater infiltration along white matter tracts. Detecting this post-bevacizumab tumor burden in glioblastoma patients is a radiographic challenge that will require the use of different radiographic modalities than those that have been used in the past to detect tumor recurrence. For example, magnetic resonance spectroscopy (MRS), which detects tumor by its hypermetabolic profile, may fail to detect the less cellular dense infiltrative tumor recurrence seen after bevacizumab treatment, perhaps due to limitations in how small the voxel resolution can be. On the other hand, cerebral perfusion MRI which reveals reduced blood flow after successful bevacizumab treatment [13], can show elevated blood flow in the setting of tumor recurrence after bevacizumab treatment, an example of which is shown in Fig. **3**. However, even elevated blood volume on cerebral perfusion MRI is not 100% specific for tumor recurrence after bevacizumab treatment, as shown in Fig. **4**. Thus, future research will be needed to develop more advanced imaging modalities with greater sensitivity and specificity at detecting glioblastoma recurrence in the era of anti-angiogenic treatments like bevacizumab. In the meantime, studies of existing imaging modalities will be needed to determine which imaging algorithm(s) should be relied upon under different circumstances in order to best identify recurrent tumor after bevacizumab treatment of glioblastoma.

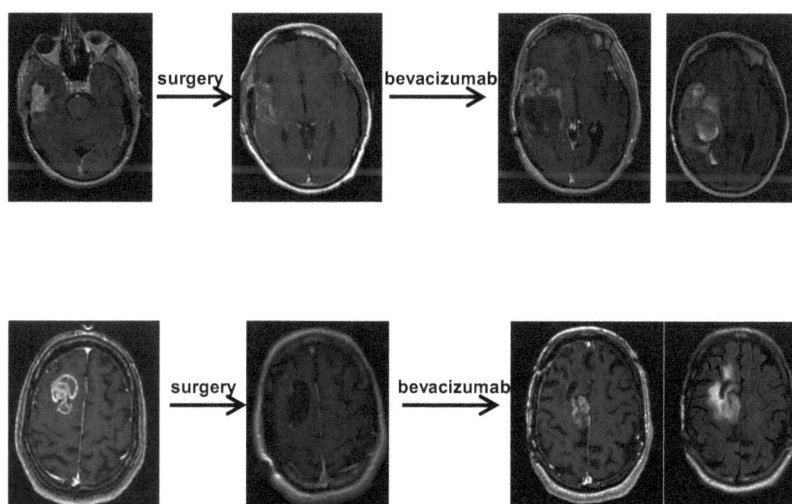

Figure 1: FLAIR bright infiltrative abnormality seen after bevacizumab treatment of glioblastoma. Two examples of glioblastomas seen on T1 gadolinium-enhanced axial images before initial resection, followed by postoperative T1 gadonlium-

enhanced images showing large resection cavities containing blood products, followed by the development of minimal adjacent enhancement but extensive surrounding FLAIR bright abnormality 6 to 9 months after starting bevacizumab treatment.

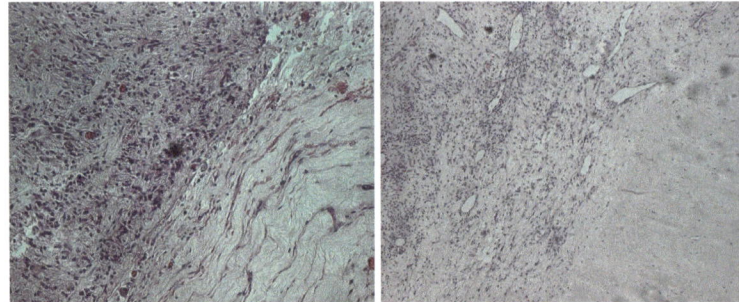

Figure 2: Tissue taken from FLAIR bright non-enhancing abnormality seen after bevacizumab treatment of glioblastoma shows infiltrating glioblastoma cells. Hematoxylin and eosin staining of tissue taken from the FLAIR bright non-enhancing abnormality in 2 patients whose glioblastomas were treated with bevacizumab for 6 months. Absolute magnification is 200x.

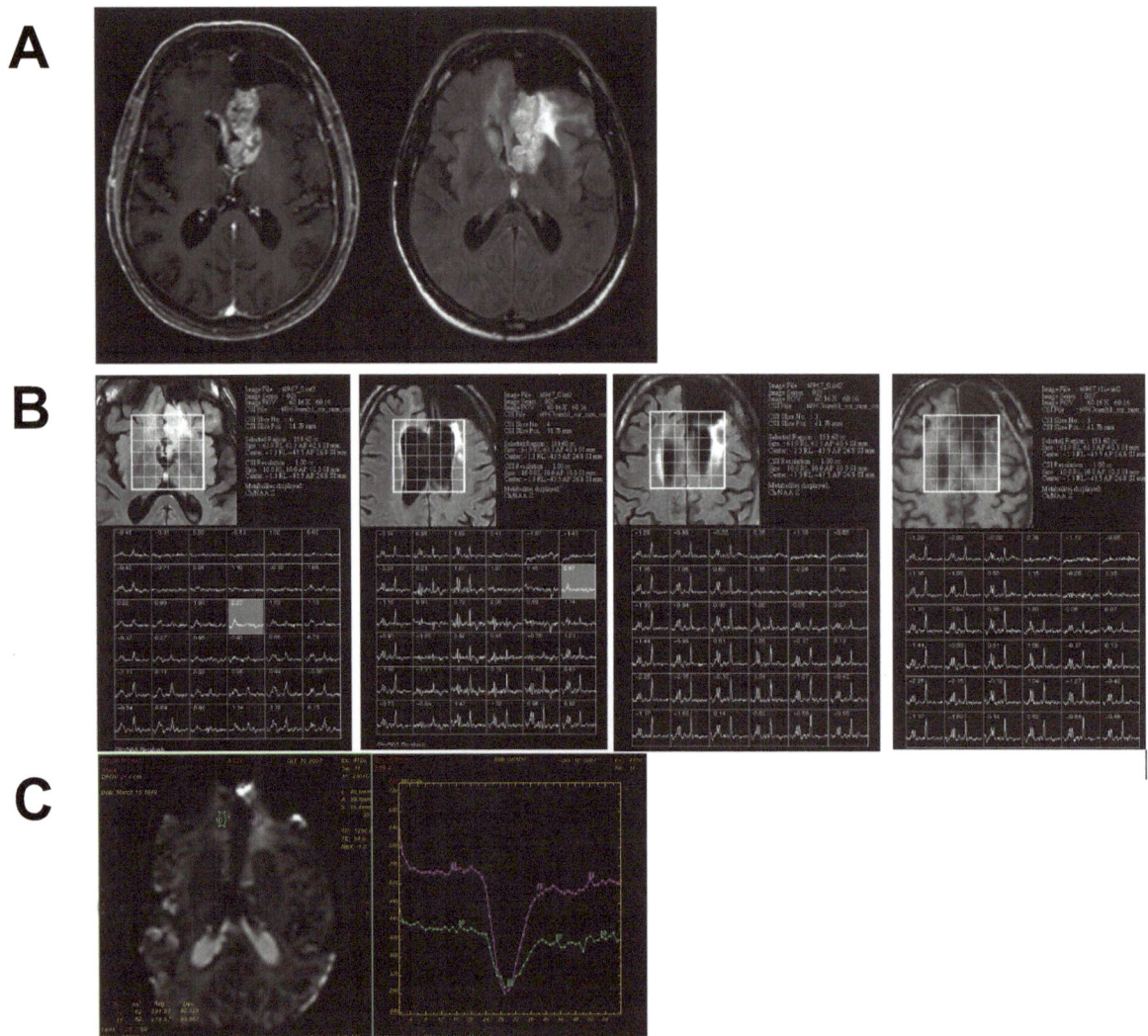

Figure 3: Advanced imaging modalities can generate conflicting results in attempting to identify glioblastoma recurrence after bevacizumab treatment. Three months after stopping bevacizumab treatment and three years after external beam radiotherapy, this patient developed a FLAIR bright infiltrative enhancing abnormality (A) whose MRS profile (B) was unremarkable, but cereberal perfusion sequence showed elevated blood volume (C),

consistent with recurrence. At surgery, recurrent infiltrative tumor was identified, without any associated radiation necrosis.

NEUROSURGICAL MANAGEMENT OF RADIOGRAPHIC CHANGES AFTER BEVACIZUMAB TREATMENT

Once this radiographic appearance develops after bevacizumab treatment, there are not many effective chemotherapy options that can target these infiltrating tumor cells. One of the few clinical trials of an agent that could theoretically target infiltrating glioblastoma cells was a phase II clinical trial of cilengitide, an inhibitor of $\alpha v \beta 3$ and $\alpha v \beta 5$ integrins, and this agent proved only moderately effective [14]. Neurosurgical options are also limited. At our institution, of the first 75 patients with recurrent glioblastomas treated with bevacizumab after undergoing their second craniotomy for surgical resection, only 16% proceeded to a third craniotomy, compared to 26% of patients with recurrent glioblastomas not treated with bevacizumab after undergoing their second craniotomy (unpublished observations), underscoring that neurosurgeons do not regard this diffuse FLAIR bright non-enhancing abnormality seen after bevacizumab treatment of glioblastoma as disease that would benefit from neurosurgical debulking. These 12 craniotomies on patients who experienced radiographic progression during bevacizumab treatment occurred an average of 31 days after their last bevacizumab dose (range 15-49 days). There were no postoperative hemorrhages in these 12 cases. While our preference is to wait 4 weeks between the last bevacizumab dose and surgery, in one case symptomatic progression led to surgery 15 days after the last bevacizumab dose, with no postoperative hemorrhage in this case as well. One of 12 patients (8%) had a perioperaitve thromboembolic complication within 30 days of craniotomy. Sutures were removed after 14 days, as is our standard practice after repeat craniotomy, and there were no wound infections or wound dehiscences. Six patients were started on subcutaneous lovenox 40 mg once a day for deep venous thrombosis prophylaxis because they failed to start mobilizing by postoperative day two. Three patients whose scalp tissues looked unusually thin at surgery were prescribed a wound-healing cocktail of vitamin A tablets (10,000 IU daily), vitamin C tablets (500 mg, taken twice daily), and zinc tablets (220 mg daily) for a total of 10 days.

The accelerated FDA approval of bevacizumab in treating recurrent glioblastoma occurred before a large multicenter randomized phase III clinical trial could be conducted to comprehensively analyze the true therapeutic benefit of bevacizumab. Such a trial is currently underway and will help determine, in all patients as well as in patient and tumor subsets, whether the development of an invasive non-enhancing phenotype after bevacizumab treatment with limited neurosurgical and chemotherapy options offsets any therapeutic benefit of bevacizumab, as compared to conventional DNA damaging chemotherapies, which bevacizumab will likely be compared to in a phase III clinical trial, or experimental treatments like immunotherapy or oncolytic viruses, which at the time of radiographic progression still leave behind tumor with potential neurosurgical or chemotherapy options. This randomized analysis of bevacizumab will be vital to conduct in a timely fashion because the accelerated FDA approval will lead to rapid widespread use of bevacizumab in treating recurrent glioblastomas as well as off-label use of bevacizumab in treating newly diagnosed glioblastomas, and it will be essential to determine whether there are any glioblastoma patients who are inappropriate to treat with bevacizumab. Interestingly, in initial patient subgroup analyses conducted as part of the nonrandomized phase II clinical trials, bevacizumab has proven particularly effective in treating recurrent gliomas in the elderly [6], suggesting a biologic difference in the level of VEGF dependence in glioblastomas in elderly patients, and suggesting a potential role for bevacizumab therapy in the care of this subpopulation with an otherwise particularly poor prognosis, and potentially avoiding the morbidity of repeat craniotomy in this population.

USE OF BEVACIZUMAB TO TREAT SYMPTOMATIC RADIATION NECROSIS

After radiotherapy, glioblastomas frequently develop enhancing lesions that prove upon resection to contain treatment-related inflammatory or cytotoxic effects. This phenomenon of radiation necrosis occurs 3 months to 2 years after radiotherapy and its incidence has been reported to be 3 to 24% [15,16]. The clinical course for radiation necrosis is highly variable. Patients can present with focal deficits, increased intracranial pressure, or can be asymptomatic [17]. Radiation necrosis often necessitates surgical resection due to mass effect or due to diagnostic uncertainty because the radiographic appearance can resemble progression of tumor burden even when more advanced imaging modalities such as magnetic resonance spectroscopy (MRS) or perfusion are used, as illustrated in Fig. **4**. Unfortunately, glioblastoma patients that have undergone treatment experience significant risk anytime they undergo surgery, and the morbidity of surgically resecting radiation necrosis has been reported to be 54% in one series, including pulmonary embolism and wound infection [18]. Recently, bevacizumab has been shown to improve the symptom control of patients with radiation necrosis after radiotherapy for malignant gliomas, and to reduce daily dexamethasone dose by 8.6 mg within 8 weeks of starting bevacizumab [19,20]. However, because these studies were not randomized with a control arm of radiation necrosis patients not treated with bevacizumab and because radiation necrosis often spontaneously resolves, the contribution of bevacizumab versus natural history remains unclear.

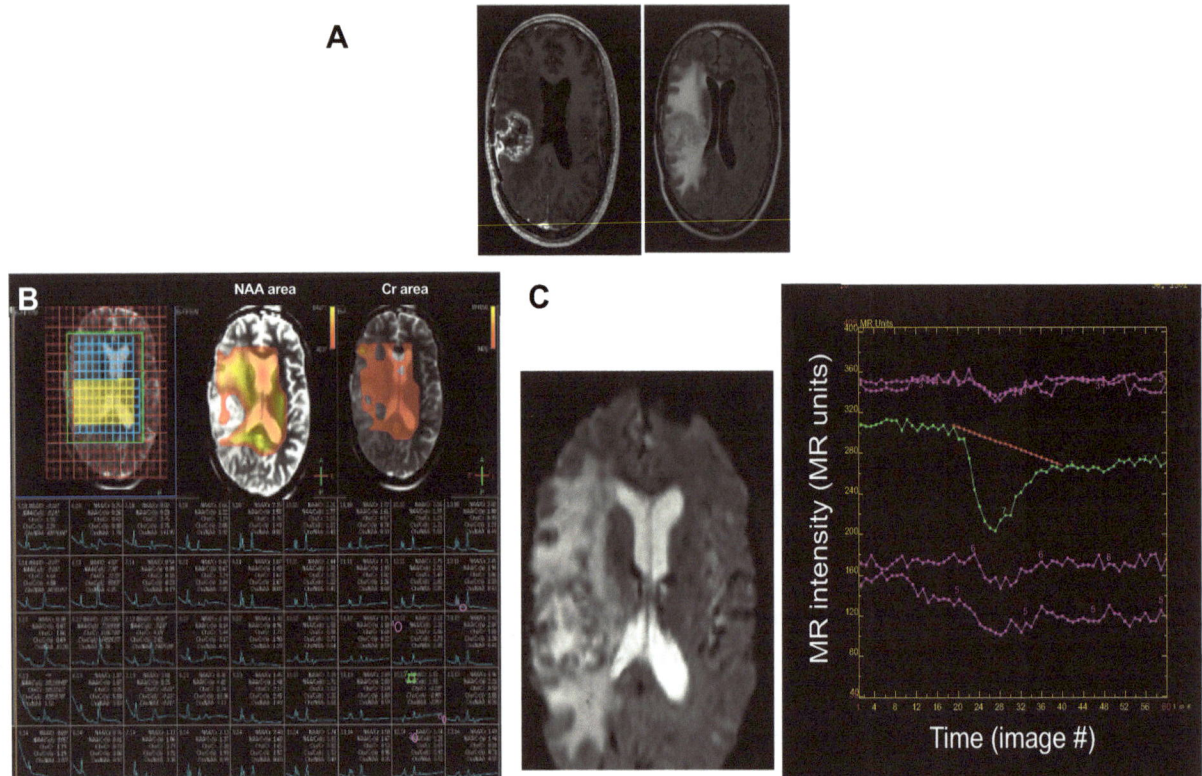

Figure 4: Advanced imaging modalities can fail to differentiate glioblastoma treatment effect from tumor progression, particularly after bevacizumab treatment. One year after external beam fractionated radiotherapy, six months after stopping bevacizumab treatment, and three months after receiving 5 fractions of cyberknife radiosurgery to an enhancing abnormality, this patient with a glioblastoma developed: (A) a progressive FLAIR bright infiltrative enhancing abnormality; with (B) 3D MRS showing the spectroscopic profiles (from left to right in each voxel: choline, creatine, and NAA) of multiple voxels in each axial image, and revealing evidence of underlying tumor metabolism with decreased NAA and elevated choline; and (C) elevated blood volume by cerebral perfusion MRI sequence. At surgery, 95% radiation necrosis was identified, refuting the imaging findings seen in MRS and perfusion.

USE OF BEVACIZUMAB TO PROMOTE THE EFFICACY OF RADIOTHERAPY AND CHEMOTHERAPY IN GLIOBLASTOMAS

Although bevacizumab itself likely exerts tumoricidal effects because bevacizumab-induced devascularization leads to tumor cell death and because VEGF increases tumor cell survival [21], the initial appeal of bevacizumab therapy of glioblastomas was as a way of augmenting the efficacy of radiotherapy and chemotherapy. This hypothesis was based on preclinical studies suggesting that anti-vascular agents "normalize" glioma vessels and hence decrease vascular permeability [22-24] . This normalization improves intratumoral temozolomide distribution in human glioma xenografts after anti-VEGF treatment [25]. Furthermore, in a murine model, this vascular normalization caused by anti-VEGF treatment is a transient "normalization window" during which radiation sensitivity is maximized [21,24]. This window is characterized by: (1) increased glioma oxygenation, a means of improving radiation sensitivity; (2) increased pericyte coverage of glioma vessels; and (3) degradation of the pathologically thick basement membrane via metalloproteinase activation, which decreases vascular permeability [24]. These findings correlate with reports that bevacizumab increases radiotherapy efficacy [21,25]. These findings, combined with the ability described above of bevacizumab to treat symptomatic radiation necrosis, also support the notion that an anti-VEGF antibody like bevacizumab could be an ideal option free of the morbidity of surgical resection but capable of controlling symptoms of radiation necrosis and exerting a concomitant anti-tumor effect.

These preclinical and early clinical findings led to a phase I clinical trial in patients with recurrent glioblastoma combining bevacizumab with 30 Gy of hypofractionated stereotactic radiotherapy in five fractions after the first cycle of bevacizumab, which led to a median overall survival of 12.5 months, with no associated toxicity [13].

CONCLUSIONS

The significant impact of bevacizumab on vascular permeability and cerebral edema have led to encouraging results in glioblastoma treatment, as assessed by progression free survival and overall survival in recurrent glioblastoma patients treated in phase II clinical trials. These findings have led to the accelerated FDA approval of avastin in recurrent glioblastoma treatment. The increasing use of bevacizumab in glioblastoma treatment will help many glioblastoma patients, but may also lead to increased tumor infiltration in a manner with limited chemotherapy or neurosurgical options. Determining whether there are subsets of glioblastomas that are more or less responsive to bevacizumab and identifying radiographic features or serum biomarkers predictive of the radiographic patterns that sometimes develop after multiple cycles of bevacizumab treatment and are difficult to treat with neurosurgery or chemotherapy will be vital in order to use this new treatment in the most effective manner possible. Bevacizumab treatment may also improve symptoms of radiation necrosis, without the associated side effects of dexamethasone and without the morbidity of neurosurgery in this setting.

REFERENCES

[1]　Vredenburgh JJ, Desjardins A, Herndon JE, 2nd, *et al.* Phase II trial of bevacizumab and irinotecan in recurrent malignant glioma. Clin Cancer Res 2007; 13:1253-1259.

[2]　Vredenburgh JJ, Desjardins A, Herndon JE, 2nd, *et al.* Bevacizumab plus irinotecan in recurrent glioblastoma multiforme. J Clin Oncol 2007; 25:4722-4729.

[3]　Nalluri SR, Chu D, Keresztes R, *et al.* Risk of Venous Thromboembolism With the Angiogenesis Inhibitor Bevacizumab in Cancer Patients: A Meta-analysis. JAMA 2008; 300:2277-2285.

[4]　Kreisl TN, Kim L, Moore K, *et al.* Phase II trial of single-agent bevacizumab followed by bevacizumab plus irinotecan at tumor progression in recurrent glioblastoma. J Clin Oncol 2009; 27:740-745.

[5]　Ananthnarayan S, Bahng J, Roring J, *et al.* Time course of imaging changes of GBM during extended bevacizumab treatment. J Neurooncol 2008; 88:339-347.

[6]　Nghiemphu PL, Liu W, Lee Y, *et al.* Bevacizumab and chemotherapy for recurrent glioblastoma: a single-institution experience. Neurology 2009; 72:1217-1222.

[7]　Levin VA, Crafts DC, Norman DM, *et al.* Criteria for evaluating patients undergoing chemotherapy for malignant brain tumors. J Neurosurg 1977; 47:329-335.

[8]　Macdonald DR, Cascino TL, Schold SC, Jr., *et al.* Response criteria for phase II studies of supratentorial malignant glioma. J Clin Oncol 1990; 8:1277-1280.

[9]　van den Bent MJ, Vogelbaum MA, Wen PY, Macdonald DR, Chang SM. End point assessment in gliomas: novel treatments limit usefulness of classical Macdonald's Criteria. J Clin Oncol 2009; 27:2905-2908.

[10]　Norden AD, Young GS, Setayesh K, *et al.* Bevacizumab for recurrent malignant gliomas: efficacy, toxicity, and patterns of recurrence. Neurology 2008; 70:779-787.

[11]　Zuniga RM, Torcuator R, Jain R, *et al.* Efficacy, safety and patterns of response and recurrence in patients with recurrent high-grade gliomas treated with bevacizumab plus irinotecan. J Neurooncol 2009; 91:329-336.

[12]　Paez-Ribes M, Allen E, Hudock J, *et al.* Antiangiogenic therapy elicits malignant progression of tumors to increased local invasion and distant metastasis. Cancer Cell 2009; 15:220-231.

[13]　Gutin PH, Iwamoto FM, Beal K, *et al.* Safety and Efficacy of Bevacizumab with Hypofractionated Stereotactic Irradiation for Recurrent Malignant Gliomas. Int J Radiat Oncol Biol Phys 2009.

[14]　Reardon DA, Fink KL, Mikkelsen T, *et al.* Randomized phase II study of cilengitide, an integrin-targeting arginine-glycine-aspartic acid peptide, in recurrent glioblastoma multiforme. J Clin Oncol 2008; 26:5610-5617.

[15] Ruben JD, Dally M, Bailey M, *et al.* Cerebral radiation necrosis: incidence, outcomes, and risk factors with emphasis on radiation parameters and chemotherapy. Int J Radiat Oncol Biol Phys 2006; 65:499-508.

[16] Zeng QS, Li CF, Zhang K, *et al.* Multivoxel 3D proton MR spectroscopy in the distinction of recurrent glioma from radiation injury. J Neurooncol 2007; 84:63-69.

[17] Brandsma D, Stalpers L, Taal W, *et al.* Clinical features, mechanisms, and management of pseudoprogression in malignant gliomas. Lancet Oncol 2008; 9:453-461.

[18] McPherson CM, Warnick RE. Results of contemporary surgical management of radiation necrosis using frameless stereotaxis and intraoperative magnetic resonance imaging. J Neurooncol 2004; 68:41-47.

[19] Gonzalez J, Kumar AJ, Conrad CA, Levin VA. Effect of bevacizumab on radiation necrosis of the brain. Int J Radiat Oncol Biol Phys 2007; 67:323-326.

[20] Torcuator R, Zuniga R, Mohan YS, *et al.* Initial experience with bevacizumab treatment for biopsy confirmed cerebral radiation necrosis. J Neurooncol 2009.

[21] Gupta VK, Jaskowiak NT, Beckett MA, *et al.* Vascular endothelial growth factor enhances endothelial cell survival and tumor radioresistance. Cancer J 2002; 8:47-54.

[22] Batchelor TT, Sorensen AG, di Tomaso E, *et al.* AZD2171, a pan-VEGF receptor tyrosine kinase inhibitor, normalizes tumor vasculature and alleviates edema in glioblastoma patients. Cancer Cell 2007; 11:83-95.

[23] Dings RP, Loren M, Heun H, *et al.* Scheduling of radiation with angiogenesis inhibitors anginex and Avastin improves therapeutic outcome via vessel normalization. Clin Cancer Res 2007; 13:3395-3402.

[24] Winkler F, Kozin SV, Tong RT, *et al.* Kinetics of vascular normalization by VEGFR2 blockade governs brain tumor response to radiation: role of oxygenation, angiopoietin-1, and matrix metalloproteinases. Cancer Cell 2004; 6:553-563.

[25] Zhou Q, Guo P, Gallo JM. Impact of angiogenesis inhibition by sunitinib on tumor distribution of temozolomide. Clin Cancer Res 2008; 14:1540-1549.

[26] Lai A, Filka E, McGibbon B, *et al.* Phase II pilot study of bevacizumab in combination with temozolomide and regional radiation therapy for up-front treatment of patients with newly diagnosed glioblastoma multiforme: interim analysis of safety and tolerability. Int J Radiat Oncol Biol Phys 2008; 71:1372-1380

CHAPTER 17

Neurosurgical Implications of Avastin

Gazanfar Rahmathulla[1] and Michael A. Vogelbaum[2,*]

[1]Brain Tumor and NeuroOncology Center, Cleveland Clinic, [2]Brain Tumor and Neuro-Oncology Center and Center for Translational Therapeutics, Department of Neurological Surgery, Cleveland Clinic / Neurological Institute, 9500 Euclid Ave. Cleveland, OH 44195

Abstract: Malignant gliomas are optimally managed with maximal surgical resection followed by radiation and chemotherapy. Drug delivery challenges and chemoresistance limits the efficacy of standard chemotherapeutic agents. Understanding glioma biology has led to the development of a variety newer molecular targeting agents which have begun to show exciting preliminary results. Bevacizumab (Avastin) is one such drug likely to play a key role in malignant glioma therapy. We review the current literature in regard to the use of bevacizumab and its adverse effects in neurosurgical patients.

INTRODUCTION

Malignant gliomas are the most common type of primary brain tumors and remain the most challenging to treat. The median survival rates remain less than 15 months with current optimal management which includes surgery and chemoradiotherapy [1,2]. GBMs are characterized histologically by the presence of neovascularization, necrosis and diffuse infiltration. Conventional chemotherapy targets tumor cells and is limited by the highly infiltrative nature of glioma cells, poor drug penetration across the blood-brain and the blood-tumor barriers, and genetically heterogeneous cell populations making them chemoresistant. Recent studies also demonstrate there are cancer stem cells involved in glioma initiation, progression and resistance to treatment, and that these cells may have unique biological properties which are not as amenable to conventional and some new, targeted therapies [3,4,5]. Targeting angiogenesis is a more recently applied strategy and one which may overcome some of the barriers to treatment noted above, as non-neoplastic endothelial cells, and not tumor cells, are the primary target [6,7]. The process of angiogenesis involves complex interaction between glioma, stromal and endothelial cells mediated by a number of factors and signaling pathways [8]. Vascular endothelial growth factor (VEGF) is a critical regulator of angiogenesis, highly expressed in GBMs and has emerged as an important therapeutic target.

Bevacizumab (Avastin; Genentech, South San Francisco, CA), a recombinant human neutralizing monoclonal antibody of VEGF, has been recently approved by the US food and drug administration (FDA) for treatment of progressive GBMs. It binds VEGF and prevents its interaction with receptors on the cell surface. Bevacizumab has an estimated half-life range of 11 to 50 days with a median of 21 days [9]. VEGF in addition to being a major mediator of angiogenesis also stimulates vascular permeability, recruits progenitor cells from bone marrow, promotes monocyte chemotaxis, plays a role in regulation of vasomotor tone and blood pressure and regulates immune and anti-inflammatory cells. It is also a trophic factor for neurons and insufficient levels could contribute to neurodegeneration [10]. Phase 2 clinical trials in the treatment of GBMs have demonstrated remarkable tumor response and prolonged survival compared with historic controls [11,12]. There is a potent anti-edema effect as well, allowing steroid doses to be significantly reduced [13].

Emerging data suggests a unique pattern of adverse events associated with bevacizumab treatment, requiring careful patient selection and monitoring while using bevacizumab in neurosurgical practice [14,15]. Bevacizumab is associated with an increased risk of bleeding and wound complications, with spontaneous opening of the craniotomy wound being reported as late as 2-6 months following therapy with bevacizumab [16]. Delaying the use of bevacizumab by 4-6 weeks, following surgery, may be sufficient to prevent these complications [17]. In patients

*Address correspondence to Michael A. Vogelbaum: Center for Translational Therapeutics, Department of Neurological Surgery, Cleveland Clinic / Neurological Institute, 9500 Euclid Ave. Cleveland, OH 44195; Email: vogelbm@ccf.org

who have wound problems such as subgaleal collections, wound breakdown and infections, they have been successfully treated with debridement and cranioplasty.

Intracranial hemorrhages, which can range from being minor to life threatening, may occur in ≤3% of patients and a prior intratumoral hemorrhage is generally considered to be a relative contraindication to therapy [18,19]. In the phase II trial using bevacizumab for recurrent gliomas conducted by Vredenburgh and colleagues, no intracranial hemorrhages were seen in their patients, who were not on any prior anticoagulant therapy. Norden *et al.* in their cohort of 55 patients, found 2 patients with asymptomatic intracranial hemorrhages and 2 patients with grade 1-2 hemorrhages.

Other common systemic side effects are fatigue, hypertension, proteinuria, epistaxis, and rarely skin toxicity [20]. Hypertension is one of the most common adverse effects observed in patients receiving systemic anti-VEGF therapy. In studies using bevacizumab for renal cell cancer, the incidence of hypertension was as high as 32%, with 11 to 16% having grade 3 hypertension requiring intensive antihypertensive treatment [21]. Neurosurgical patients have to be carefully monitored and appropriately treated for hypertension which is a common and dose limiting toxicity [22]. In addition to this the risk of deep vein thrombosis, pulmonary embolism and stroke in a high risk population is further increased [23]. Accumulated data reveals the addition of bevacizumab to chemotherapy increases the risk of arterial thrombosis, and independent risk factors being age over 65 years and a history of previous clots [24]. The risk of proteinuria with bevacizumab is approximately 25%, and monitoring is essential as nephrotic syndrome, although rare could occur and if proteinuria is more than 2 grams bevacizumab should be discontinued [25]. The risk of developing GI perforations in patients with malignant gliomas treated with bevacizumab is around 0.6 to 2.5% [26]. Rare CNS side effects which have been reported include a reversible posterior leukoencephalopathy, seizures, disequilibrium and ataxia. The various studies investigating Bevacizumab have been listed in Table **1**.

Table 1: Studies investigating Bevacizumab in surgical patients

Author (Yr)	Cancer	No. patients	Complications	Therapy	Incidence
Hurwitz *et al.* (2004) [27]	Colon	N = 80	Wound healing / bleeding	Cx + Bev	3%
D' Angelica *et al.* (2007) [28]	Colon	N = 64	Wound healing	Cx + Bev (pre) Cx + Bev (post)	38% 31%
Kabbinavar *et al.* (2003) [29]	Colon	N = 104 N = 100	Proteinuria Arterial thromboembolic event	Cx + Bev (5mg/kg or 10mg/kg) Cx + Bev	23% & 28% 10%
Johnson *et al.* (2004) [30]	Lung	N = 99 N = 66	Proteinuria Arterial thromboembolic event	Cx + Bev (7.5mg/kg or 15mg/kg) Cx +_ Bev	21% & 42% 4.5%
Escuduer (2007) [31]	Renal	N= 649	Proteinuria	Cx + Bev	18%
Sandler *et al.* (2008) [32]	Lung	N = 878	Hypertension	Cx + Bev	7%
Saltz *et al.* (2008) [33]	Colon	N = 1401	Hypertension	Cx + Bev	8%
Scappatici *et al.* (2007) [34]	Colon	N = 1745	Arterial thrombosis Venous thrombosis	Cx + Bev Cx + Bev	4% 10%
Vredenburgh *et al.* (2007) [11]	Glioma	N = 32	Ischemic stroke DVT/pulmonary emboli	Cx + Bev Cx + Bev	0.03% 0.09%
Bokstein *et al.* (2008) [35]	Glioma	N = 20	Epistaxis grade 2 Fatigue Hypertension	Cx + Bev Cx + Bev Cx + Bev	5% 15% 5%
Vredenburgh *et al.* (2007) [18]	Glioma	`N = 35	CNS hemorrhage Thromboembolic complications Grade 2 fatigue	Cx + Bev Cx + Bev Cx + Bev	3% 11% 11%

Cx = Cytotoxic chemotherapy Bev = Bevacizumab

A number of questions regarding the role of systemic antiangiogenic therapies like bevacizumab need to be answered. Future medical treatment of glioblastomas will require a combination of drugs directed at multiple targets. Is there a role for bevacizumab or similar systemic anti-angiogenic therapies concomitant with chemoradiotherapy following the first surgery? Gutin *et al.* reported their results of bevacizumab with re-irradiation for selected cases of recurrent glioblastomas and showed an objective response rate of 74% and a median PFS and OS of 7 and 10 months, with no grade IV/V toxicity [35]. These are similar to the results of Vredenburgh et al, indicating that bevacizumab can be used in conjunction with radiation therapy. Narayan *et al.* used bevacizumab in conjunction with chemoradiation in patients with newly diagnosed GBM and had a radiologic response rate of 86%, and 1 year PFS and OS rates were 59.3 and 86.7% respectively [36]. Their study indicates the feasibility of using bevacizumab in conjunction with chemoradiotherapy, and clearly further trials with larger sample sizes will provide definitive evidence of the role of systemic antiangiogenic therapy. Of concern, though is that wound healing problems may be potentiated in using combination therapy of bevacizumab with RT/chemotherapy [37,38].

There is also interest in the use of bevacizumab as an alternative to surgery in patients with tumor progression with mass effect and edema. The rationale for using bevacizumab in this situation seems sound, as clinical and radiologic evidence from published studies has shown significant reduction in edema and mass effect associated with tumor control. The true efficacy of this approach can only be answered by conducting well designed and powered clinical trials in a cohort of patients where a second surgery may not be feasible.

CONCLUSIONS

As bevacizumab becomes more widely used in neurosurgical oncology, it is important to be aware of the complications. With increasing experience, additional safety concerns may arise and will require subsequent development of guidelines for their management. Although the results of these initial studies remain encouraging, malignant gliomas eventually progress due to their resistance to current drug therapies. Targeting glioblastoma stem cells, development of drugs that block invasion of glioma cells, immunotherapy and combinations of these approaches remain ongoing challenges for neuro-oncologists.

REFERENCES

[1]   Furnari FB, Fenton T, Bachoo RM *et al.* Malignant astrocytic gliomas: genetics, biology, and paths to treatment. Genes Dev 2007;21:2683-2710.

[2]   Wen PY, Kesari S. Malignant gliomas in adults. N Eng J Med 2008;359:492-507.

[3]   Omay SB, Vogelbaum MA. Current concepts and newer developments in the treatment of malignant gliomas. Indian J Cancer. 2009 Apr-Jun;46(2):88-95.

[4]   Dirks PB. Brain tumor stem cells: bringing order to the chaos of brain cancer. J Clin Oncol 2008;26:2916-2924.

[5]   Dietrich J, Imitola J, Kesari S. Mechanisms of disease: the role of stem cells in the biology and treatment of gliomas. Nat Clin Pract Oncology 2008;5:393-404.

[6]   Jain RK, di Tomaso E, Duda DG, *et al.* Angiogenesis in brain tumors. Nat Rev Neuroscie 2007,8:610-622.

[7]   Kesari S, Ramakrishna N, Sauvageot C, *et al.* Targeted molecular therapy of malignant gliomas. Curr Oncol Rep Jan 2006;8(1):58-70.

[8]   Gerstner ER, Sorensen AG, Jain RK, *et al.* Anti-Vascular endothelial growth factor therapy for malignant glioma. Current Neurology and Neuroscience Reports 2009;9:254-262.

[9]   Gordon MS, Margolin K, Talpaz M, *et al.* Phase I safety and pharmacokinetic study of human recombinant anti-vascular endothelial growth factor in patients with advanced cancer. J Clin Oncol 2001;19:843-850.

[10]   Greenburg DA, Jin K. From angiogenesis to neuropathology. Nature 2005;438(7070):954-9

[11]   Vredenburgh JJ, Desjardins A, Herndon JE II, *et al.* Phase II trial of bevacizmab and irinotecan in recurrent malignant glioma. Clin Cancer Res 2007;13:1253-1259

[12]   Chen W, Delaloye S, Silverman DH, *et al.* Predicting treatment response of malignant gliomas to Bevacizumab and irinotecan by imaging proliferation with 18[F] fluorothymidine positron emission tomography: A pilot study. J Clin Oncology 2007;25:4714-4721

[13]   Batchelor TT, Sorensen AG, di Tomaso E, *et al.* AZD2171, a pan VEGF receptor tyrosine kinase inhibitor, normalizes tumor vasculature and alleviates edema in glioblastoma patients. Cancer Cell 2007;11:83-95.

[14] Verheul HM, Pinedo HM. Possible molecular mechanisms involved in the toxicity of angiogenesis inhibition. Nat Rev Cancer 2007;7:475-485.

[15] Eskens FA, Verweij J. The clinical toxicity profile of vascular endothelial growth factor (VEGF) and vascular endothelial growth factor receptor (VEGFR) targeting angiogenesis inhibitors; a review. Eur J Cancer 2006;42:3127-3139.

[16] Chamberlain MC. Bevacizumab plus irinotecan in recurrent glioblastoma. J of Clin Onc 2008;26:1012-1013.

[17] Gordon CR, Rojavin Y, Patel M, *et al.* A review on Bevacizumab and surgical wound healing – An important warning to all surgeons. Annals of Plastic Surgery 2009;62(6):707-709.

[18] Vredenburgh JJ, Desjardins A, Herndon JE 2nd, *et al.* Bevacizumab plus irinotecan in recurrent glioblastoma multiforme. J Clin Oncol 2007;25:4722-4729.

[19] Cloughesy TF, Prados MD, Wen PY, *et al.* A phase II, randomized, noncomparative clinical trial of the effect of bevacizuman (BV) alone or in combination with irinotecan (CPT) on 6-month progression free survival (PFS6) in recurrent, treatment-refractory glioblastoma (GBM) [abstract]. J Clin Oncol 2008;26:2010b.

[20] Dietrich J, Norden AD, Wen PY. Emerging antiangiogenic treatments for gliomas – efficacy and safety issues. Curr Opin Neurol 2008;21(6);736-744.

[21] Zhu X, Wu S, Dahut WL, Parikh CR. Risks of proteinuria and hypertension with Bevacizumab, an antibody against vascular endothelial growth factor: Systemic review and meta-analysis. Am J kidney disease 2007;49:186-193.

[22] Gressett SM, Shah SR. Intricacies of Bevacizumab-Induced toxicities and their management. The Annals of Pharmacotherapy, March 2009;43:490-500.

[23] Semrad TJ, O'Donell R, Wun T, *et al.* Epidemiology of venous thromboembolism in 9489 patients with malignant gliomas. J Neurosurg 2007;106:601-608.

[24] Nalluri SR, Shu D, Keresztes R, *et al.* Risk of venous thromboembolism with the angiogenesis inhibitor Bevacizumab in cancer patients: a meta-analysis.JAMA 2008;300:2277-2285.

[25] Eremina V, Jefferson JA, Kowalewska J *et al.* VEGF inhibition and renal thrombotic microangiopathy.N Eng J Medicine 2008;358:1129-1136

[26] Norden AD, Drappatz J, Ciampa AS, *et al.* Colon perforation during antiangiogenic therapy for malignant gliomas. Neuro-oncology, Feb 2009:92-95.

[27] Hurwitz H, Fehrenbacher L, Novotny W, *et al.* Bevacizumab plus irinotecan,fluorouracil and leucovorin fpr metastatic colorectal cancer. N Eng J Med. 2004;350:2335-2342.

[28] D'Angelica M, Kornpart P, Gonen M, *et al.* Lack of evidence for increased morbidity after hepatectomy with perioperative use of Bevacizumab: a matched case-control study. Ann Surg Oncol. 2007;14:759-765.

[29] Kabbinavar F, Hurwitz HI, Fehrenbacher L, *et al.* Phase II randomized trial comparing Bevacizumab plus fluorouracil (FU)/leucovorin(LV) with FU/LV alone in patients with metastatic colorectal cancer. J Clin Oncol 2003;21:60-65.

[30] Johnson DH, Fehrenbacher L, Novotny WF *et al.* Randomized phase II trial comparing Bevacizumab plus carboplatin and paclitaxel alone in previously untreated locally advanced or metastatic non-small lung cell cancer. J Clin Oncol 2004;22:2184-2191.

[31] Escudier B, Pluzanska A, Koralewski P, *et al.* Bevacizumab plus interferon alfa-2a for treatment of metastatic renal cell carcinoma: a randomized, double-blind phase III trial. Lancet 2007;370:2103-2111.

[32] Sandler A, Gray R, Perry MC *et al.* Paclitaxel-carboplatin alone or with Bevacizumab for non-small cell lung cancer. N Eng J Med. 2006;355:2542-50.

[33] Saltz LB, Clarke S, Diaz-Rubio E *et al.* Bevacizumab in combination of oxaliplatin-based chemotherapy as first-line therapy in metastatic colorectal; a randomized phase III study. J Clin Oncol. 2008;26:2013-2019.

[34] Scappatici FA, Skillings JR, Holden SN, *et al.* Arterial thrombo-embolic events in patients with metastatic carcinoma treated with chemotherapy and Bevacizumab. J Natl Cancer Inst. 2007;99:1232-1239.

[35] Bokstein F, Shpigel S, Blumenthal DT. Treatment with Bevacizumab and Irinotecan for Recurrent High-Grade Glial Tumors. Cancer. 2008;112(10):2267-73

[36] Gutin P, Mohile N, Lymberis S *et al.* Safety and efficacy of Bevacizumab as a radiosensitizer in malignant glioma: Stereotactic re-irradiation for recurrence as a pilot for adjuvant treatment [abstract]. J Clin Oncol 2007;69(Suppl 20):2028A

[37] Narayan A, Golfinos JG, Fischer I, Shahzad R *et al.* Feasibility of using Bevacizumab with radiation therapy and temozolomide in newly diagnosed high-grade glioma.Int J Radiation Onc Biol Physics 2008;Vol72(2):383-389

[38] Lai A, Filka E, McGibbon B, *et al.* Phase II pilot study of Bevacizumab in combination with temozolomide and regional radiotherapy for up-front treatment of patients with newly diagnosed glioblastoma multiforme: interim analysis of safety and tolerability. Int J Radiation Oncol Biol Physics 2008;71(5):1372-1380.

CHAPTER 18

Novel Applications for Bevacizumab and other Angiogenic Inhibitors

Marc C. Chamberlain*

Department of Neurology and Neurological Surgery, Division of Neuro-Oncology, University of Washington, Fred Hutchinson Cancer Research Center, Seattle Cancer Care Alliance, 825 Eastlake Avenue E, POB 19023, MS G4940, Seattle, WA 98109-1023

Abstract: Background: Angiogenesis is a common theme in cancer and accordingly, antiangiogenic therapies are increasingly utilized for the treatment of cancer including cancers of the central nervous system (CNS). At present, proof of principle of antiangiogenic therapy for CNS tumors has only been realized for recurrent glioblastoma (GBM). Methods: A literature review of the use of bevacizumab and other antiangiogenic therapies in neuro-oncology apart from the treatment of recurrent GBM. Results: Several potential applications for antiangiogenic therapy are suggested by the limited literature presently available including; recurrent anaplastic gliomas, elderly newly diagnosed GBM, unresectable high-grade gliomas with significant mass effect requiring high dose steroid (up-front therapy), radiation necrosis with mass effect, pseudoprogression requiring surgical intervention, highly angiogenic non-glioma primary brain tumors (i.e. vestibular schwannomas, meningioma, hemangiopericytoma, hemangioblastoma), brain metastases in bevacizumab responsive cancers (i.e. renal cell, ovarian, breast and non-small cell lung cancers), up-front treatment of newly diagnosed GBM, radiation optic neuropathy and treatment of selected intracranial sarcomas. Conclusions: Bevacizumab and other angiogenic inhibitory therapies appear to have the potential to treat a variety of brain tumors and brain tumor treatment-related conditions such as pseudoprogression and radiation necrosis. To date; however, these novel applications of angiogenesis inhibitors remain conjectural given that majority of data is retrospective or exploratory.

INTRODUCTION

Since the introduction of bevacizumab as a novel treatment for recurrent glioblastoma (GBM) and subsequent demonstration of efficacy and safety in both retrospective and prospective clinical trials, the FDA recently approved single agent bevacizumab for recurrent GBM based on two prospective studies [1-8]. Simultaneous with the utilization of bevacizumab for recurrent GBM, a number of investigators have explored novel neuro-oncology uses for antiangiogenic therapy (primarily bevacizumab) outside of the currently approved recurrent GBM indication [9-31]. Table **1** is an outline of potential novel applications of antiangiogenic therapy that provide the infrastructure for this review. This review admittedly is conjectural and hypothesis generating given the limited data that exists for angiogenic inhibitor (AI)-based central nervous system (CNS) therapy outside of recurrent GBM.

Table 1: Novel Applications for Antiangiogenic Therapy

■ Recurrent anaplastic gliomas [10, 13-16]
■ Elderly newly diagnosed GBM [33]
■ Unresectable high-grade gliomas with significant mass effect requiring high dose steroid [25]
■ Radiation necrosis with mass effect [27, 27, 30, 31]
■ Pseudoprogression requiring surgical intervention [40-43]
■ Highly angiogenic non-glioma primary brain tumors [24, 28]
■ Brain metastases in bevacizumab responsive cancers [18]
■ Up-front treatment of glioblastoma [19-22, 32]
■ Radiation optic neuropathy [48]
■ Treatment of selected intracranial sarcomas [49-51]

GLIOBLASTOMA

Potentially five new indications for GBM can be envisioned amongst which one is already in formal trials. Based on

*Address correspondence to Marc C Chamberlain:** Department of Neurology and Neurological Surgery, Division of Neuro-Oncology, University of Washington, Fred Hutchinson Cancer Research Center, Seattle Cancer Care Alliance, 825 Eastlake Avenue E, POB 19023, MS G4940, Seattle, WA 98109-1023; Tel: (206) 288-8280; Fax: (206) 288-2000; E-mail: chambemc@u.washington.edu

the efficacy of bevacizumab in recurrent GBM, it is not surprising that bevacizumab was moved forward into the front-line treatment of GBM. Initial studies at UCLA, NYU, University of Chicago and Duke have suggested the feasibility and safety of such an approach when combined with the standard concurrent and sequential temozolomide (TMZ) regimen (the European Organization for Research and Treatment of Cancer/ National Cancer Institute, Canada [EORTC/NCIC] platform) for newly diagnosed GBM [19-22]. Less clear from the early single-arm phase 2 data presented by UCLA is whether a survival benefit is seen in patients treated with every 2-week bevacizumab concurrent with chemo-radiation followed by post-radiotherapy TMZ [19]. As this was a hypothesis generating trial, the control and comparator group of patients were derived from patients treated according to the standard EORTC/NCIC platform at UCLA. Median survival was similar between these groups of patients (21 vs. 20 months). In part this similarity in outcome may reflect the utility of bevacizumab as salvage therapy for patients treated with EORTC/NCIC platform as well as an overall improvement in the management of patients treated with standard up-front therapy. Lastly, up-front bevacizumab likely selects for resistant tumor clonogens (non-vascular endothelial growth factor [VEGF] dependent) in a defined interval as antiangiogenic therapies appear to have a comparatively short therapeutic window during which tumor vasculature is normalized [12,33-36].

Nonetheless, two large double-blinded randomized phase 3 trials have commenced to define the role of bevacizumab in the up-front treatment of patient with newly diagnosed GBM (Chapter 8). Both trials are similar in design with patients randomized to intravenous bevacizumab or placebo given every 2-weeks beginning 2-3 weeks after initiation of concurrent TMZ and radiotherapy (RT). Intravenous bevacizumab or placebo continues every 2-weeks post-radiotherapy as well with post-radiotherapy TMZ. Patients will be assessed for MGMT promoter methylation status *a priori* but methylguanine methyltransferase (MGMT) status will not affect randomization assignment.

Another novel use of bevacizumab and potentially other AI is administration to elderly patients with newly diagnosed GBM. Elderly patients are defined as patients greater than 70 years of age for whom there is no standard of care. Elderly patients constitute 20% of all GBM and were excluded from participation in the EORTC/NCIC trial. Consequently, the best treatment for this subpopulation is unknown and treatment is based on best clinical judgment. Patients independent in activities of daily living and otherwise physiologically fit are often offered the EORTC/NCIC platform notwithstanding the lack of evidence and data suggesting the regimen is less effective in patients of advanced age. Alternatively, elderly patients may be treated with hypofractionated RT only or with primary TMZ-based chemotherapy and deferred RT. The NCIC is conducting a trial in newly diagnosed patients with GBM comparing hypofractionated RT with or without TMZ. In addition, the German Cancer Study Group NOA is evaluating a trial (NOA-08) for elderly GBM patients comparing up-front dose dense TMZ (7/14 schedule) to standard RT and at recurrence, crossover to the alternative therapy. Another proposed use of AI would be combining primary TMZ with bevacizumab in elderly patients with newly diagnosed GBM. Nghiemphu reported that VEGF expression increases as a function of age in patients with GBM as does radiographic response, progression free and overall survival [33]. This emerging data indicates a potentially age dependent response to AI where heretofore anti-GBM therapies have been less effective.

Another challenging subpopulation of newly diagnosed GBM patients is patients with large unresectable tumors as a result of tumor location in eloquent regions of brain and for whom large doses of steroids are required to control peritumoral edema and mass effect. Patients such as these are difficult to treat and often can not complete RT due to clinical decompensation related to tumor size or steroid-related morbid side effects i.e. proximal myopathy, skin fragility, Cushingnoid habitus and diabetes. Anecdotally, patients with this constellation of findings have been treated with up-front bevacizumab and chemo-radiation resulting in control of peritumoral edema related mass effect, either marked reduction or discontinuance of steroids and completion of RT [25]. In addition, performance status in these patients often improves dramatically resulting in an improved quality of life.

Pseudoprogression is an increasingly common clinical issue based in part upon more effective up-front therapy for GBM [40-43]. Pseudoprogression is seen in 20-30% of all newly diagnosed GBM patients treated with the EORTC/NCIC platform, is more common in MGMT deficient tumors, mostly but not exclusively seen within 3 months of initial surgery, represents a treatment-related disruption of the blood brain barrier and is difficult to differentiate from true disease progression radiographically regardless if anatomic or functional imaging-based [40-43]. Consequently, an operational definition has been utilized to define pseudoprogression as apparent radiographic disease progression that improves with continuation of planned post-RT therapy. A subset of pseudoprogression develops sufficient mass effect that surgical intervention is warranted [40]. It is in this group that administration of bevacizumab may obviate surgery by lessening mass effect and improving peritumoral edema. Unclear at present is the duration of bevacizumab therapy that is required however treatment is likely to be relatively short and similar to that prescribed for radiation necrosis (Chapter 11).

ANAPLASTIC GLIOMAS

As discussed in Chapter 20, there is emerging retrospective single institution data for the utility of bevacizumab in the treatment of recurrent anaplastic gliomas (AG) [1,3,5,6,9,10,13-16]. With two exceptions, these studies have utilized combinatorial therapy and treated predominantly with bevacizumab and CPT-11 (irinotecan, Camptosar). Based on the five studies reported to date using bevacizumab for recurrent AG response (n=140 patients), rates vary with complete response to bevacizumab plus therapy in 0-20% (median 10%), partial response in 34-68% (median 52%) and stable disease in 5-59% (median 16%) of patients (44, 49). Survival varies as well (median 28 weeks; 6-month progression free 32-68%, median 55%). These results require validation and it would seem rationale at this time to consider a prospective trial for recurrent AG in patients previously treated with TMZ and RT. Notwithstanding the improved response to bevacizumab seen in recurrent AG, as with GBM, how best to determine response with AI therapy is problematic as current response criteria are based on measuring tumor as defined by contrast enhancement. Similar to radiographic interpretation in AI-based therapy and GBM, interpreting response with agents that normalize the blood brain barrier is difficult and creates new challenges in evaluating response rates and time to progression for AG as well [44,45]. To date, survival in patients with recurrent AG treated with bevacizumab does not appear to be improved over past therapies. Bevacizumab treated 12-month progression free survival ranges from 16-23% compared to TMZ for recurrent TMZ-naïve recurrent AG median overall survival of 13.6 months and in an aggregate series of 8 phase II trials for recurrent AG (pre-TMZ) from the MD Anderson Cancer Center, median overall survival was 47 weeks [46,47]. In part this data may reflect the age dependent response to bevacizumab therapy as mentioned above in addition to the fact that the majority of trials treating recurrent AG with bevacizumab have previously utilized and failed TMZ-based chemotherapy [23].

RADIATION NECROSIS

Radiation injury to brain is not uncommon and manifests as acute, early- and late-delayed radiation injury. One form of late-delayed injury, radiation necrosis, presents as an intracranial mass not easily differentiated from recurrent and progressive disease radiographically [26,27,30,31]. Definitive diagnosis may require obtaining tissue and mass effect may necessitate surgical resection. Several case reports suggest patients with symptomatic intracranial radiation necrosis benefit from bevacizumab treatment by decreasing peritumoral edema, improving mass effect, hastening recovery from this treatment-related injury and obviating surgical intervention [27,30,31]. The natural history of radiation necrosis in the majority of patients is slow improvement after an initial worsening though the time course is measured in months. Steroids are most often used to ameliorate neurologic symptoms that accompany radiation necrosis and when clinically indicated, surgery is used to ameliorate mass effect. However the prolonged time course of radiation necrosis necessitates significant steroid exposure and commonly is associated with steroid-related morbidity and declining quality of life. Bevacizumab rapidly normalizes blood brain barrier disruption due to radiation injury thereby markedly diminishing the time required for recovery from injury [27,30,31]. Bevacizumab by rapidly diminishing edema associated with radiation necrosis obviates the need for steroids and spares patients steroid-related side effects. As well, bevacizumab appears to provide a long duration of effect following a relatively short course of therapy. Treatment beyond 3-4 cycles of bevacizumab appears unnecessary and may result in ischemic injury if bevacizumab therapy is prolonged due to over-normalization of injured brain vasculature. A single case report has described similar benefit of bevacizumab in a patient with spinal cord radiation-induced myelitis [26]. Another interesting application of bevacizumab is for radiation optic neuropathy where the administration of bevacizumab is intra-vitreous [48]. A prospective trial using bevacizumab for intracranial radiation necrosis is nearing completion and is discussed in Chapter 19.

HIGHLY ANGIOGENIC NON-GLIOMA PRIMARY BRAIN TUMORS

The use of bevacizumab outside of gliomas at present is relatively unexplored for primary brain tumors [24,28]. Highly vascular tumors such as meningioma, hemangioblastoma and hemangiopericytoma would appear rationale targets for AI therapy. A recent report described a small case series (n=10) suggests that bevacizumab may be an effective therapy for vestibular schwannomas not otherwise candidates for surgery or radiotherapy [28]. Unlike gliomas, radiographic response suggests a cytotoxic mechanism of action with apparent and measurable shrinkage of tumor. However and similar to gliomas, the appropriate dose, schedule and duration of bevacizumab treatment are yet to be defined. In another small case series, modest benefit of bevacizumab therapy was seen in patients with recurrent intracranial ependymoma [24]. What is lacking at present is data from prospective phase 2 trials establishing new indications for bevacizumab in the treatment of recurrent primary brain tumors not GBM.

BRAIN METASTASES

The initial reluctance to use bevacizumab for intracranial disease (and for primary brain tumors in particular) was based on a report of intracranial hemorrhage in a patient with hepatocellular carcinoma and occult brain metastases in a phase 1 trial [44,45]. Consequently, patients with CNS metastases were routinely excluded from most late-stage bevacizumab clinical trials. In a recent report, the safety of bevacizumab in patients with CNS metastases was confirmed by comparing 187 patients with brain metastases (half treated with bevacizumab; half not receiving bevacizumab) treated on 13 randomized clinical trials [18]. Approximately 3.3% of patients with CNS metastases treated with bevacizumab manifested a Grade 4 intracranial hemorrhage compared to 1% in the non-bevacizumab treated group. In addition, in two open-label trials in patients with non-small cell lung cancer and treated brain metastases (n=87), only a single patient (1%) developed a grade 2 intracranial hemorrhage. In this retrospective review, the rates of intracranial hemorrhage are low in bevacizumab treated patients and not dissimilar to historical controls [18]. Further studies are likely to confirm the safety of bevacizumab in this patient population and perhaps engender studies of bevacizumab in patients with CNS metastases and bevacizumab responsive cancers such as renal cell, ovarian, non-small cell lung, breast and colorectal cancers.

INTRACRANIAL SARCOMAS

Primary intracranial sarcomas are rare CNS malignancies and most often are treated with surgery and radiotherapy. Recurrence is not uncommon and current chemotherapy, in particular doxorubicin and ifosfamide, results in very modest responses of relatively short duration. Consequently new targeted therapies are of interest and AI therapy has demonstrated some early favorable responses in mixed sarcoma histology phase 2 trials [48-50]. Sorafenib (Nexavar) and sunitinib (Sutent) appear to have activity in angiosarcomas and leiomyosarcomas [49-51]. Sorafenib as well appears to have activity in chordoma and solitary fibrous tumors (hemangiopericytoma) [50]. Pazopanib, a multi-kinase AI, has activity against leiomyosarcoma [51]. At present there are no trials specifically for intracranial sarcomas but emerging data suggests AI therapy may be effective in some mesenchymal-derived intracranial tumors.

CONCLUSIONS

In summary, bevacizumab and other AI therapies appear to have the potential to treat a variety of brain tumors and brain tumor treatment-related conditions such as pseudoprogression and radiation necrosis. To date however these novel applications of AI therapy remain conjectural given that majority of data is retrospective or exploratory based on early phase 2 trials. Most mature for new applications of bevacizumab and brain tumors are the newly diagnosed GBM upfront trials (RTOG in the United States and Roche Pharmaceuticals in Europe, both having opened this year) as well as a prospective intracranial radiation necrosis trial. The need for multi-institutional prospective trials evaluating the role of bevacizumab and other AI therapies for the treatment of recurrent AG for example is acute given the generally poor prognosis seen following recurrence. Such trials would likely better define the treatment of recurrent AG and potentially lead to an approved indication of bevacizumab for recurrent AG. As well, collaborative trials for uncommon tumors like recurrent and refractory meningioma and chordoma would be welcome and would represent a paradigm shift in the neuro-oncology community focus on gliomas. The limited therapeutic tools available to treat intracranial radiation necrosis and radiation refractory brain metastases further represent an unmet need for which AI therapy may prove valuable.

REFERENCES

[1]   Stark-Vance V. Bevacizumab and CPT-11 in the treatment of relapsed malignant glioma. Neuro-Oncology 2005;7(3):369.

[2]   Vredenburgh JJ, Desjardins A, Herndon JE, *et al.* Bevacizumab plus irinotecan in recurrent glioblastoma multiforme. J Clin Oncol 2007;25(30):4722-4729.

[3]   Norden AD, Young GS, Setayesh K, *et al.* Bevacizumab for recurrent malignant glioma: efficacy, toxicity and patterns of recurrence. Neurology. 2008;70:779-787.

[4]   Cloughesy T, Prados MD, Mikkelsen T, *et al.* A phase 2 randomized non-comparative clinical trial of the effect of bevacizumab alone or in combination with irinotecan on 6-month progression free survival in recurrent treatment refractory glioblastoma. J Clin Oncol. 2008;26:91s (Abstract).

[5]   Bokstein F, Shpigel S, Blumenthal DTl. Treatment with bevacizumab and irinotecan for recurrent high-grade glial tumors. Cancer 2008; 112 (10): 2267-2273.

[6]   Raizer JJ, Gallot L, Cohn R, *et al.* A phase II safety study of bevacizumab in patients with multiple recurrent or progressive malignant gliomas. J Clin Oncol, 2007; 25 (18S), 2007: 2079 (abstract).

[7]   Kreisl TN, Kim L, Moore K, *et al.* Phase II trial of single agent bevacizumab followed by bevacizumab plus irinotecan at tumor progression in recurrent glioblastoma. J Clin Oncol 2009;27: 740-745.

[8]   Chamberlain MC, Johnston S. Salvage therapy with single agent bevacizumab for recurrent glioblastoma. J Neurooncol 2009c. [Epub ahead of print].

[9]   Pope WB, Lai A, Nghiemphu P, Mischel P, Cloughesy TF. MRI in patients with high-grade gliomas treated with bevacizumab and chemotherapy. Neurology 66 (8); 1258-1260, 2006.

[10]   Vredenburgh JJ, Desjardins A, Herndon JE II, *et al.* Phase II trial of bevacizumab and irinotecan in recurrent malignant glioma. Clin Cancer Res 2007;13(4):1253-59.

[11]   Chen C, Silverman DHS, Geist C, *et al.* Predicting treatment response of malignant gliomas to bevacizumab and irinotecan by imaging proliferation with [18F] fluorothymidine positron emission tomography: a pilot study. J Clin Oncol 2007;25(30):4714-4721.

[12]   Batchelor TT, Sorensen AG, di Tomaso E, *et al.* AZD2171, a Pan-VEGF receptor tyrosine kinase inhibitor, normalizes tumor vasculature and alleviates edema in glioblastoma patients. Cancer Cell. 2007;11:83-95.

[13]   Tallibert S, Vincent LA, Granger B, *et al.* Bevacizumab and irinotecan for recurrent oligodendroglial tumors. Neurology 2009; 72:1601-1606.

[14]   Chamberlain MC, Johnston S. Salvage chemotherapy with bevacizumab for recurrent alkylator-refractory anaplastic astrocytoma. J Neurooncol 2009; 91: 359–367.

[15]   Chamberlain MC, Johnston S. Bevacizumab for recurrent alkylator-refractory anaplastic oligodendroglioma. Cancer 2009; 115: 1734-43.

[16]   Desjardins A, Reardon DA, Herndon JE, *et al.* Bevacizumab plus irinotecan in recurrent WHO grade 3 malignant gliomas. Clin Cancer Res 2008; 14: 7068–7073.

[17]   Nghiemphu PL, Green RM, Pope WB, *et al.* Safety of anticoagulation use and bevacizumab in patients with glioma. Neuro Oncol. 2008;10:355–360.

[18]   Rohr UP, Augustus S, Lassere SF, Compton P, Huang J, Hoffman F. Safety of bevacizumab in patients with metastases to the central nervous system. J Clin Oncol 2009; 27 (15S), 88s (abstract).

[19]   Lai A, Nghiemphu P, Green R, *et al.* Phase II trial of bevacizumab in combination with temozolomide and regional radiation therapy for up-front treatment of patients with newly diagnosed glioblastoma multiforme. J Clin Oncol 2009; 27 (15S), 86s (abstract).

[20]   Nicholas MK, Lucas RV, Arzbaecher J, *et al.* Bevacizumab in combination with temozolomide in the adjuvant treatment of newly diagnosed glioblastoma multiforme; preliminary results of a phase 2 study. J Clin Oncol 2009; 27 (15S), 91s (abstract).

[21]   Gruber ML, Raza S, Gruber D, Narayana A. Bevacizumab in combination with radiotherapy plus concomitant and adjuvant temozolomide for newly diagnosed glioblastoma: update progression free survival, overall survival and toxicity. J Clin Oncol 2009; 27 (15S), 91s (abstract).

[22]   Vredenburgh J, Desjardins A, Reardon D, *et al.* Safety and efficacy of the addition of bevacizumab to temozolomide and radiation therapy followed by bevacizumab, temozolomide and irinotecan for newly diagnosed glioblastoma multiforme. J Clin Oncol 2009; 27 (15S), 90s (abstract).

[23]   Nghiemphu PL, Liu W, Lee Y, *et al.* Bevacizumab and chemotherapy for recurrent glioblastoma: a single-institution experience. Neurology 2009;72:1217–1222.

[24]   Green RM, Cloughesy T, Stupp R, *et al.* Bevacizumab for recurrent ependymoma. J Clin Oncol 2009;27:15s. (Abstract).

[25]   Peters K, Desjardins A, Reardon DA, *et al.* Temozolomide (TMZ) and bevacizumab (BV) as initial treatment for unresectable or multifocal glioblastoma multiforme (GBM). J Clin Oncol 2009;27:15s (Abstract).

[26]   Greenberg BM, Blakeley JO. Bevacizumab for the treatment of radiation myelopathy. Neurology 2009;72 (11): A30. (Abstract).

[27]   Gonzalez J, Kumar AJ, Conrad CA, *et al.* Effect of bevacizumab on radiation necrosis of the brain. Int J Radiat Oncol Biol Phys. 2007;67:323–326.

[28]   Plotkin S, Stemmer-Rachamimov A, Barker F, *et al.* Hearing improvement after bevacizumab in patients with neurofibromatosis Type 2. NEJM 2009 ; 361(4) :358-67.

[29]   Reardon D, Desjardins A, Vredenburgh JJ, *et al.* Bevacizumab plus etoposide among recurrent malignant glioma patients: Phase II study final results. J Clin Oncol 2009;27:15s (Abstract).

[30]   Torcuator R, Zuniga R, Mohan YS, *et al.* Initial experience with bevacizumab treatment for biopsy confirmed cerebral radiation necrosis. J Neurooncol 2009 [epub ahead of print].

[31]   Wong ET, Huberman M, Lu XQ, *et al.* Bevacizumab reverses cerebral radiation necrosis. J Clin Oncol 2008;26:5649–5650

[32]   Stupp R, Mason WP, Van Den Bent MJ, *et al.* Concomitant and adjuvant temozolomide and radiotherapy for newly diagnosed glioblastoma multiforme. Conclusive results of a randomized phase III trial by the EORTC Brain & RT Groups and NCIC Clinical Trial Groups. J Clin Oncol 22: 1s, 2004.

[33]   Bergers G, Hanahan D. Modes of resistance to anti-angiogenic therapy. Nat Rev Cancer 2008;8:592–603.

[34]   Kerbel RS. Tumor angiogenesis. N Engl J Med 2008;358:2039–2049.

[35]   Jain RK. Normalization of tumor vasculature: an emerging concept in antiangiogenic therapy. Science 2005;307:58–62.

[36]   Jain RK, di Tomaso E, Duda DG, *et al.* Angiogenesis in brain tumors. Nat Rev Neurosci 2007; 8:610–622.

[37]   Chamberlain MC, Chalmers L. A pilot study of primary temozolomide chemotherapy and deferred radiotherapy in elderly patients with glioblastoma. J Neuro-Oncology 2007;82(2):207-209.

[38]   Glantz M, Chamberlain MC, Liu Q, Litofsky NS, Recht LD. Temozolomide as an alternative to irradiation for elderly patients with newly diagnosed malignant gliomas. Cancer 2003;97:2262-2266.

[39]   Roa W, Brasher PM, Bauman G, Anthes M, Bruera E, Chan A, Fisher B, Fulton D, Glavita S, ho C, Husain S, Murtha A, Petruk K, Stewart D, Tai P, Urtasun R, Chirncross JG, Forsyth P. Abbreviated course of radiation therapy in older patients with glioblastoma multiforme: a prospective randomized clinical trial. J Clin Oncol 22 (9):1583-8, 2004.

[40]   Chamberlain MC, Glantz MJ, Chalmers L, Sloan A. Early necrosis following temodar and radiotherapy in patients with glioblastoma. J Neuro-Oncology 2007;82(1):81-83.

[41]   Brandsma D, Stalpers L, Taal W, *et al.* Clinical features, mechanisms, and management of pseudoprogression in malignant gliomas. Lancet Oncol 9:453-61, 2008

[42]   Taal W, Brandsma D, de Bruin HG, *et al.* Incidence of early pseudo-progression in a cohort of malignant glioma patients treated with chemoirradiation with temozolomide. Cancer 113:405-10, 2008

[43]   Brandes AA, Franceschi E, Tosoni A, *et al.* MGMT promoter methylation status can predict the incidence and outcome of pseudoprogression after concomitant radiochemotherapy in newly diagnosed glioblastoma patients. J Clin Oncol 26:2192-7, 2008

[44]   Reardon DA, Wen PY, Desjardins A, *et al.* Glioblastoma multiforme: an emerging paradigm of anti-VEGF therapy. Expert Opin Biol Ther 2008;8:541–553.

[45]   Dietrich J, Norden AD, Wen PY. Emerging antiangiogenic treatments for gliomas – efficacy and safety issues. Curr Opin Neurol 2008;21:736–744.

[46]   Yung WK, Prados MD, Yaya-Tur R, Rosenfeld SS, Brada M, *et al.* Multicenter Phase II trial of temozolomide in patients with anaplastic astrocytoma or anaplastic oligoastrocytoma at first relapse. J Clin Oncol 17: 2762-2771, 1999.

[47]   Wong ET, Hess KR, Gleason MJ, *et al.* Outcomes and prognostic factors in recurrent glioma patients enrolled onto phase II clinical trials. J Clin Oncol 17: 2572-2578, 1999.

[48]   Finger PT. Anti-VEGF bevacizumab (Avastin®) for radiation optic neuropathy. Amer J Ophthalmology 2007;143(2):335-8.

[49]   George S, Merriam P, Maki R, *et al.* Multicenter phase 2 trial of sunitinib in the treatment of non-gastrointestinal stromal sarcomas. J Clin Oncol 2009; 27 (19):3154-3160.

[50]   Maki R, D'Adamo D, Keohan M, *et al.* Phase 2 study of sorafenib in patients with metastatic or recurrent sarcomas. J Clin Oncol 2009; 27 (19):3133-3140.

[51]   Sleijfer S, Ray-Coquard I, Papai Z, *et al.* Pazopanib, a multikinase angiogenesis inhibitor, in patients with relapsed or refractory advanced soft tissue sarcoma: A phase 2 study from the European Organization for Research and Treatment of Cancer: Soft tissue and bone sarcoma group (EORTC study 62043). J Clin Oncol 2009; 27 (19):3126-3132.

CHAPTER 19

Role of Avastin for Treatment of Central Nervous System Radiation Necrosis

Jing Wu and Victor A. Levin*

Department of Neuro-Oncology, The University of Texas MD Anderson Cancer Center, Houston, Texas

Abstract: Radiation therapy continues to be a common therapy for most primary central nervous system (CNS) tumors, tumors that metastasize to the CNS, and tumors of the head and neck. Radiation injury is an inevitable side effect in many of these cases. Understanding the pathophysiology and clinical manifestation of different stages of radiation injury is crucial for developing methods to maximally mitigate radiation injury. In this chapter, we discuss the classification of radiation injury and emphasize the potential mechanisms of radiation necrosis. More importantly, our clinical experience and ongoing clinical studies of treatment for radiation necrosis are discussed. Hopefully, these efforts will substantially assist the field of treatment of radiation necrosis to move forward.

INTRODUCTION

Radiation therapy remains an important component in treating primary and metastatic cancers in the head, neck and central nervous system (CNS). When radiation therapy is used for primary brain tumors, normal adjacent brain tissue receives variable amounts of radiation dose as well. Similarly, when head and neck tumors are treated with extracranial radiation, variable amounts of radiation may reach the normal brain. In both circumstances, the potential for radiation-induced injury of normal brain tissue becomes the dose-limiting factor. Since radiotherapy, alone or combination with chemotherapy, continues to be widely used, it is important to develop methods to protect normal tissues in the CNS from radiation injury and/or to mitigate the damaging effects. To that end, understanding the pathogenesis of radiation-induced CNS injury is crucial for developing rational clinical trials that may lead to effective treatments for radiation injury and protective strategies to reduce or prevent such injury.

CLASSIFICATION AND CLINICAL MANIFESTATION OF RADIATION INJURY TO CNS

Classically, radiation-induced injury has been divided into 3 phases: acute reaction, early delayed reaction, and late delayed reaction [1]. Acute reaction usually happens within a few weeks of initiating radiation therapy and is thought to be caused by radiation-induced cerebral edema. Headache, nausea, and somnolence may occur. These symptoms are usually very minor with a conventional schedule of 1.8-2.0 Gy per day, 5 days per week to a total dose of 60 Gy [1]. Even hyperfractionated schedules, in which the patient receives 1.2 Gy twice a day to a total dose of 81.6 Gy, and accelerated schedules, in which the patient receives 1.6 Gy twice a day to a total dose of 49 to 70.4 Gy have been used to treat patients without much acute reaction as long as corticosteroid prophylaxis is used. While acute tolerance of the brain to doses as high as 6 Gy has been reported, fraction sizes over 7.5 Gy have been associated with severe acute reactions, from severe headache and pyrexia to cerebral herniation and death [2,3].

Early delayed reaction appears within a few weeks up to 3 months following the completion of radiation therapy is thought to be caused, in part, by transient interruptions of myelin synthesis secondary to radiation injury to the oligodendrocytes. It may occur after radiation for benign or malignant brain tumors and is usually marked by transient neurological deterioration, increased somnolence, and worsening of tumor-related neurological deficits. Some think it is related to the location of the underlying brain tumor, the dose of radiation, and the volume of the irradiated brain tissue [1]. It was first described clinically by Rider in 1963 [4]. Two patients who had received radiation therapy for extracranial lesions developed cerebellar and brain stem symptoms 10 weeks after treatment. Complete and spontaneous recovery was found in both patients 10-12 weeks later. Other reports have presented similar cases that were all marked by transient course and spontaneous recovery [5,6]. This phenomenon of transient early delayed radiation-induced clinical and radiographic worsening is often referred to as "pseudoprogression."

---

*Address correspondence to Victor A. Levin:** Department of Neuro-Oncology, The University of Texas M. D. Anderson Cancer Center, Houston, TX 77030; Email: vlevin49@comcast.net

With concurrent chemotherapy, subacute radiation effects can occur earlier and even more frequently. In a study of 85 patients with malignant gliomas who received daily temozolomide chemotherapy with irradiation, 21% of the patients developed pseudoprogression [7]. However, in another study, only 9% of the patients with malignant gliomas who received radiotherapy only were found to have pseudoprogression [8]. Another study showed more frequent pseudoprogression in patients given O^6-methyl guanine-DNA methyl transferase methylation [9]. This finding could partially explain the difference in individual sensitivity to pseudoprogression. Neither the size of the radiated tumor volume nor the patients' ages were found to be related to the incidence of pseudoprogression [7] suggesting that there may be genetic predisposing factors. Unfortunately, a genetic basis to explain radiation toxicity to the CNS has not yet been elucidated.

Late delayed radiation reaction typically occurs 6 months to 3 years after radiation therapy, although it has been reported in biopsy-proven cases as early as 3 months and as late as 13 years after the completion of radiation therapy [10,11]. Its manifestation can range from asymptomatic white matter lesions to pituitary-hypothalamus dysfunction and necrosis with progressive neurological dysfunction. The pathogenesis of late delayed reaction has been attributed to vascular endothelial injury [12-15] and the direct effect of radiation on glial cells [16,17]. Unlike acute and early delayed reactions, which usually spontaneously recover or can be mitigated by corticosteroid prophylaxis, late delayed reactions are usually irreversible and can progress over time to include destructive necrosis and small vessel strokes. The outcome of late delayed reaction varies from focal neurological deficits to death, depending on the region and volume of brain that has been irradiated. Following large-volume or whole brain irradiation, a computed tomography may reveal diffuse hypodense areas in the white matter, and T2-weighted magnetic resonance imaging (MRI) might show diffuse hyperintense signal in the periventricular white matter. These white matter lesions can increase in size and may progress to more severe effects, such as radiation necrosis.

PATHOLOGY OF RADIATION NECROSIS

Delayed radiation necrosis may follow radiation therapy to an intracranial tumor or any other tumor when the brain or spinal cord is included in the treatment field. In contrast to the necrosis caused by chemotherapy, which occurs primarily in the tumor lesions themselves, radiation-induced necrosis mainly appears in the white matter. In the early stage of delayed necrosis, nonspecific swollen gyri can be grossly observed in intact brain specimens and typical hemorrhagic coagulation necrosis. Histologically, the most characteristic abnormality associated with radiation necrosis is the exudation of an amorphous, eosinophilic, and structureless substance that is positive for fibrin in immunohistochemical staining. The abnormality becomes diagnostic of radiation necrosis when the fibrin exudates and forms hypocellular laminae at the gray-white matter junction. This zone abnormality can further extend into the deep layer of the gray matter. Calcification occurs in this zone over time and makes a distinctive radiographic appearance. In the brain parenchyma, the coalescing foci of necrosis in the white matter have a granular eosinophilic feature that distinguishes them from infarction. As lesions transform from the subacute to chronic stage, some necrotic foci evolve into multiple cysts through the invasion and activity of macrophages. In the acute stage of radiation necrosis, vascular proliferation also occurs. Over weeks to months the vascular change evolves and the acute fibrin-positive substance exudates while fibrinoid necrosis is replaced by telangiectasia and vascular thickening with atypia or missing endothelial cells. In the brainstem, the lesions most frequently appear in the base of the pons, where the crossing fibers are located. Microscopically, central coagulation necrosis and dystrophic calcification are surrounded by eosinophilic swollen axons. In the spinal cord, delayed radiation necrosis is characterized by fibrinoid necrosis and coagulation necrosis in the white matter [18,19].

PSEUDOPROGRESSION AND RADIATION NECROSIS

As discussed earlier, pseudoprogression describes a clinical phenomenon that mimics tumor progression radiographically during the early delayed reaction period. Typically, increased contrast enhancement appears near the brain tumor a few weeks after radiation therapy is initiated. Patients may or may not have clinical deterioration and may have an increase in edema evident on T2-weighted fluid attenuated inversion recovery (FLAIR) images. As noted, these lesions usually resolve over time without treatment other than corticosteroids. Histologically, pseudoprogression is best viewed as a point on the continuum between early demyelination and radiation-induced necrosis. As such, it should be considered an early delayed reaction, although at times it may have some of the attributes of a late delayed reaction. While in clinical practice, these two terms, radiation necrosis vs.

pseudoprogression may be used interchangeably, in our opinion, early delayed reaction conveys more information about the process and helps to distinguish this clinical entity from other reasons for tumor expansion such as cell division and tumor growth. Generally, early delayed radiation injury occurs within 1 to 3 months after completion of radiation therapy and is normally distinguishable from late delayed radiation injury, which is true radiation necrosis, with its attendant vascular changes, necrotic tissue, and edema adjacent to the damaged area.

The incidence of radiation necrosis has not been strongly linked to any consistent cause and is somewhat sporadic. However, it has been shown to have some relationship to radiation dose per fraction, total dose administered, and overall treatment duration [1,20]. In a study of 139 patients with primary brain tumors who received radiation therapy at 1.8-2.0 Gy per fraction, for a total of at least 45 Gy, only 5% of the patients developed radiation necrosis [21]. When the fraction size is less than 1.8 Gy, the incidence of radiation necrosis directly correlates with the total dose: A total dose of more than 64.8 Gy significantly increases the chance of developing radiation necrosis [22]. Sheline and colleagues reviewed 80 cases of radiation necrosis in the literature. Of those, 68 were histologically confirmed as radiation necrosis, 4 cases occurred in patients radiated for extracranial tumors and the remaining 8 cases represented instances where the tumor sites were in distant from the new lesions. The reported doses received by these patients were converted into megavoltage rad equivalents (MREs). For each patient, MREs were plotted against the number of treatments on a double logarithmic scale. An isoeffect line was drawn such that most of the patients with radiation necrosis were represented by points on or above the line. The slope of the line was 0.44, defining the lower limits for radiation necrosis of the brain. This slope of the isoeffect line is consistent with data for spinal cord necrosis in humans and rats [23]. Based on the slope of that isoeffect line, the Ellis formula (24), which is used to calculate the threshold of radiation necrosis, was modified to $neuret = D \times N^{-0.41} \times T^{-0.03}$ (D, total dose in MRE; N, number of fraction; T, total time in days). According to this formula, the threshold for radiation necrosis is 1000-1100 neuret. The most common radiation schedule that we used for glioblastoma, 200 cGy per fraction, 5 days a week to a total dose of 60 Gy, is about 1080 neuret by this equation [23].

MECHANISMS OF RADIATION NECROSIS

The mechanisms responsible for radiation necrosis are not completely understood. Vascular and parenchymal hypothesis have been proposed. In addition, cytokines and reactive oxygen species (ROS) have been found to be involved in the process at the molecular level.

VASCULAR HYPOTHESIS

The vascular hypothesis argues that white matter necrosis is secondary to the ischemia caused by the vascular damage in a late delayed reaction. Vascular abnormalities, including vessel dilatation, nuclear enlargement in endothelial cells, endothelial cell atypia, blood-brain barrier (BBB) breakdown, fibrinoid deposits, and telangectasia, are found in the radiation-damaged tissues [15,25]. The vascular hypothesis is also supported by a study of boron neutron capture therapy [26] that demonstrated that white matter necrosis in rat spinal cords appeared to be caused by radiation delivered to the vasculature. Since studies in rat models have shown that white matter necrosis can take months to develop after vasculature abnormalities have initiated [14,15], other pathophysiological changes that directly cause radiation necrosis remain possible. Furthermore, radiation-induced necrosis has been reported in the absence of vascular changes [20,27]. Therefore, endothelial cell loss and vascular damage are sufficient, but may not be necessary, to cause radiation-induced necrosis.

PARENCHYMAL HYPOTHESIS

The parenchymal hypothesis of the mechanism underpinning radiation necrosis focuses on the loss of oligodendrocytes. In an early delayed reaction, demyelination secondary to the loss of oligodendrocytes is predominant. This parenchymal theory is supported by the identification of O-2A progenitor cells [17], which are the precursors of oligodendrocytes, and the finding that the reproductive capacity of O-2A progenitor cells was largely reduced by radiation of the brain and spinal cord in rat models [17,18-20]. Unlike the vascular hypothesis, theparenchymal hypothesis explains the selectivity of white matter in radiation necrosis. However, a few studies showed that the demyelination mainly accounts for the early stage of radiation injury, but has not been linked to delayed reactions such as radiation necrosis [27,31]. In addition, another neurological entity, multiple sclerosis, which is also caused by oligodendrocyte loss, does not necessarily have similar necrosis as a feature. Therefore, factors aside from endothelial cell injury and oligodendrocyte loss are very likely to be required in causing radiation-induced necrosis.

OTHER COMPONENTS IN THE CNS NETWORK

Given the highly integrated nature of the CNS, failure of cell-cell interactions may significantly contribute to any radiation injury. Interaction between astrocytes and endothelial cells in the maintenance of BBB is a good example of this hypothesis.

Astrocytes are the most populous cell type in the mammalian CNS, making up more than half the glial cells and more than 10 times the number of neurons [32]. They can regulate the response of vasculature, neurons, and oligodendrocytes by secreting cytokines, protease, and growth factors [33,34]. In addition, astrocytes are also found to have critical roles in responding to CNS injury and protecting neurons, oligodendrocytes, and endothelial cells from oxidative injury [35-40]. This function is evidenced by a dose-dependent increase in astrocytes in rat and mouse brains after irradiation [14,41]. Astrocytes are also identified as the vascular endothelial growth factor (VEGF) and hypoxia-induced factor (HIF)-expressing cells in rat spinal cords after exposure to radiation [42]. This expression could initiate of the cascade effect of radiation necrosis.

Microglia constitute about 10% of all the glial cells and are involved in the inflammatory reaction in the brain [43,44]. They are capable of proliferation, phagocytosis, and exacerbating responses to injury by secreting ROS, lipid metabolites, and hydrolytic enzymes [45,46]. Increased numbers of microglial cells have been reported in the brain tissues of mice, rats, and dogs, as well as human spinal cord tissue, after irradiation [41, 47-49]. This evidence supports the potential role of microglia in radiation-induced injury.

Although recent data suggest radiation-induced neuronal DNA damage leads to late delayed radiation injury, cognitive dysfunction rather than frank necrosis is the more likely outcome [50].

MOLECULAR COMPONENTS OF RADIATION-INDUCED NECROSIS

ROS include oxygen ions, free radicals, and organic and inorganic peroxide. They are highly reactive and cause oxidative damage to tissues. Tissue hypoxia secondary to vascular damage caused by radiation injury promotes the production of proinflammatory cytokines and subsequently ROS [51]. The brain has low levels of antioxidants, including superoxide dismutase, catalase, and glutathione peroxidase [52]. This deficiency makes the CNS tissue highly susceptible to oxidative injury, especially the myelin sheath, which contains high levels of acids that can be peroxidated [53]. To overcome the difficulty in measuring ROS, investigators have used Hmox1, formerly known as HO-1, as a surrogate marker of oxidative stress [54]. Although Hmox1 expression is normally low, increased expression has been found in the rat cervical spinal cord after irradiation but well before the onset of myelopathy [50]. However, another study found that lipid peroxidation played no role in late delayed radiation injury in the white matter of rat cervical spinal cords [55]. Although it is highly reasonable to speculate that ROS are involved in radiation necrosis, more direct evidence and full elucidation of the involved mechanisms are warranted.

Alteration of cytokines has also been proposed as a possible mechanism of radiation necrosis [56,57]. In cerebral radiation necrosis, increased macrophage cell infiltration, interlukine 6 (IL-6) immunoreactivity, and tumor necrosis factor (TNF) α have been observed [58]. Radiation also affects cytokines' gene expression in microglia [59]. During BBB breakdown, the inflammatory cells could cross to the extravascular space, causing further inflammatory response. Overproduction of the inflammatory response and inflammation related to various cytokine secretions can possibly perpetuate a vicious cycle of necrosis. Such an event could potentially explain why some cases of radiation-induced necrosis progress relentlessly and even recur after surgical resection.

VEGF IN RADIATION NECROSIS

The VEGF family consists of 5 glycoproteins, VEGFA, VEGFB, VEGFC, and VEGFD and the placenta growth factor [60]. The receptors of VEGF are 3 group receptor tyrosine kinases with similar structures, VEGFR1,

VEGFR2, and VEGFR3. VEGFR2 is the key regulator of angiogenesis and its expression is restricted mainly to the vasculature. VEGFR1 is also expressed mainly in the vasculature but is sometimes expressed in other types of cells [61]. Wu and colleagues demonstrated the expression of VEGFR1 in the human tumor cells [62]. VEGF can regulate vascular tone and lead to vessel dilation by inducing nitric oxide, prostacyclin, and other soluble factors [63]. VEGF has been found to induce micro-vessel permeability and cause edema [64,65] in normal brain tissue as well as in the endothelial cell monolayers *in vitro* [66]. Increased VEGF expression has been found at the mRNA and protein levels in the white matter following radiation therapy. The distribution of cells positive for VEGF expression largely correlates with the degree of BBB disruption and tissue hypoxia [67]. The increased expression has been found to be associated with only BBB disruption in late delayed reaction, not early delayed reaction. Hypoxia can also trigger VEGF expression [68]. In a rat model of myelopathy, researchers found a significant increase in the number of cells expressing HIF1α, VEGF, and Glut 1 (another HIF1α-targeted gene) after delivering 17 Gy to the cervical spinal cord [42]. Interestingly, there is evidence that VEGF-mediated increased vascular permeability does not require ligand-receptor binding [42,69]. Indeed, two studies suggest that VEGF-mediated increased permeability is associated with altering occluding and zonula occluden 1 (ZO-1), the interaction protein that maintains the BBB's integrity [70,71]. However, the underlying mechanisms of VEGF-mediated effects on necrosis are not completely clear.

TREATMENT OF RADIATION NECROSIS

There is no proven and uniformly effective treatment for radiation necrosis in the CNS. Steroids, antiplatelet agents, anticoagulants, hyperbaric oxygen, and high-dose vitamins have all been used to treat radiation necrosis, although the evidence is not sufficient to make either a routine treatment [72-76]. Although no large controlled clinical trials have been conducted to test treating radiation necrosis with anticoagulants, clinical improvement has been reported with heparin and warfarin sodium [77]. Cyclooxygenase-2 inhibitors have been found to be useful in treating radiation necrosis [78], and surgery has also been used in symptomatic cases. Given the large amount of evidence suggesting that VEGF is involved in later stages of radiation injury, targeting VEGF has recently been tested for treating radiation necrosis, with encouraging results.

EXPERIENCE WITH BEVACIZUMAB TREATMENT

The first and most popular anti-VEGF agent is bevacizumab, a humanized monoclonal antibody that binds to VEGF. Gonzales *et al.* treated 8 patients with radiation necrosis with bevacizumab at 5mg/kg/2-week or 7.5mg/kg/3-week's schedule [79]. This study showed a reduction in the volume of both FLAIR (by a mean of 60%) and contrast-enhanced (by a mean of 48%) abnormalities. At the same time, the average daily reduction in dexamethasone was more than 8 mg. A retrospective review of 6 patients with biopsy-proven radiation necrosis treated with bevacizumab reported 79% of reduction in the volume of the contrast-enhanced lesion and a 49% of reduction in the volume of the hyper-intense lesion in FLAIR images [80]. Treatment with bevacizumab was also reported in the study of a patient who had received radiation therapy for nasopharyngeal carcinoma and developed radiation necrosis in the temporal lobe. The enhancement which was considered for radiation necrosis was gone after she was treated with bevacizumab at 5mg/kg every 2weeks for four doses [81].

Although bevacizumab has been successful in treating radiation necrosis, none of the evidence to date has come from controlled trials. At the time of this writing, one such study, a randomized double-blind placebo controlled trial of bevacizumab for the treatment of radiation necrosis of CNS has been launched through the NCI (Levin et al, unpublished data, 2009). Thirteen patients with histologically proven World Health Organization grade 2 or 3 primary brain tumors or head and neck cancers who received cranial radiation with evidence of progressive radiation necrosis and neurological signs and/or symptoms were available for response determination. They received either placebo or bevacizumab at 7.5 mg/kg every 3 weeks for 2 treatments. Magnetic resonance imaging (MRI) of the brain was performed 3 weeks after the second dose. Patients failing whose tumors progressed on placebo were allowed to cross over to receive bevacizumab. All patients, including those who crossed over, were given 4 treatments with bevacizumab and responded to the treatment, with reductions in neurological signs and symptoms, T2-weighted FLAIR volume (-89%), and contrast-enhanced volume (-63%), while none of the patients improved while receiving placebo. A typical patient progressing on oral dexamethasone and then responding to bevacizumab is shown in Fig. **1**. With this first prospective randomized controlled clinical trial, we believe that class-one evidence for bevacizumab treatment of radiation necrosis will be demonstrated. From the interim analysis of the 11 patients who received bevacizumab, we have found that 6 experienced adverse events. In 3 cases, the adverse events were ischemic changes and neurological deficits, depending on the location of the infarct. We considered all ischemic changes to be instances of small vessel thrombosis. Interestingly, 1 patient who received placebo also had developed an ischemic change that was detected at the week 24 visit. Since small vessel occlusions could be caused by radiation injury, the ischemic changes observed in this study could have been partially potentiated by bevacizumab administration in someone already at risk. Three patients developed serious adverse events, including pulmonary embolism secondary to deep venous thrombosis, aspiration pneumonia, and superior sagittal sinus thrombosis.

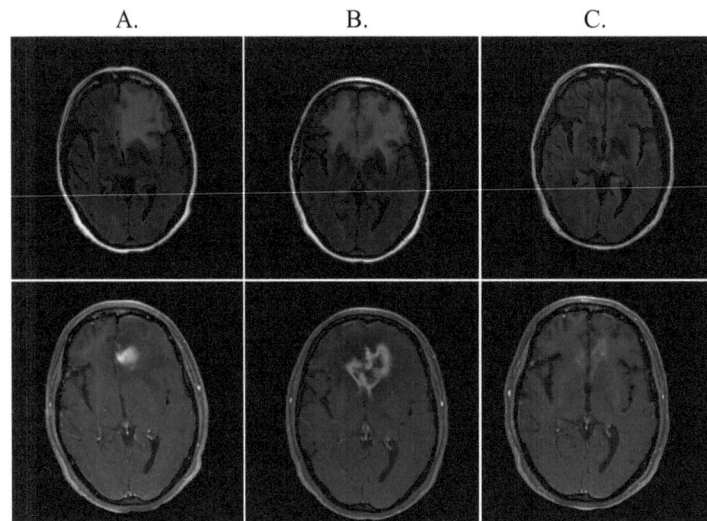

Figure 1: An example of a patient with cerebral radiation necrosis who received bevacezumab. A. MRI that initially performed supported diagnosis of radiation necrosis. B. MRI after 6 weeks of dexamethasone. C. MRI 12 weeks later after patient received four cycles of bevacizumab at 3-week intervals. MRI was done at 3 weeks after the fourth bevacizumab treatment. In both series, the upper set of MRI shows T2 FLAIR and lower set shows Gd-contrast T1 images.

Based on our clinical trial experience, the dose of bevacizumab in treating radiation necrosis need not be higher than 7.5mg/kg intravenously every 3 weeks for 4 treatments to control progressive radiation necrosis. Our study was not designed to determine whether a lower dosage of bevacizumab and/or a longer administration interval would produce the same benefit.

Anecdotal cases brought to our attention have been cases of brainstem radiation necrosis and cervical cord radiation myelopathy that responded to bevacizumab. There is no logical reason why bevacizumab would not be expected to work equally well in treating radiation necrosis at other locations in CNS. The only proviso to this statement is that it appears to work best when the process of radiation necrosis is active. This is logical since that is the period during which VEGF production by damaged astrocytes is most likely to occur.

FUTURE TREATMENT OPPORTUNITIES FOR RADIATION NECROSIS

Radiation necrosis is a serious complication of primary and secondary CNS tumors as well as head and neck cancers when radiation therapy is required. Unfortunately, late deterioration from radiation necrosis rather than the tumor itself is not an uncommon phenomenon; therefore, effective therapy for radiation necrosis is an extremely important topic in the field of neuro-oncology.

A large but somewhat inconclusive effort has been made to identify effective treatments for radiation necrosis. In all cases, treatment was based on the speculative mechanisms of radiation necrosis. Why did these logical approaches fail? The reason for the lack of effective treatments for radiation necrosis is probably twofold: an incomplete understanding of the mechanisms of radiation necrosis and the need for concerted effort by clinicians, laboratory scientists, and the pharmaceutical industry. Today, we may be a step closer to lessening the impact of radiation necrosis on the CNS; however, more pieces of the puzzle need to be discovered to fully understand the pathophysiology of radiation necrosis and better modulate its consequences on the health and well-being of patients.

Radiation necrosis is a dynamic process and can be perpetuated in a vicious cycle. It may start with vascular injury, where endothelial cell damage plays a crucial role. The upregulation of VEGF may directly result from radiation itself or be secondary to hypoxia caused by endothelial cell injury and subsequent BBB breakdown. Upregulated VEGF, together with increased levels of cytokines, ROS, and thrombocytes, will further potentiate tissue damage and may lead to radiation necrosis. VEGF is therefore an attractive target in the development of radiation necrosis, playing its role at different stages of the process of radiation injury.

After carefully reviewing the literature on radiation necrosis and analyzing our experiences in treating radiation necrosis with bevacizumab, we believe bevacizumab is an effective agent. However, we believe opportunities exist to improve on its value and possibly reduce its neurotoxicity by combining it with low-dose anticoagulation and anti-inflammatory agents. The dose response of bevacizumab in treating radiation necrosis is also worthy of study; studies in appropriate animal models would likely facilitate this line of inquiry. Last, since VEGF can be upregulated by radiation therapy and hypoxia, we believe that a combination of anti-VEGF agents shortly after radiation therapy may reduce the risk of radiation necrosis in the long run.

ACKNOWLEDGEMENTS

The authors would like to thank Markeda L. Wade for editorial assistance.

REFERENCES

[1]   Leibel S, Sheline, G. Tolerance of the Brain and Spinal Cord to Conventional irradiation. In: Gutin P LS, Sheline G, editor. Radiaiton injury to the nervous system. New York: Raven Press; 1991. p. 239-56.

[2]   Young DF, Posner JB, Chu F, *et al.* Rapid-course radiation therapy of cerebral metastases: results and complications. Cancer. 1974 Oct;34(4):1069-76.

[3]   Hindo WA, DeTrana FA, 3rd, Lee MS, *et al.* Large dose increment irradiation in treatment of cerebral metastases. Cancer. 1970 Jul;26(1):138-41.

[4]   Rider WD. Radiation damage to the brain--a new syndrome. J Can Assoc Radiol. 1963 Jun;14:67-9.

[5]   Hoffman WF, Levin VA, Wilson CB. Evaluation of malignant glioma patients during the postirradiation period. J Neurosurg. 1979 May;50(5):624-8.

[6]   Wilson CB, Crafts D, Levin V. Brain tumors: criteria of response and definition of recurrence. Natl Cancer Inst Monogr. 1977 Dec;46:197-203.

[7]   Taal W, Brandsma D, de Bruin HG, *et al.* Incidence of early pseudo-progression in a cohort of malignant glioma patients treated with chemoirradiation with temozolomide. Cancer. 2008 Jul 15;113(2):405-10.

[8]   de Wit MC, de Bruin HG, Eijkenboom W, *et al.* Immediate post-radiotherapy changes in malignant glioma can mimic tumor progression. Neurology. 2004 Aug 10;63(3):535-7.

[9]   Brandes AA, Tosoni A, Franceschi E, *et al.* Recurrence pattern after temozolomide concomitant with and adjuvant to radiotherapy in newly diagnosed patients with glioblastoma: correlation With MGMT promoter methylation status. J Clin Oncol. 2009 Mar 10;27(8):1275-9.

[10] Kumar AJ, Leeds NE, Fuller GN, *et al.* Malignant gliomas: MR imaging spectrum of radiation therapy- and chemotherapy-induced necrosis of the brain after treatment. Radiology. 2000 Nov;217(2):377-84.

[11] Brandsma D, Stalpers L, Taal W, *et al.* Clinical features, mechanisms, and management of pseudoprogression in malignant gliomas. Lancet Oncol. 2008 May;9(5):453-61.

[12] Martins AN, Johnston JS, Henry JM, *et al.* Delayed radiation necrosis of the brain. J Neurosurg. 1977 Sep;47(3):336-45.

[13] Yoshii Y, Phillips TL. Late vascular effects of whole brain X-irradiation in the mouse. Acta Neurochir (Wien). 1982;64(1-2):87-102.

[14] Calvo W, Hopewell JW, Reinhold HS, Yeung TK. Time- and dose-related changes in the white matter of the rat brain after single doses of X rays. Br J Radiol. 1988 Nov;61(731):1043-52.

[15] Reinhold HS, Calvo W, Hopewell JW, van der Berg AP. Development of blood vessel-related radiation damage in the fimbria of the central nervous system. Int J Radiat Oncol Biol Phys. 1990 Jan;18(1):37-42.

[16] Manz HJ, Woolley PV, 3rd, Ornitz RD. Delayed radiation necrosis of brainstem related to fast neutron beam irradiation: case report and literature review. Cancer. 1979 Aug;44(2):473-9.

[17] Raff MC, Miller RH, Noble M. A glial progenitor cell that develops *in vitro* into an astrocyte or an oligodendrocyte depending on culture medium. Nature. 1983 Jun 2-8;303(5916):390-6.

[18] Malamud N, Boldrey EB, Welch WK, Fadell EJ. Necrosis of brain and spinal cord following x-ray therapy. J Neurosurg. 1954 Jul;11(4):353-62.

[19] Palmer JJ. Radiation myelopathy. Brain. 1972;95(1):109-22.

[20] Schultheiss TE, Stephens LC. Invited review: permanent radiation myelopathy. Br J Radiol. 1992 Sep;65(777):737-53.

[21] Marks JE, Baglan RJ, Prassad SC, Blank WF. Cerebral radionecrosis: incidence and risk in relation to dose, time, fractionation and volume. Int J Radiat Oncol Biol Phys. 1981 Feb;7(2):243-52.

[22] Leibel SA, Sheline GE. Radiation therapy for neoplasms of the brain. J Neurosurg. 1987 Jan;66(1):1-22.

[23] Sheline GE, Wara WM, Smith V. Therapeutic irradiation and brain injury. Int J Radiat Oncol Biol Phys. 1980 Sep;6(9):1215-28.

[24] Ellis F. Dose, time and fractionation: a clinical hypothesis. Clin Radiol. 1969 Jan;20(1):1-7.

[25] Burger PC, Boyko, O.B. The pathology of central nervous system radiation injury. In: Gutin P LS, Sheline G, editor. Radiation injury to the nervous system. New York: Raven Press; 1991. p. 191-208.

[26] Morris GM, Coderre JA, Bywaters A, *et al.* Boron neutron capture irradiation of the rat spinal cord: histopathological evidence of a vascular-mediated pathogenesis. Radiat Res. 1996 Sep;146(3):313-20.

[27] Mastaglia FL, McDonald WI, Watson JV, *et al.* Effects of x-radiation on the spinal cord: an experimental study of the morphological changes in central nerve fibres. Brain. 1976 Mar;99(1):101-22.

[28] van der Maazen RW, Kleiboer BJ, Verhagen I, *et al.* Irradiation *in vitro* discriminates between different O-2A progenitor cell subpopulations in the perinatal central nervous system of rats. Radiat Res. 1991 Oct;128(1):64-72.

[29] van der Maazen RW, Kleiboer BJ, Verhagen I, *et al.* Repair capacity of adult rat glial progenitor cells determined by an *in vitro* clonogenic assay after *in vitro* or *in vivo* fractionated irradiation. Int J Radiat Biol. 1993 May;63(5):661-6.

[30] van der Maazen RW, Verhagen I, Kleiboer BJ, *et al.* Radiosensitivity of glial progenitor cells of the perinatal and adult rat optic nerve studied by an *in vitro* clonogenic assay. Radiother Oncol. 1991 Apr;20(4):258-64.

[31] Hornsey S, Myers R, Coultas PG, Rogers MA, White A. Turnover of proliferative cells in the spinal cord after X irradiation and its relation to time-dependent repair of radiation damage. Br J Radiol. 1981 Dec;54(648):1081-5.

[32] Hansson E. Astroglia from defined brain regions as studied with primary cultures. Prog Neurobiol. 1988;30(5):369-97.

[33] Muller HW, Junghans U, Kappler J. Astroglial neurotrophic and neurite-promoting factors. Pharmacol Ther. 1995 Jan;65(1):1-18.

[34] Song H, Stevens CF, Gage FH. Astroglia induce neurogenesis from adult neural stem cells. Nature. 2002 May 2;417(6884):39-44.

[35] Hong-Brown LQ, Brown CR. Cytokine and insulin regulation of alpha 2 macroglobulin, angiotensinogen, and hsp 70 in primary cultured astrocytes. Glia. 1994 Nov;12(3):211-8.

[36] Ijichi A, Sakuma S, Tofilon PJ. Hypoxia-induced vascular endothelial growth factor expression in normal rat astrocyte cultures. Glia. 1995 Jun;14(2):87-93.

[37] Iwata-Ichikawa E, Kondo Y, Miyazaki I, *et al.* Glial cells protect neurons against oxidative stress via transcriptional up-regulation of the glutathione synthesis. J Neurochem. 1999 Jun;72(6):2334-44.

[38] Janzer RC, Raff MC. Astrocytes induce blood-brain barrier properties in endothelial cells. Nature. 1987 Jan 15-21;325(6101):253-7.

[39] Schroeter ML, Mertsch K, Giese H, *et al.* Astrocytes enhance radical defence in capillary endothelial cells constituting the blood-brain barrier. FEBS Lett. 1999 Apr 23;449(2-3):241-4.

[40] Wilson JX. Antioxidant defense of the brain: a role for astrocytes. Can J Physiol Pharmacol. 1997 Oct-Nov;75(10-11):1149-63.

[41] Chiang CS, McBride WH, Withers HR. Radiation-induced astrocytic and microglial responses in mouse brain. Radiother Oncol. 1993 Oct;29(1):60-8.

[42] Nordal RA, Nagy A, Pintilie M, Wong CS. Hypoxia and hypoxia-inducible factor-1 target genes in central nervous system radiation injury: a role for vascular endothelial growth factor. Clin Cancer Res. 2004 May 15;10(10):3342-53.

[43] Thomas WE. Brain macrophages: evaluation of microglia and their functions. Brain Res Brain Res Rev. 1992 Jan-Apr;17(1):61-74.

[44] Vaughan DW, Peters A. Neuroglial cells in the cerebral cortex of rats from young adulthood to old age: an electron microscope study. J Neurocytol. 1974 Oct;3(4):405-29.

[45] Giulian D, Chen J, Ingeman JE, George JK, Noponen M. The role of mononuclear phagocytes in wound healing after traumatic injury to adult mammalian brain. J Neurosci. 1989 Dec;9(12):4416-29.

[46] Stoll G, Jander S. The role of microglia and macrophages in the pathophysiology of the CNS. Prog Neurobiol. 1999 Jun;58(3):233-47.

[47]   Mildenberger M, Beach TG, McGeer EG, Ludgate CM. An animal model of prophylactic cranial irradiation: histologic effects at acute, early and delayed stages. Int J Radiat Oncol Biol Phys. 1990 May;18(5):1051-60.

[48]   Nakagawa M, Bellinzona M, Seilhan TM, *et al.* Microglial responses after focal radiation-induced injury are affected by alpha-difluoromethylornithine. Int J Radiat Oncol Biol Phys. 1996 Aug 1;36(1):113-23.

[49]   Schultheiss TE, Stephens LC, Maor MH. Analysis of the histopathology of radiation myelopathy. Int J Radiat Oncol Biol Phys. 1988 Jan;14(1):27-32.

[50]   Tofilon PJ, Fike JR. The radioresponse of the central nervous system: a dynamic process. Radiat Res. 2000 Apr;153(4):357-70.

[51]   Kim JH, Brown SL, Jenrow KA, Ryu S. Mechanisms of radiation-induced brain toxicity and implications for future clinical trials. J Neurooncol. 2008 May;87(3):279-86.

[52]   Dringen R, Gutterer JM, Hirrlinger J. Glutathione metabolism in brain metabolic interaction between astrocytes and neurons in the defense against reactive oxygen species. Eur J Biochem. 2000 Aug;267(16):4912-6.

[53]   Smith KJ, Kapoor R, Felts PA. Demyelination: the role of reactive oxygen and nitrogen species. Brain Pathol. 1999 Jan;9(1):69-92.

[54]   Applegate LA, Luscher P, Tyrrell RM. Induction of heme oxygenase: a general response to oxidant stress in cultured mammalian cells. Cancer Res. 1991 Feb 1;51(3):974-8.

[55]   Gutin PH, Levin KJ, McDermott MW, *et al.* Lipid peroxidation does not appear to be a factor in late radiation injury of the cervical spinal cord of rats. Int J Radiat Oncol Biol Phys. 1993 Jan;25(1):67-72.

[56]   Belka C, Budach W, Kortmann RD, Bamberg M. Radiation induced CNS toxicity--molecular and cellular mechanisms. Br J Cancer. 2001 Nov 2;85(9):1233-9.

[57]   Yoshii Y. Pathological review of late cerebral radionecrosis. Brain Tumor Pathol. 2008;25(2):51-8.

[58]   Kureshi SA, Hofman FM, Schneider JH, *et al.* Cytokine expression in radiation-induced delayed cerebral injury. Neurosurgery. 1994 Nov;35(5):822-9; discussion 9-30.

[59]   Hayakawa K, Borchardt PE, Sakuma S, *et al.* Microglial cytokine gene induction after irradiation is affected by morphologic differentiation. Radiat Med. 1997 Nov-Dec;15(6):405-10.

[60]   Hicklin DJ, Ellis LM. Role of the vascular endothelial growth factor pathway in tumor growth and angiogenesis. J Clin Oncol. 2005 Feb 10;23(5):1011-27.

[61]   Ellis LM, Hicklin DJ. VEGF-targeted therapy: mechanisms of anti-tumour activity. Nat Rev Cancer. 2008 Aug;8(8):579-91.

[62]   Wu Y, Hooper AT, Zhong Z, *et al.* The vascular endothelial growth factor receptor (VEGFR-1) supports growth and survival of human breast carcinoma. Int J Cancer. 2006 Oct 1;119(7):1519-29.

[63]   Curiel TJ, Cheng P, Mottram P, *et al.* Dendritic cell subsets differentially regulate angiogenesis in human ovarian cancer. Cancer Res. 2004 Aug 15;64(16):5535-8.

[64]   Proescholdt MA, Heiss JD, Walbridge S, *et al.* Vascular endothelial growth factor (VEGF) modulates vascular permeability and inflammation in rat brain. J Neuropathol Exp Neurol. 1999 Jun;58(6):613-27.

[65]   van Bruggen N, Thibodeaux H, Palmer JT, *et al.* VEGF antagonism reduces edema formation and tissue damage after ischemia/reperfusion injury in the mouse brain. J Clin Invest. 1999 Dec;104(11):1613-20.

[66]   Wang W, Merrill MJ, Borchardt RT. Vascular endothelial growth factor affects permeability of brain microvessel endothelial cells in vitro. Am J Physiol. 1996 Dec;271(6 Pt 1):C1973-80.

[67]   Li YQ, Ballinger JR, Nordal RA, *et al.* Hypoxia in radiation-induced blood-spinal cord barrier breakdown. Cancer Res. 2001 Apr 15;61(8):3348-54.

[68]   Dibbens JA, Miller DL, Damert A, *et al.* Hypoxic regulation of vascular endothelial growth factor mRNA stability requires the cooperation of multiple RNA elements. Mol Biol Cell. 1999 Apr;10(4):907-19.

[69]   Stacker SA, Vitali A, Caesar C, *et al.* A mutant form of vascular endothelial growth factor (VEGF) that lacks VEGF receptor-2 activation retains the ability to induce vascular permeability. J Biol Chem. 1999 Dec 3;274(49):34884-92.

[70]   Fischer S, Clauss M, Wiesnet M, *et al.* Hypoxia induces permeability in brain microvessel endothelial cells via VEGF and NO. Am J Physiol. 1999 Apr;276(4 Pt 1):C812-20.

[71]   Wang W, Dentler WL, Borchardt RT. VEGF increases BMEC monolayer permeability by affecting occludin expression and tight junction assembly. Am J Physiol Heart Circ Physiol. 2001 Jan;280(1):H434-40.

[72]   Chuba PJ, Aronin P, Bhambhani K, *et al.* Hyperbaric oxygen therapy for radiation-induced brain injury in children. Cancer. 1997 Nov 15;80(10):2005-12.

[73]   Hart GB, Mainous EG. The treatment of radiation necrosis with hyperbaric oxygen (OHP). Cancer. 1976 Jun;37(6):2580-5.

[74]   Kohshi K, Imada H, Nomoto S, *et al.* Successful treatment of radiation-induced brain necrosis by hyperbaric oxygen therapy. J Neurol Sci. 2003 May 15;209(1-2):115-7.

[75] Leber KA, Eder HG, Kovac H, *et al.* Treatment of cerebral radionecrosis by hyperbaric oxygen therapy. Stereotact Funct Neurosurg. 1998 Oct;70 Suppl 1:229-36.

[76] Levin V, Leibel, S., Gutin, P. Neoplasmas of the Central Nervous System. In: DeVita V, Hellman, S., Rosenberg., S., editor. Cancer : principles & practice of oncology 6th ed. Philadelphia: Lippincott Williams & Wilkins; 2001. p. 2100-60.

[77] Glantz MJ, Burger PC, Friedman AH, *et al.* Treatment of radiation-induced nervous system injury with heparin and warfarin. Neurology. 1994 Nov;44(11):2020-7.

[78] Khan RB, Krasin MJ, Kasow K, Leung W. Cyclooxygenase-2 inhibition to treat radiation-induced brain necrosis and edema. J Pediatr Hematol Oncol. 2004 Apr;26(4):253-5.

[79] Gonzalez J, Kumar AJ, Conrad CA, Levin VA. Effect of bevacizumab on radiation necrosis of the brain. Int J Radiat Oncol Biol Phys. 2007 Feb 1;67(2):323-6.

[80] Torcuator R, Zuniga R, Mohan YS, *et al.* Initial experience with bevacizumab treatment for biopsy confirmed cerebral radiation necrosis. J Neurooncol. 2009 Aug;94(1):63-8.

[81] Wong ET, Huberman M, Lu XQ, Mahadevan A. Bevacizumab reverses cerebral radiation necrosis. J Clin Oncol. 2008 Dec 1;26(34):5649-50.

CHAPTER 20

Salvage Chemotherapy with Bevacizumab for Recurrent Anaplastic Glioma

Marc C. Chamberlain[*]

Department of Neurology and Neurological Surgery, Division of Neuro-Oncology, University of Washington, Fred Hutchinson Cancer Research Center, Seattle Cancer Care Alliance, 825 Eastlake Avenue E, POB 19023, MS G4940, Seattle, WA 98109-1023

Abstract: <u>Background</u>: The treatment of recurrent anaplastic glioma (AG) like all high-grade gliomas (HGG) is problematic, as only partially effective therapeutic modalities are available and there is a lack of a standard therapy for recurrence. <u>Methods</u>: A literature review of the use of bevacizumab for recurrent HGG including five studies involving recurrent AG. <u>Results</u>: In the 5 studies of bevacizumab for the treatment of recurrent AG (n=140 patients) neuroradiographic response rates were as follows; complete response 0-20%, partial response 34-68% (median 52%), and stable disease 5-59% (median 16%). Median overall survival was 28 weeks (range 18-35 weeks) and progression free survival at 6- and 12-months was 55% (range 32-68%) and 23% (16-39%) respectively. <u>Conclusions</u>: Bevacizumab therapy appears to increase response of recurrent AG by 2-fold and 6-month progression free survival by 1.5 fold without a clear benefit with respect to overall survival. Toxicity of bevacizumab therapy is manageable and most often comprised of hypertension, proteinuria and fatigue. To date, there are no multi-institutional prospective trials evaluating the role of bevacizumab for the treatment of recurrent AG notwithstanding the increasingly common use of bevacizumab for this indication.

INTRODUCTION

The treatment of recurrent anaplastic glioma (AG) like all high-grade gliomas (HGG) is problematic, as only partially effective therapeutic modalities are available and there is a lack of a standard therapy for recurrence. These therapies include chemotherapy, radioactive implants, stereotactic radiotherapies, targeted therapy and re-operation [1-28]. Chemotherapy for recurrent HGG is of modest benefit, primarily because response to chemotherapy is of limited duration. In an analysis of eight institutional phase 2 studies of chemotherapy for recurrent high-grade gliomas, Wong reported that response rates in recurrent anaplastic gliomas were 14% and progression free survival at 6 months was 31% [13]. Those drugs most active are the nitrosoureas, such as Carmustine (BCNU) and Lomustine (CCNU), in addition to temozolomide (TMZ), procarbazine, cis-retinoic acid, irinotecan (CPT-11) and platinum compounds [1, 2, 4, 5, 10, 11, 12, 14, 17, 23-27, 29-38]. Bevacizumab, with or without CPT-11, has activity in recurrent glioblastoma (GBM) and a small data set exists for activity as well in recurrent anaplastic gliomas [39-52].

How best to manage recurrent AG remains ill-defined notwithstanding a variety of studies. Most studies however are small nonrandomized trials comparing outcome to historical controls. Only a minority of patients with recurrent AG are candidates for image-verified complete or near complete re-resection followed by Gliadel implantation [26]. Therefore, the majority of patients if desirous of further therapy are offered chemotherapy. PCV (procarbazine, CCNU and vincristine) has been used in TMZ refractory anaplastic oligodendroglial tumors in an EORTC trial with response rates of 17% and 6-PFS of 25% [38].

Although multiple antiangiogenic strategies are being explored, with respect to anti-glioma based therapy, only two have entered clinical practice, ligand-based antagonist therapy utilizing monoclonal antibodies such as bevacizumab and receptor-based antagonist with tyrosine kinase inhibitors such as AZD2171 [39-53]. The use of bevacizumab is based upon several concepts; inhibition of new vessel growth, induction of endothelial cell apoptosis, blockade of hematopoietic and endothelial precursor cell migration and incorporation into the tumor vasculature, interruption of VEGF signaling leading to sensitization or reversal of cytotoxic drug resistance, improvement in cytotoxic drug vascular access through vascular normalization and decrease in tumor interstitial pressure, direct effects on glioma cells, immune modulation permitting dendritic cell maturation and counteracting VEGF or bone marrow derived cell

*Address correspondence to Marc C Chamberlain:** Department of Neurology and Neurological Surgery, Division of Neuro-Oncology, University of Washington, Fred Hutchinson Cancer Research Center, Seattle Cancer Care Alliance, 825 Eastlake Avenue E, POB 19023, MS G4940, Seattle, WA 98109-1023; Tel: (206) 288-8280; Fax: (206) 288-2000; E-mail: chambemc@u.washington.edu

Thomas C. Chen (Ed)

up-regulation seen as a consequence of genotoxic therapy, so called induced vasculogenic rebound. Although the use of bevacizumab in the treatment of recurrent AG has been predominantly with cytotoxic chemotherapy (CPT-11 or carboplatin), this combinatorial rationale is compelling for non-neural cancers for example colorectal, non-small cell lung and breast cancer though has not been convincingly demonstrated for HGG [45].

BEVACIZUMAB FOR RECURRENT ANAPLASTIC GLIOMAS

The available data for antiangiogenic therapy in HGG is most robust for ligand-based VEGF antagonism and is based on several single institution studies, many of which are retrospective [39-52]. With two exceptions, these studies have utilized combinatorial therapy and treated predominantly GBM (amongst a total of 344 patients treated, 45 [13%] were AG). Data regarding response rates and survival for AG treated with bevacizumab are difficult to determine as outcome is often reported for both GBM and AG (Table 1). Based on the two largest studies using bevacizumab for recurrent AG response rates vary with complete response to bevacizumab plus therapy in 0%, partial response in 34-67% and stable disease in 25-30% of patients (44, 49). Progression free survival varies as well (median 30 weeks; PFS-6 32-56%). These results with bevacizumab can be compared to TMZ for recurrent TMZ-naïve AG (response rate 35%; PFS-6 44%; median overall survival 13.6 months) and an aggregate series of 8 phase II trials for recurrent AG (pre-TMZ) from the MD Anderson Cancer Center [response rate 14%, PFS-6 31%, median overall survival 47 weeks] [13, 16]. In another retrospective study and compared to the above mentioned historical controls, bevacizumab only therapy improved both response rate (64%) and PFS-6 (60%) in patients with recurrent alkylator-refractory anaplastic astrocytoma but had no clear survival benefit (median overall survival 9 months) [47]. In a second and similar retrospective study, bevacizumab only therapy improved both response rate (68%) and PFS-6 (68%) in patients with recurrent alkylator refractory anaplastic oligodendroglial tumors but had no clear survival benefit (median overall survival 8 months) [48]. Tallibert et al treated 25 patients with recurrent anaplastic oligodendroglial tumors (7 patients [28%] with WHO grade 2 tumors that appeared to have de-differentiated by neuroradiology into grade 3 tumors) with bevacizumab and irinotecan [50]. Whether transformation into higher grade gliomas can be determined by anatomic MR imaging is arguable. Also whether low-grade gliomas respond to bevacizumab is uncertain though available data suggests response only in contrast enhancing gliomas. Non-enhancing tumors or tumor compartments appear not to respond to bevacizumab reflecting independence of vascular endothelial growth factor mediated angiogenesis. Furthermore, disease progression following response to bevacizumab in HGG most often appears as increasing nonenhancing tumor as reflected by increased MRI FLAIR signal [44, 45, 47, 48]. Nonetheless, the Tallibert study reported a 72% neuroradiographic complete and partial response, a median overall survival of 4.6 months and a PFS-6 of 42% in patients with recurrent anaplastic oligodendroglial tumors. An expected and anti-glioma independent activity of bevacizumab based on VEGF antagonism is that of marked improvement in peritumoral edema. In the majority of patients, approximately two thirds, a reduction in steroid dose is achieved and nearly a third of patients are able to discontinue steroids altogether. This steroid sparing effect in many patients results in a marked improvement in steroid related side effects as well as a corresponding improvement in quality of life.

Table 1: Bevacizumab in Recurrent Anaplastic Glioma

Author (reference	Tumor	Number	Gr3+ toxicity	Response			Survival		
				CR	PR	SD	Median	6-mo	12-mo
Norden [44]	AG	35	41%	34%		59%	24 wks	32%	NS
Desjardins [49]	AG	33	33%	9%	52%	33%	35 wks	55%	39%
Chamberlain [47]	AA	25	28%	0%	64%	8%	29 wks	60%	16%
Chamberlain 48]	AO	22	41%	0%	68%	5%	28 wks	68%	23%
Tallibert [46]	AO/ AOA	25	50%	20%	52%	16%	4.6 mo	42%	NS

TOXICITY

In these various studies of bevacizumab for recurrent AG, toxicity of bevacizumab have been modest and comprised primarily of low-grade bleeding (epistaxis, vaginal, or oral cavity), proteinuria, impaired wound healing and hypertension [39-52]. The majority of antiangiogenic side effects appear to be a consequence of on-target actions of this class of agents and reflect disruption of VEGF in normal tissue. Rare serious side effects include gastrointestinal perforation, intratumoral hemorrhage and craniotomy or central venous line wound dehiscence (each approximately with a 1% incidence). The high incidence of deep vein thrombosis and pulmonary embolism in patients with HGG confounds separation as an independent toxicity of antiangiogenic therapies though antiangiogenic therapy may aggravate this thrombogenic predisposition [54-57]. In addition, a retrospective review of bevacizumab plus therapy in patients with recurrent HGG suggests that concurrent use of anticoagulation appears safe without an apparent increased risk of hemorrhage [44, 58].

CONCLUSION

In summary, bevacizumab therapy appears to increase response of recurrent AG by 2-fold and 6-month progression free survival by 1.5 fold without a clear benefit with respect to overall survival. Nonetheless, how to determine radiographic response following bevacizumab (and other antiangiogenic therapies) is challenging due to the normalization of the disrupted blood brain barrier by bevacizumab that results in a marked diminution in the contrast enhancing component of HGG. Therefore traditional outcome measures such as response rate and progression free survival are confounded by improvement in blood brain barrier disruption achieved by bevacizumab. These issues as well are challenging with respect to determining time to bevacizumab failure as re-emergence of contrast enhancement is often a late phenomenon in patients treated with bevacizumab. More often seen is incremental worsening of T2W or FLAIR signal by MRI, MRI parameters not easily quantified and often appreciated retrospectively in patients failing bevacizumab. Notwithstanding the limited literature, based on these data and historical comparisons, bevacizumab (as either a single agent or combined with CPT-11) has become the current treatment of choice for recurrent AG (Table **1**). In a phase II study of bevacizumab with or without CPT-11 in patients with recurrent GBM (the only prospective randomized non-comparative parallel designed bevacizumab trial in recurrent gliomas) results suggest similar outcomes between treatment arms raising the question what added value is provided by CPT-11 [45]. Further supporting this position is the recent FDA approval of bevacizumab as a single agent for recurrent GBM based on two prospective trials [45,52]. Not yet clear is the optimal partner (either a cytotoxic chemotherapy or targeted agent) for bevacizumab in the treatment of recurrent high-grade gliomas though future investigational trials are likely to clarify this issue. Unlike the majority of solid tumors treated to date with bevacizumab, high-grade gliomas are unique (as are ovarian and kidney cancer) in demonstrating single agent anti-tumoral activity for recurrent disease. Toxicity of bevacizumab therapy is manageable and most often comprised of hypertension, proteinuria and fatigue. Rarely, intracranial hemorrhage, wound dehiscence, bowl perforation and arteriovenous thrombosis occur as side effects of bevacizumab therapy that may prove challenging to manage clinically. At present, Grade 1 intracranial hemorrhage does not necessitate discontinuance of bevacizumab therapy though higher grades of hemorrhage mandate cessation. Arteriovenous thrombosis may be managed with concurrent anticoagulation and continuation of bevacizumab therapy [58]. Wound dehiscence and bowl perforation usually requires discontinuance of bevacizumab to permit surgical repair. To date, there are no multi-institutional prospective trials evaluating the role of bevacizumab for the treatment of recurrent AG. Such trials would better define the treatment of recurrent AG and potentially lead to an approved indication of bevacizumab for recurrent AG.

REFERENCES

[1]   The Medical Research Council Brain Tumor Working Party: Randomized trial of procarbazine, lomustine, and vincristine in the adjuvant treatment of high-grade astrocytoma: A Medical research Council Trial. J Clin Oncol 2000;19: 509-518.

[2]   Prados, MD, Scott, C, Curran, WJ, *et al.* Procarbazine, lomustine, and vincristine (PCV) chemotherapy for anaplastic astrocytoma: A retrospective review of Radiation Therapy Oncology Group protocols comparing survival with carmustine or PCVadjuvant chemotherapy. J Clin Oncol 1999; 17:3389-3395.

[3]   Westphal, M, Hilt, DC, Bortey, E., *et al.* A phase 3 trial of local chemotherapy with biodegradable Carmustine (BCNU) wafers (Gliadel wafers) in patients with primary malignant glioma. Neuro-Oncology 2003; 5(2):79-88.

[4]   Grossman, SA, O'Neill, A, Grunnet, M, Mehta, M, *et al.* Phase III study comparing three cycles of infusional carmustine and cisplatin followed by radiation therapy with radiation therapy and concurrent carmustine in patients with newly diagnosed supratentorial glioblastoma multiforme: Eastern Cooperative Oncology Group Trial 2394. J Clin Oncol 2003; 21:1485-1491.

[5]   Prados MD, Levin V. Biology and treatment of malignant glioma. Sem Oncology 2000; 27 (Suppl 3):1-10.

[6]   Gutin PH, Prados MD, Phillips TL, *et al.* External irradiation followed by an interstitial high activity iodine-125 implant "boost" in the initial treatment of malignant gliomas: NCOG Study 6G82-2. Int J Radiat Oncol Biol Phys 1991; 21:601.

[7]   Kornblith PD, Welch WC, Bradley MK. The future of therapy for glioblastoma. Surg Neurol 1993;39:538-543.

[8]   Loeffler JS, Alexander E, Shea WM, *et al.* Radiosurgery as part of the initial management of patients with malignant gliomas. J Clin Oncol 1992;10(9):1379-85.

[9]   Prados MD, Gutin PH, Phillips TL, *et al.* Interstitial brachytherapy for newly diagnosed patients with malignant gliomas: The UCSF experience. Int J Radiat Oncol Biol Phys 1992; 24:593.

[10]   Levin VA, Silver P, Hannigan J, *et al.* Superiority of post-radiotherapy adjuvant chemotherapy with CCNU, procarbazine, and vincristine (PCV) over BCNU for anaplastic gliomas: NCOG 6G61 final report. Int J Radiat Oncol Biol Phys 1990; 18: 321-324.

[11]   Stewart LA: Chemotherapy in adult high-grade glioma: A systemic review and meta-analysis of individual patient data from 12 randomized trials. Lancet 2002; 359:1011-1018.

[12]   Fine HA, Dear KB, Loeffler JS, *et al.* Meta-analysis of radiation therapy and without chemotherapy for malignant gliomas in adults. Cancer 1993; 71: 2585-2597.

[13]   Wong ET, Hess KR, Gleason MJ, *et al.* Outcomes and prognostic factors in recurrent glioma patients enrolled onto phase II clinical trials. J Clin Oncol 1999; 17: 2572-2578.

[14]   Yung WKA, Mechtler L, Gleason MJ. Intravenous carboplatin for recurrent malignant gliomas: A phase II study. J Clin Oncol 1991; 9:860.

[15]   Allen JC, Walker R, Luks E, *et al.* Carboplatin and recurrent childhood brain tumors. J Clin Oncol 1987; 5:759-763.

[16]   Yung WK, Prados MD, Yaya-Tur R, Rosenfeld SS, Brada M, *et al.* Multicenter Phase II trial of temozolomide in patients with anaplastic astrocytoma or anaplastic oligoastrocytoma at first relapse. J Clin Oncol 1999; 17: 2762-2771.

[17]   See SJ, Levin VA, Yung A, *et al.* 13-*cis*-Retinoic acid in the treatment of recurrent glioblastoma multiforme. Neuro-Oncol 2004; 6: 253-258.

[18]   Allen JC, Helson L: High-dose cyclophosphamide chemotherapy for recurrent CNS tumors in children. J Neurosurg 1981; 55: 749-756.

[19]   Longee, DC, Friedman, HS, Albright, RE, Burger, PC, *et al.* Treatment of patients with recurrent gliomas with cyclophosphamide and vincristine. J Neurosurg 1990; 72: 583-588.

[20]   Chamberlain MC, Tsao-Wei D. Recurrent glioblastoma multiforme: Salvage therapy with cyclophosphamide. Cancer 2004; 100:1213-1220.

[21]   21. Macdonald DR, Cascino TL, Schold SC, *et al.* Response criteria for phase II studies of supratentorial malignant glioma. J Clin Oncol 1990; 8:1277-1280.

[22]   Prados MD, Gutin PH, Phillips TL, *et al.* Highly anaplastic astrocytoma: A review of 357 patients treated between 1977 and 1989. Int J Radiat Oncol Biol Phys 1992; 23: 3-8.

[23]   Tortosa A, Vinolas N, Villa S, Verger E, Gil JM, *et al.* Prognostic implications of clinical, radiologic, and pathologic features in patients with anaplastic gliomas. Cancer 2003; 97:1063-1071.

[24]   Chamberlain M, Glantz MJ. Salvage chemotherapy with CPT-11 for recurrent temozolomide-refractory 1p19q co-deleted anaplastic oligodendroglioma J Neuro-Oncology 2008; 89(2):231-8.

[25]   Mirimanof RO, Gorlia T, Mason W, *et al.* Radiotherapy and temozolomide for newly diagnosed glioblastoma: recursive partitioning analysis of the EORTC 26981/22981-NCIC CE3 phase III randomized trial. J Clin Oncol 2006; 24(16):2563-9.

[26]   Brem H, Piantadosi S, Burger PC, Walker M, Selker R, *et al.* Placebo-controlled trial of safety and efficacy of intraoperative controlled delivery by biodegradable polymers of chemotherapy for recurrent gliomas. The Lancet 1995; 345:1008-1012.

[27]   Jaeckle KA, Hess KR, Yung A, *et al.* Phase II evaluation of temozolomide and 13-cis-retinoic acid for the treatment of recurrent and progressive malignant glioma: a North American Brain Tumor Consortium study. J Clin Oncol 2003; 21:2305-2311.

[28]   Voges J, Reszka R, Grossman A, Dittmar C, Richter R., *et al.* Image-guided convection-enhanced delivery and gene therapy of glioblastoma. Ann Neurol 2003; 54: 479-487.

[29]   Batchelor TT, Gilbert MR, Supko JG, *et al.* Phase 2 study of weekly irinotecan in adults with recurrent malignant glioma: Final report of NABTT 97-11. Neuro-Oncology 2004; 6: 21-27.

[30]   Buckner JC, Reid JM, Wright K, *et al.* Irinotecan in the treatment of glioma patients: Current and future studies of the North Cancer Central treatment Group. Cancer 2003; 97:2352-2358.

[31]   Chamberlain MC. Salvage chemotherapy with CPT-11 for recurrent glioblastoma. J Neurooncol. 2002; 56:183-188.

[32]   Cloughesy TF, Filka E, Kuhn J, *et al.* Two studies evaluating irinotecan treatment for recurrent malignant glioma using an every 3-week regimen. Cancer 2003; 97: 2381-2386.

[33]   Friedman HS, Petros WP, Friedman AH, *et al.* Irinotecan therapy in adults with progressive malignant glioma. J Clin Oncol 1999; 17:1516-1525.

[34]   Prados MD, Yung WKA, Jaeckle KA, *et al.* Phase 1 trial of irinotecan (CPT-11) in patients with recurrent malignant glioma: A North American Brain Tumor Consortium study. Neuro-Oncology 2004; 6: 44-54.

[35]   Prados MD, Lamborn K, Yung WKA, *et al.* A Phase 2 trail of irinotecan (CPT-11) in patients with recurrent malignant glioma: A North American Brain Tumor Consortium study. Neuro-Oncol 2006;82:189-193.

[36]   Soffieti R, Nobile M, Rida F, *et al.* Second-line treatment with carboplatin for recurrent or progressive oligodendroglial tumors after PCV chemotherapy: a phase II study. Cancer 2004; 15:807-813.

[37]   Brandes AA, Basso U, Vastola F, *et al.* Carboplatin and teniposide as third-line chemotherapy in patients with recurrent oligodendroma or oligoastrocytoma: a phase II study. Ann Oncol 2003; 14:1727-1731.

[38]   Triebels VH, Taphoorn, Brandes AA, *et al.* Salvage PCV chemotherapy for temozolomide resistant oligodendrogliomas. Neurology 2004; 63: 904-906.

[39]   Stark-Vance V. Bevacizumab and CPT-11 in the treatment of relapsed malignant glioma. Neuro-Oncology 2005;7(3):369.

[40]   Pope WB, Lai A, Nghiemphu P, Mischel P, Cloughesy TF. MRI in patients with high-grade gliomas treated with bevacizumab and chemotherapy. Neurology 2006; 66 (8); 1258-1260.

[41]   Vredenburgh JJ, Desjardins A, Herndon JE II, Dowell JM, Reardon DA, Quinn JA, *et al.* Phase II trial of bevacizumab and irinotecan in recurrent malignant glioma. Clin Cancer Res 2007;13(4):1253-59.

[42]   Vredenburgh JJ, Desjardins A, Herndon JE, *et al.* Bevacizumab plus irinotecan in recurrent glioblastoma multiforme. J Clin Oncol 2007;25(30):4722-4729.

[43]   Chen C, Silverman DHS, Geist C, *et al.* Predicting treatment response of malignant gliomas to bevacizumab and irinotecan by imaging proliferation with [18F] fluorothymidine positron emission tomography: a pilot study. J Clin Oncol 2007;25(30):4714-4721.

[44]   Norden AD, Young GS, Setayesh K, *et al.* Bevacizumab for recurrent malignant glioma: efficacy, toxicity and patterns of recurrence. Neurology. 2008;70:779-787.

[45]   Cloughesy T, Prados MD, Mikkelsen T, *et al.* A phase 2 randomized non-comparative clinical trial of the effect of bevacizumab alone or in combination with irinotecan on 6-month progression free survival in recurrent treatment refractory glioblastoma. J Clin Oncol. 2008;26:91s (Abstract).

[46]   Tallibert S, Vincent LA, Granger B, *et al.* Bevacizumab and irinotecan for recurrent oligodendroglial tumors. Neurology 2009; 72: 1601-1606.

[47]   Chamberlain MC, Johnston S. Salvage chemotherapy with bevacizumab for recurrent alkylator-refractory anaplastic astrocytoma. J Neurooncol 2009; 91: 359–367.

[48]   Chamberlain MC, Johnston S. Bevacizumab for recurrent alkylator-refractory anaplastic oligodendroglioma. Cancer 2009; 115: 1734-43.

[49]   Desjardins A II, Reardon DA, Herndon JE, *et al.* Bevacizumab plus irinotecan in recurrent WHO grade 3 malignant gliomas. Clin Cancer Res 2008; 14: 7068–7073.

[50]   Bokstein F, Shpigel S, Blumenthal DTl. Treatment with bevacizumab and irinotecan for recurrent high-grade glial tumors. Cancer 2008; 112 (10):2267-2273.

[51]   Raizer JJ,Gallot L, Cohn R, *et al.* A phase II safety study of bevacizumab in patients with multiple recurrent or progressive malignant gliomas. J Clin Oncol, 2007; 25 (18S), 2079 (abstract).

[52]   Kreisl TN, Kim L, Moore K, *et al.* Phase II trial of single agent bevacizumab followed by bevacizumab plus irinotecan at tumor progression in recurrent glioblastoma. J Clin Oncol 2009;27(5):740-5.

[53]   Batchelor TT, Sorensen AG, di Tomaso E, *et al.* AZD2171, a Pan-VEGF receptor tyrosine kinase inhibitor, normalizes tumor vasculature and alleviates edema in glioblastoma patients. Cancer Cell 2007;11:83-95.

[54]   Brandes AA, Scelzi E, Salmistraro G, *et al.* Incidence of risk of thromboembolism during treatment of high-grade gliomas: a prospective study. Eur J Cancer. 1997; 33:1592-6.

[55]   Marras LC, Geerts WH, Perry JR. The risk of venous thromboembolism is increased throughout the course of malignant glioma: an evidence-based review. Cancer. 2000; 89:640-6.

[56]   Semrad TJ, O'Donnell R, Wun T, *et al.* Epidemiology of venous thromboembolism in 9489 patients with malignant glioma. J Neurosurg. 2007; l06(4):601-8.

[57]   Simanek R, Vormittag R, Hassler M, *et al.* Venous thromboembolism and survival in patients with high-grade glioma. Neuro Oncol 2007; 9(2):89-95.

[58]   Nghiemphu PL, Green RM, Pope WB, Lai A, Cloughsey TF. Safety of bevacizumab for anticoagulated patients with high grade gliomas. Neuro Oncol 2008; 10(3):355-60.

CHAPTER 21

Bevacizumab for Recurrent Glioma – A Personal View

Roger Stupp*

Centre Hospitalier Universitaire Vaudois and University of Lausanne, Departments of Oncology and Neurosurgery

Abstract: Treatment of recurrent glioma remains a therapeutic challenge. Unprecedented high response rates associated with rapid clinical improvement have been observed. Despite the absence of definitive data and while definitive trial has not even been started, regulatory approval was requested. And while the United States Food and Drug Administration granted accelerated approval based on 2 small uncontrolled phase II trials, the European Medicines Agency rejected the application.

INTRODUCTION

A large number of questions remain open: what is the right dose and schedule of bevacizumab in glioblastoma, when should a patient be treated (early in the disease course or only in the presence of substantial perilesional edema), should bevacizumab be used as a single agent or in combination with cytotoxic therapy? Is bevacizumab prolonging survival, or is it a mainly an anti-inflammatory effect that leads to temporary symptomatic improvement? With the early approval based on immature data the way is paved for uncritical, potentially dangerous use of an undoubtfully useful agent in the armamentarium against recurrent glioma.

Recently the Food and Drug Administration (FDA) approved bevacizumab (Avastin®, Genentech, South San Francisco, CA and Roche, Basel, Switzerland), a monoclonal antibody against vascular endothelial growth factor (VEGF) for the treatment of recurrent glioblastoma. Despite this rapid approval, numerous questions remain. Optimal dose, frequency of administration, and anti-tumor efficacy await investigation and confirmation. The available and limited evidence started in 2005 when a practicing neuro-oncologist reported on 21 patients with recurrent malignant glioma treated with irinotecan and bevacizumab using a regimen that had previously been established for colorectal cancer [1]. Objective responses were observed in almost half of the patients, while virtually all patients had some clinical or radiological improvement.

Subsequently the combination of bevacizumab and irinotecan was prospectively evaluated in uncontrolled clinical trials for recurrent glioma [2,3,4]. Unlike the initial report, the dose of bevacizumab was doubled to 10 mg/kg every 2 weeks, while irinotecan was also given every 2 weeks rather then weekly (Table 1). Again high response rates and a clinical benefit in the great majority of patients were observed. Subsequent investigations evaluated modifications of the irinotecan schedules (either every 2 weeks or weekly x 4 every 6 weeks) with escalated doses for patients on enzyme-inducing antiepileptic drugs. However, the bevacizumab dose was kept at an escalated dose intensity of 5 mg/kg/week, given either every 2 (10 mg/kg) or occasionally every 3 weeks (15 mg/kg).

Table 1: Reports of bevacizumab in recurrent glioma.

Author/ref.	N pts	Bevacizumab	CPT11	RR	PFS6	OS	Remarks
Stark-Vance [1]	21	5 mg/kg q14d	125 mg/m2 weekly x4 q 6wks	43%	NR	NR	Retrospective. Various glioma histol. Hemorrh.
Vredenburgh [3]	35	15 mg/kg q21d	125 mg/m2 d1+8, q21d	57% (39; 74)	46% (32; 66)	9.8 mo (8.2; 14.0)	Academic trial, bev provided by Genentech 2 diff. dosing schedules

*Address correspondence to Roger Stupp: Department of Neurosurgery, University Hospital (CHUV), Rue du Bugnon 46, CH-1011 Lausanne / Switzerland; Tel: +41-21-314-0156; Fax: +41-21-314-0737; E-mail: Roger.Stupp@chuv.ch

Thomas C. Chen (Ed)

Table 1: cont....							
Bokstein [27]	20	5 mg/kg	125 mg/m2 q14d	47% (NR)	25% (NR)	7.0 mo (1.7; 16.0)	Retrospecive, commercial drug supply.
Kreisl [28]	48	10 mg/kg q 14d	added after PD	35% (NR)	29% (18; 48%)	7.2 (4.9; 12.6)	NCI trial
Friedman [6]	82	10 mg/kg q14d	added after PD	28% (19;40)	43% (30; 56%)	9.2 mo (8.2; 10.7)	Randomized phase II, Genentech-sponsored
	85	10 mg/kg q 14d	125 mg/m2 q14d	38% (27; 51)	50% (37; 64%)	8.7 mo (7.8; 10.9)	
Nghiemphu, [29]	44	5 mg/kg q14d	125 mg/m q14d (most pts)	NR	41% (NR)	9.0 (NR)	Retrospective, commercial drug supply
Poulsen [30]	27	10 mg/kg q 14d	125 mg/m2 q 14d	30% (14; 57)	40% (16; 67)	6.5 mo (3.0; 10.0)	Retrospective, drug supply not described

RR; response rate (Macdonald criteria)
CPT11; irinotecan, doses for pts on enzyme-inducing antiepileptic drugs: 340 mg/m2.
PFS6; progression-free survival at 6 months, OS; overall survival, q14d; every 2 weeks (14 days)
NR; not reported, PD; progressive disease

Toxicity was of major concern particularly intratumoral hemorrhage when bevacizumab was introduced for the treatment of brain tumors. Hemorrhagic and thromboembolic complications as well as hypertension are well-known complications of bevacizumab administered for non-CNS cancers, with fatal consequences if occurring in the brain [5]. In recurrent glioma spontaneous intracranial bleeding may occur even in the absence of anti-VEGF therapy. In the pivotal trial of bevacizumab in patients with glioblastoma, 46 and 66% $\geq$ grade 3 adverse events were reported for bevacizumab alone or bevacizumab and irinotecan, although some adverse events may have been not directly related to the therapy [6]. In the bevacizumab alone treated patients, hypertension was reported in 30% (severe in 8%) and fatigue in 45% of patients. Intracranial hemorrhage occurred in 3 patients (1%), thromboembolic event in 6% of patients. Intestinal perforation and wound healing problems have been described [7-9].

Throughout all the reports, the initial observation of high radiological response rates and temporary clinical improvement was confirmed. Despite this radiological and clinical efficacy a definitive prolongation of overall survival remains to be demonstrated [10]. The reported survival times of 8-9 months correspond to what has been reported as median survival after progression for patients treated with radiotherapy alone, or radiotherapy and concomitant temozolomide before the availability of bevacizumab [11].

THE LAUSANNE EXPERIENCE

Our own experience with bevacizumab in Lausanne confirms the results of the reported clinical trials. Since 2006 we have treated over 70 patients suffering from recurrent glioma with bevacizumab. However, our treatment strategy was slightly different:

a) Bevacizumab was only added very late in the treatment course, in patients with a substantial mass effect and edema requiring high-doses of steroids.

b) Bevacizumab was always given in combination with a cytotoxic agent, usually with irinotecan.

c) Most patients were started on single agent irinotecan and bevacizumab was added only at tumor progression.

d) A lower dose of bevacizumab was used with a simplified dosing regimen of 400 mg total dose (equivalent to 1 vial) every 2 weeks, corresponding in an average patient to a dose of approximately 5-6 mg/kg (dose intensity of approximately 2.5 mg/kg per week).

e) Irinotecan was administered at increasing doses of 125-180 mg/m^2, in analogy with regimens used in colorectal cancer.

f) In patients progressing while receiving bevacizumab and irinotecan, the treatment with bevacizumab was continued and combined with another cytotoxic agent.

The bevacizumab was commercially supplied and in the majority paid patients insurance and in approximately one fourth of patients' bevacizumab was provided free of charge by Roche (Switzerland) after refusal by insurance. Although no formal analysis of our results has been conducted yet, our preliminary experience confirms the observations made in the prospective clinical trials – high response rates, albeit sometimes short-lived, and a lower than expected incidence of complications. Minor bleeding has been observed in 2 patients, a fatal cerebral hemorrhage occurred in one patient undergoing surgery several weeks after bevacizumab discontinuation. The majority of our patients had substantial peritumoral edema at treatment start, and clinical improvement could be evident as quickly as 48 hours after administration of bevacizumab [12,13]. It allowed us to rapidly taper and often entirely omit corticosteroids. In accordance with other reports, progressive patients under bevacizumab only poorly responded to a third-line salvage therapy. Clinical progression has been observed in the absence of evident tumor progression on T1-gadolinium-enhanced magnetic resonance imaging (MRI). However careful analysis of the T2-weighted sequences often showed tumor extension without disruption of the blood-brain barrier [14,15].

CLINICAL EFFICACY AND DRUG APPROVAL

In May 2009 bevacizumab received accelerated approval after an unanimous vote of the Oncology Drug Advisory Committee (ODAC) based on the high response rates seen in two prospective controlled phase II trials of 20-26% and a response duration of 4 months that were believed to translate into a meaningful clinical benefit [16]. However, the limitations of radiological response alone as assessed by MRI based on contrast enhancement has been recognized for over 2 decades [17]. The established World Health Organization (WHO) response criteria had been adapted over 20 years ago to reflect changes of the blood-brain barrier when high-doses of corticosteroids are used [17]. These so-called Macdonald criteria are currently being revisited by an international panel of brain tumor experts in order to account for changed imaging with novel antiangiogenic therapies [18]. The substantial differences in response rates when independently assessed by the investigators (39% and 46% for bevacizumab and bevacizumab with irinotecan, respectively) [19], by a sponsor mandated central radiological review (28% and 38%) [6] and finally by the FDA (20% and 26%) [16] illustrates the difficulties and limitations of this endpoint. The true response rate remains thus undetermined. Some decrease in tumor size from baseline has been observed in the great majority of patients and likely better reflects what is considered by clinicians a substantial benefit (waterfall plot in) [6].

The available data of bevacizumab for recurrent glioblastoma does not allow any statement about prolongation of survival. This is a result of the limited prospective clinical trials, lack of randomization to a non-bevacizumab containing treatment arm and the failure to assess overall survival as the primary endpoint. The pivotal prospective randomized phase II trial evaluated the rate of patients being alive and free of progression at 6 months (PFS6), a surrogate endpoint that was considered meaningful in the era before antiangiogenic agents modified radiographic interpretation of response [20]. In addition the data as presented to the FDA and recently published remains immature, with a minimum follow-up of only 6 months and just half of the patients having died at the time of analysis [6].

Consequently, we are left with more questions than answers. Should bevacizumab be used as a single agent, or in combination with a cytotoxic agent? The randomized phase II trial suggests that time to tumor progression is prolonged with a combined therapy with irinotecan. For how long should the bevacizumab therapy be given? Long-term side effects and risks of bevacizumab therapy are unknown. Prolonged administration of bevacizumab may induce dose-dependent hypertension and possibly increase the risk of intracranial hemorrhage in brain tumor patients. Recent clinical experience suggests induction of a more aggressive and diffusely invasive tumor phenotype as a mechanism of escape to anti-VEGF therapy [10,21-23].

The present FDA labeled indication for bevacizumab in patients with recurrent glioblastoma is to continue treatment until tumor progression. However, salvage therapy after failure of bevacizumab has been particularly challenging, no drug or regimen either alone or in combination with bevacizumab has demonstrated identifiable activity. The clinical course after progression on bevacizumab-containing regimen has been particularly dramatic, and discontinuation of bevacizumab may cause a rebound with rapid increasing peritumoral edema.

With the accelerated approval of bevacizumab for recurrent glioblastoma, many answers to the above mentioned questions will be delayed and likely some questions will remain unanswered. Finally, randomized controlled clinical trials have been launched, however only in combination with chemoradiotherapy in newly diagnosed glioblastoma. VEGF pathway inhibition in combination with radiotherapy follows an entirely different rational [24]. Definitive data will not be available before another 3-4 years at least.

PERSONAL COMMENT

Based on clinical experience, bevacizumab is without doubt a useful drug in many neuro-oncological clinical situations, including recurrent malignant glioma. Nevertheless, it is disappointing that over 3 years less than 300 patients were accrued in prospective clinical trials, while thousands of patients were treated off-label. The data of the only pivotal randomized but uncontrolled phase II (!) trial – bevacizumab in both arms - focuses on inappropriate endpoints (progression and response rate), a mature survival update 2-years after initial database closure has still not be released (?!).

At first overview, the approval of bevacizumab may be good news for the patients and clinicians treating recurrent malignant glioma. And indeed, we have been regularly prescribing bevacizumab since 2006. However, its uncritical use, the early administration at first recurrence without proper clinical trials will hamper new glioma drug development. Its efficacy may be primarily related to a vasculature normalizing and anti-inflammatory steroid-like effect. This may be equally of value but has a different rational and indication for use than an agent with anti-glioma efficacy [12,13,25,26]. Consequently a rebound of contrast enhancement after discontinuation of bevacizumab may occur, due to the long biological half-live of the monoclonal antibody this may be observed as late 6-8 weeks following the last dose. New and potentially active investigational agents to be tested after bevacizumab failure, risk to be discontinued early as a consequence of the slowly waning steroid-like effect of the previously prescribed bevacizumab, while not perhaps having a an adequate opportunity to exhibit inherent anti-tumor efficacy. Understandably, withholding a proven effective second-line salvage therapy such as bevacizumab for 2 months while investigating an alternative novel anti-glioma therapy, may be problematic for patients and clinicians given the rapidly progressive nature of the disease. The more invasive glioma phenotype observed after bevacizumab is an additional obstacle to subsequent treatments [10,21-23].

All prospective trials evaluating bevacizumab reported to date have been conducted in the United States. The twice as high a dose of bevacizumab compared to colorectal and non-small cell lung cancer was chosen without sufficient, if any clinical data to suggest that the higher doses translate into increased efficacy. One cannot rule out that the high dose of bevacizumab actually increases toxicity and complication rate, independent of the not inconsiderable economical impact.

For clinical drug trials in Europe in non-approved indications, experimental drug must be provided free of charge due to the restrictive nature of national formularies. However, other than industry, there is no funding agency willing and capable to provide the agents, and at the current prices of new drugs, European neuro-oncologist are entirely dependent on collaboration with industry. Until very recently, Roche who hold the rights outside the US did not wish to pursue any development of bevacizumab in glioma, and was thus unwilling to provide any bevacizumab for use within clinical trials. In my opinion, it would have been prudent not to apply for market approval in Europe before proper trials in recurrent glioblastoma are conducted. Interestingly, the majority of ongoing trials evaluating bevacizumab in recurrent glioma (Table 2) are still conducted only in the United States. All these trials have a primary endpoint that is recognized among experts to be inadequate, and none of the trials has a control arm. The high dose of bevacizumab, when compared to dosing in other cancers, is now considered standard despite of lack of trials exploring dose in recurrent glioma.

In Europe randomized controlled phase II trials evaluating bevacizumab have been proposed. A planned Dutch trial will compare bevacizumab as a single agent versus bevacizumab and lomustine (CCNU) in recurrent GBM, with PFS as the primary endpoint. A proposed EORTC trial aims at clarifying the optimal timing of the introduction of an antiangiogenic agent. Lomustine at first recurrence followed by the addition of bevacizumab at subsequent progression would be compared to bevacizumab with lomustine added at progression, evaluating overall survival as the primary endpoint, and progression-free survival, quality of life, pattern of failures as secondary endpoints. The combination of temozolomide and bevacizumab versus temozolomide is proposed to evaluate recurrence in patients with grade II and grade III astrocytoma. Limited support from Roche for these academically sponsored trials have been acquired, however the use of progression-free survival has given rise to some controversy between the drug maker and investigators.

Table 2: Ongoing or recently completed trials of bevacizumab alone or in combination for recurrent glioma: abstracted from clinicaltrials.gov (accessed on 16. September 2009)

Bevacizumab	Combination partner	Planned no pts	1° endpoint	Sponsor	Remarks
	Single agent bevacizumab	88	PFS6	NCI	
	Single agent bevacizumab	35	PFS6	Northwestern	
	Temsirolimus	NR	PFS	Righshospitalet, Copenhagen	
	Erlotinib	56		Duke	
	Dasatinib	95	PFS6	NCCTG/NCI	Not yet recruiting
	Sorafenib	53	PFS6	NCCTG	
	Enzastaurin	120	PFS	Eli Lilly	
	Enzastaurin	80	PFS6	NCI	
	Tandutanib	80	PFS6	NCI	
	BCNU wafers/CPT11	50	PFS6	Duke	
	BCNU	20	PFS6	UC Davis	
10 mg/kg	CPT11	32	PFS	Seoul Cancer Ctr, Korea	
every 2 weeks	CPT11	54	NR	Righshospitalet, Copenhagen	
plus	CPT11	40	RR	NCI	
	Cetuximab/CPT11	32	NR	Righshospitalet, Copenhagen	
	CPT11 / TMZ (d1-21)	121	PFS6	RTOG	Completed, randomized phase II
	TMZ (q 2 wks)	30	PFS6	Ctr for Neuroscience, Tucson	
	TMZ metronomic	32	PFS	Duke	
	TMZ or Etoposide	48	PFS6	Duke	third line after bev/CPT11 failure
	Etoposide	59	PFS6	Duke	
	SAHA, TMZ metronomic	52	PFS6	Duke	Histone deacetylase inhibitor
	Bortezomib	64	PFS6	Duke	

Proposed controlled trials in Europe (awaiting approval by Roche†):

Bevacizumab 10 mg/kg every 2 weeks	+ CCNU / single agent bev.	NA	PFS	Dutch neuro-oncologists	Randomized phase II
	Single agent bev →PD: bev + CCNU / + CCNU →PD: bev + CCNU	NA	OS	EORTC	Randomized phase II. Awaiting approval by Roche. Early versus late introduction of bev
	+ TMZ / TMZ	NA	OS at 12 mo	EORTC	Randomized phase II looking at the combination with TMZ in recurrent grade II and III astrocytoma.

PFS; progression-free survival, PFS6, % alive and progression-free at 6 months, RR, response rate, OS, overall survival TMZ; temozolomide, CPT11; irinotecan; BCNU; carmustine, CCNU; lomustine, SAHA; suberoylanilide hydroxamic acid, bev; bevacizumab NCCTG; North Central Clinical Trials Group, NCI; National Cancer Institute, EORTC; European Organisation for Research and Treatment of Cancer, NR; not reported, Pts;patients, Ctr; center † drug supply and educational grant requested

The precedent set with the approval of bevacizumab for recurrent glioblastoma is already influencing the attitude of other drug manufacturers. Rather than conducting proper randomized phase III investigations, cheap(er) drug development strategies based on phase II trials allowing accelerated approval has been suggested. But whether these short-cuts will ultimately benefit the patients remains to be determined.

POST SCRIPTUM

During the editing this text, bevacizumab was also approved as a single agent for the first-line treatment of recurrent glioma in Switzerland, the verdict by the European Medicinal Agency (EMEA) is still pending.

REFERENCES

[1]   Stark-Vance V. Bevacizumab and CPT-11 in the treatment of relapsed malignant glioma. Neuro-Oncol. 2005;7:369 {abstr 342}.

[2]   Vredenburgh JJ, Desjardins A, Herndon JE, 2nd, *et al.* Phase II trial of bevacizumab and irinotecan in recurrent malignant glioma. Clin Cancer Res. 2007;13:1253-1259.

[3]   Vredenburgh JJ, Desjardins A, Herndon JE, 2nd, *et al.* Bevacizumab plus irinotecan in recurrent glioblastoma multiforme. J Clin Oncol. 2007;25:4722-4729.

[4]   Desjardins A, Reardon DA, Herndon JE, 2nd, *et al.* Bevacizumab plus irinotecan in recurrent WHO grade 3 malignant gliomas. Clin Cancer Res. 2008;14:7068-7073.

[5]   Gordon MS, Margolin K, Talpaz M, *et al.* Phase I safety and pharmacokinetic study of recombinant human anti-vascular endothelial growth factor in patients with advanced cancer. J Clin Oncol. 2001;19:843-850.

[6]   Friedman HS, Prados MD, Wen PY, *et al.* Bevacizumab Alone and in Combination With Irinotecan in Recurrent Glioblastoma. J Clin Oncol. 2009.

[7]   Norden AD, Drappatz J, Ciampa AS, *et al.* Colon perforation during antiangiogenic therapy for malignant glioma. Neuro Oncol. 2009;11:92-95.

[8]   Chamberlain MC. Bevacizumab plus irinotecan in recurrent glioblastoma. J Clin Oncol. 2008;26:1012-1013; author reply 1013.

[9]   Lai A, Filka E, McGibbon B, *et al.* Phase II Pilot Study of Bevacizumab in Combination With Temozolomide and Regional Radiation Therapy for Up-Front Treatment of Patients With Newly Diagnosed Glioblastoma Multiforme: Interim Analysis of Safety and Tolerability. Int J Radiat Oncol Biol Phys. 2008.

[10]   Norden AD, Drappatz J, Muzikansky A, *et al.* An exploratory survival analysis of anti-angiogenic therapy for recurrent malignant glioma. J Neurooncol. 2009;92:149-155.

[11]   Stupp R, Mason WP, van den Bent MJ, *et al.* Radiotherapy plus concomitant and adjuvant temozolomide for glioblastoma. N Engl J Med. 2005;352:987-996.

[12]   Chen W, Delaloye S, Silverman DH, *et al.* Predicting treatment response of malignant gliomas to bevacizumab and irinotecan by imaging proliferation with [18F] fluorothymidine positron emission tomography: a pilot study. J Clin Oncol. 2007;25:4714-4721.

[13]   Kamoun WS, Ley CD, Farrar CT, *et al.* Edema control by cediranib, a vascular endothelial growth factor receptor-targeted kinase inhibitor, prolongs survival despite persistent brain tumor growth in mice. J Clin Oncol. 2009;27:2542-2552.

[14]   Norden AD, Young GS, Setayesh K, *et al.* Bevacizumab for recurrent malignant gliomas: efficacy, toxicity, and patterns of recurrence. Neurology. 2008;70:779-787.

[15]   Narayana A, Kelly P, Golfinos J, *et al.* Antiangiogenic therapy using bevacizumab in recurrent high-grade glioma: impact on local control and patient survival. J Neurosurg. 2009;110:173-180.

[16]   Summary Minutes of the Oncologic Drugs Advisory Committee March 31, 2009. In: Center for Drug Evaluation and Research ed. Washington: Food and Drug Administration; 2009.

[17]   Macdonald DR, Cascino TL, Schold SC, Jr., *et al.* Response criteria for phase II studies of supratentorial malignant glioma. J Clin Oncol. 1990;8:1277-1280.

[18]   van den Bent MJ, Vogelbaum MA, Wen PY, *et al.* End point assessment in gliomas: novel treatments limit usefulness of classical Macdonald's Criteria. J Clin Oncol. 2009;27:2905-2908.

[19]   Cloughesy T, Prados M, Wen P, *et al.* A phase II, randomized, non-comparative clinical trial of the effect of bevacizumab (BV) alone or in combination with irinotecan (CPT) on 6-month progression free survival (PFS6) in recurrent, treatment-refractory glioblastoma (GBM). . Proc Am Soc Clin Oncol J Clin Oncol. 2008;26:abstr #2010b.

[20]   Wong ET, Hess KR, Gleason MJ, *et al.* Outcomes and prognostic factors in recurrent glioma patients enrolled onto phase II clinical trials. J Clin Oncol. 1999;17:2572.

[21]   Lassman A, Iwamoto F, Gutin P, *et al.* Patterns of relaps and prognosis after bevacizumab failure in recurrent glioblastoma. Proc Ann Meeting Am Soc Clin Oncol, J Clin Oncol 2008;26 (suppl):{abstact #2028}.

[22]   Ebos JM, Lee CR, Cruz-Munoz W, *et al.* Accelerated metastasis after short-term treatment with a potent inhibitor of tumor angiogenesis. Cancer Cell. 2009;15:232-239.

[23]   Paez-Ribes M, Allen E, Hudock J, *et al.* Antiangiogenic therapy elicits malignant progression of tumors to increased local invasion and distant metastasis. Cancer Cell. 2009;15:220-231.

[24]   Duda DG, Jain RK, Willett CG. Antiangiogenics: the potential role of integrating this novel treatment modality with chemoradiation for solid cancers. J Clin Oncol. 2007;25:4033-4042.

[25]   Gonzalez J, Kumar AJ, Conrad CA, *et al.* Effect of bevacizumab on radiation necrosis of the brain. Int J Radiat Oncol Biol Phys. 2007;67:323-326.

[26]   Batchelor TT, Sorensen AG, di Tomaso E, *et al.* AZD2171, a pan-VEGF receptor tyrosine kinase inhibitor, normalizes tumor vasculature and alleviates edema in glioblastoma patients. Cancer Cell. 2007;11:83-95.

[27]   Bokstein F, Shpigel S, Blumenthal DT. Treatment with bevacizumab and irinotecan for recurrent high-grade glial tumors. Cancer. 2008;112:2267-2273.

[28]   Kreisl TN, Kim L, Moore K, *et al.* Phase II trial of single-agent bevacizumab followed by bevacizumab plus irinotecan at tumor progression in recurrent glioblastoma. J Clin Oncol. 2009;27:740-745.

[29]   Nghiemphu PL, Liu W, Lee Y, *et al.* Bevacizumab and chemotherapy for recurrent glioblastoma: a single-institution experience. Neurology. 2009;72:1217-1222.

[30]   Poulsen HS, Grunnet K, Sorensen M, *et al.* Bevacizumab plus irinotecan in the treatment patients with progressive recurrent malignant brain tumours. Acta Oncol. 2009;48:52-58.

CHAPTER 22

Inhibitors of VEGF Signaling Pathways in Glioblastoma: Is the Evidence Sufficient for Widespread Use? A European Perspective

M.J. van den Bent[*]

Department Neuro-Oncology, Daniel den Hoed Cancer Center/Erasmus University Hospital Rotterdam, Rotterdam, The Netherlands

Abstract: First uncontrolled trials suggest significant activity of bevacizumab in recurrent glioblastoma. However, many questions still remain unresolved, in particular in view of the occurrence of pseudo-responses, the development of gliomatosis cerebri, the unclear impact on survival, and the high costs associated with this treatment. Further studies need to focus the early identification of responders, better combination regimen, and on the assessment of survival benefit. The widespread use of bevacizumab prior to registration may actually become an obstacle for the answering of some of these questions.

INTRODUCTION

Inhibitors of Vascular Endothelial Growth Factor signaling pathway have raised interest for the treatment of brain tumors for a long time. Early on, the relevance of VEGF signaling for the neo-angiogenesis of glioblastoma multiforme (GBM) and other high grade glioma have been recognized, and it has long been hypothesized that interfering with VEGF signaling might be a way to block tumor growth and progression. The results obtained in particular with bevacizumab in recurrent GBM with response rates between 25 and 35%, and 6 months progression free survival (6 mo PFS) rates of 40-50% resulted in considerable excitement about anti-angiogenic treatment [1,2]. Indeed, these outcome data in recurrent GBM are unparalleled. Following the first uncontrolled trials on bevacizumab and the randomized but still uncontrolled phase II study investigating bevacizumab and bevacizumab in combination with irinotecan, these treatments have been approved by the FDA in the United States for use in recurrent GBM. Of note, even prior to the approval by FDA bevacizumab was widely used in the US for recurrent GBM. The registration application to the central European registration authorities (EMEA) is as of today still pending. Nonetheless, and similar to the situation in the US, in several European countries bevacizumab is widely used for the management of recurrent GBM. The interest in angiogenesis inhibitors was further increased by the small phase II trial with cediranib, an oral VEGF tyrosine kinase receptor inhibitor. Following the first signs of activity in this trial a large and controlled phase III study has been initiated, the results of which are eagerly awaited for.

These developments mark the rapid acceptance of bevacizumab as part of the standard of care of recurrent or progressive GBM. Ongoing efforts to further establish the role of bevacizumab are mainly directed towards newly diagnosed GBM, and to a far lesser extent to recurrent disease. Two major trials in newly diagnosed GBM are in preparation, one company sponsored trial with an emphasis on European sites, and one that will be conducted by RTOG. Both trials have a very similar trial design: bevacizumab will be added to the backbone of combined chemo-irradiation with temozolomide. Both are placebo controlled trials, and in view of the widespread use of bevacizumab at the time of recurrence they will be subject to cross over at the time of recurrence. Nonetheless, most likely they will at least learn us if the early addition of bevacizumab to combined chemo-irradiation will improve survival. And those trials will generate the first survival data coming from properly designed comparative studies with a control arm without bevacizumab. The outcome of these studies is by no means certain. Undisputedly, the rationale of adding a VEGF inhibitor to combined chemo-irradiation is strong: VEGF signaling is up regulated during radiotherapy. Indeed, in some GBM models VEGF signaling was related to resistance to radiotherapy; inhibiting VEGF signaling resulted in longer lasting tumor control [3-8]. Still, in the various model systems favorable effects of blocking VEGF signaling were by no means the invariable outcome [9]. Moreover, an unresolved issue is the

*Address correspondence to M.J. van den Bent: Department Neuro-Oncology, Daniel den Hoed Cancer Center/Erasmus University Hospital Rotterdam, Rotterdam, The Netherlands; Tel +31 10 7041415; Fax +31 10 7041031; E-mail: m.vandenbent@erasmusmc.nl

Thomas C. Chen (Ed)

question whether anti-VEGF signaling drugs increases or decreases the penetration of co-medication into tumors. Theoretically, anti-VEGF agents may impede intratumoral penetration of temozolomide and other agents by decreasing the abnormal permeability of blood vessels, or may improve penetration by reducing the intratumoral pressure and through normalization of abnormal and non-functional capillary networks [10-12]. There is relatively little information available on these effects.

The unresolved question (and one that is left behind in view of the paucity of further controlled studies in recurrent disease), is to what extent the promise of anti-VEGF agents for the management of recurrent GBM has been materialized, and how these drugs should be used to achieve optimal results. Numerous reviewers have pointed at the pseudo-responses seen after treatment with VEGF signaling inhibitors. Of note, some of the groups that first identified the VEGF protein originally named the substance Vascular Permeability Factor. They noticed that this factor increased vascular permeability independent of inflammatory pathways, could cause edema, and observed that these effects could be diminished by dexamethason [13-15]. Indeed the increased leakiness of high grade glioma vessels is a major factor contributing to the signs and symptoms of high grade glioma, and not surprisingly, effective VEGF pathway signaling inhibitors also diminish the VEGF depending increased vascular leakiness. The rapid relief of signs and symptoms in some GBM patients and the rapid decrease of contrast enhancement of GBM after the initiation of treatment with VEGF signaling inhibitors give support for a non-tumoral effect of these drugs [16]. Clearly, the normalization of the abnormal vascular permeability and the restoration of the regional cerebral blood volume is responsible for the immediate relief of symptoms, and for the high response rates. These 'clinical' response rates are not to be mistaken for tumor response rates: Macdonalds criteria, the widely applied approach to assess outcome of medical treatment of high grade glioma use the area of enhancement as the way to assess response [17]. It needs to be realized however that enhancement is an aspecific phenomenon which may represent tumor activity although not necessarily so: any factor that increases or reduces permeability will affect the area of enhancement without affecting the real tumor size or activity. Indeed, it has long been recognized that steroids may interfere with the assessment of response, simply by restoring the abnormal permeability of intratumoral vessels leading to a decrease in contrast enhancement [18]. Clearly, bevacizumab and cediranib have a similar steroid-like effect, which has been coined 'pseudo-response' [19]. The obvious question is whether the effects of bevacizumab by and large resemble that of dexamethason. That might explain both the high response rate and the favorable 6 mo PFS observed in trials, but also the relative modest increase in survival suggested by the uncontrolled studies. In these studies median survival was only 9 months, compared to 6-7 months in many bluntly negative trials on recurrent GBM. Obviously, improved techniques to identify early 'true' from pseudo-responders would be of great interest. First series have suggested that PET imaging or advance MR techniques in combination with serum markers might be helpful for this, purpose true from false responders but confirmation of the results of these small studies remain necessary [20,21].

From a patient perspective, it may not matter whether the decrease of signs and symptoms is due to a pseudo or a real response: both are likely to translate into a clinical benefit. Even if these drugs bring a steroid like effect only, these effects are obtained without the unfavorable side effect profile of steroids. What need to be realized though, is the high costs of treatment with these novel drugs which adds to the burden of the increasingly costly health care in western societies.

But there are more fundamental issues with the use of bevacizumab. Several papers have given evidence of ongoing control of enhancing lesions, despite clear progression of unenhancing disease as depicted by T2 or FLAIR imaging, suggestive of the development of gliomatosis cerebri in tumors in which the possibility of neo-angiogenesis is shut of [22,23]. Apparently, in the presence of VEGF signal inhibitors glioma tumor cells start to migrate and co-opt pre-existing vessels in order to survive. There observations are in line with the absence of a true anti-tumoral effect of bevacizumab treatment. Similar findings were made in in experimental mouse models in which an increase of metastases or of local tumor invasion has been observed after treatment with angiogenesis inhibitors [24-26]. Shutting down angiogenesis appears to induce other signalling pathways within the tumor that circumvent the effects of angiogenesis inhibition. This would provide the explanation why the survival increase in GBM managed with angiogenesis inhibitors is modest at best, despite the fascinating response rates and PFS. It further emphasizes that only evaluating the contrast enhancement as a measure of outcome is insufficient, and T2 weighted and/or FLAIR MR images need to be considered.

Currently, numerous trials are ongoing in which bevacizumab is combined with other agents. Indeed, the randomized phase II study (of note, which was not designed to compare between bevacizumab and bevacizumab plus irinotecan) suggests little difference in activity between the two agents [1]. That by itself is no surprise; irinotecan has little if any single agent activity in recurrent GBM [27]. From other tumor types it is clear that anti-angiogenic treatment provides the best results if combined with active cytotoxic drugs. The many ongoing bevacizumab combination trials are however ill designed, without proper controls and thus unlikely to answer the question if outcome is improved. Another source of concern here is the occurrence of rebound edema after treatment with bevacizumab. The rapid clinical progression that may occur after the end of treatment with anti-VEGF signaling agents may interfere with studies into further treatments. This has in particular implications for the conduct of studies on other agents in relapsed GBM, and may hamper the identification of new and active drugs.

The major question that we are still facing today, if the current information about the efficacy of bevacizumab in recurrent GBM is sufficient to warrant its widespread use. Individual doctors have the responsibility to treat their patients to the best of their abilities, whatever the costs. However, on a more abstract and macro-economic level, doctors also have the responsibility to keep health care affordable and to improve the treatment of further generations. The dilemma is that what may be good for the individual may not necessarily be good neither for the society nor for the progress of medicine.

If clinical benefit is obtained with new treatments with a reasonable side effect profile and at a reasonable price – whatever that means- that treatment should be implemented as soon as possible. The question is, whether that level of evidence has been achieved. The current widespread use of bevacizumab is building on uncontrolled data, without a proper health economic analysis, without proper attempts to identify early responders, and without properly designed trials how to best use the agent. The introduction of bevacizumab even prior to the registration and without further attempts to get properly controlled data impedes on the possibility to conduct the new and necessary trials required to get the proper answers. And that those trials are needed is clear from the experience in colorectal tumors, in which disease the addition of cetuximab to a bevacizumab containing combination regimen decreased outcome [28]. Some of the trials that are currently being planned in Europe are aiming to fill in the gaps we have in our knowledge how to best use this agent. Apart from the newly diagnosed trial, currently planned trials in recurrent disease that are planned in Europa are using randomized studies to identify optimal combinations with other agents and the best timing of bevacizumab (at first relapse, at further progression), and to assess the role of bevacizumab in recurrent grade II and grade III tumors. A concern is that the widespread use of bevacizumab will hamper properly designed trials to identify active combination strategies. Unfortunately, in many areas of Europe the US experience of pre-registration wide spread use of bevacizumab prior to official registration is being repeated. This is likely to diminish the possibility to conduct these urgently needed trials.

At this point in time, one conclusion that has to be made is that the neuro-oncological community has not done a proper job in assessing if and how bevacizumab should be used in recurrent GBM. It needs to be realized though that this is to a large extent due to insufficient support and strategy from the involved pharmaceutical companies that followed a strategy primarily aiming at a rapid registration of bevacizumab for use in recurrent disease, not at how it should be used best. That underscores, that in general a research agenda driven by academic research groups as opposed to one driven by pharmaceutical companies provides more relevant clinical data.

REFERENCES

[1]   Cloughesy TF, Prados MD, Mikkelsen T, *et al.* A phase II, randomized, non-comparative clinical trial of the effect of bevacizumab (BV) alone or in combination with irinotecan (CPT) on 6-months progression free survival (PFS6) in recurrent, treatment refractory glioblastoma (GBM). Proc Am Soc Clin Oncol 26:91s-(abstract #2010b), 2008 (abstr)

[2]   Vredenburgh JJ, Desjardins A, Herndon JE, *et al.* Phase II trial of bevacizumab and irinotecan in recurrent malignant glioma. Clin Cancer Res 13:1253-1259, 2007

[3]   Gorski DH, Beckett MA, Jaskowiak NT, *et al.* Blockade of the vascular endothelial growth factor stress response increases the antitumor effects of ionizing radiation. Cancer Res 59:3374-3378, 1999

[4]   Lee C-G, Heijn M, di Tomaso E, *et al.* Anti-vascular endothelial growth factor treatment augments tumor radiation response under nromoxic or hypoxic conditions. Cancer Res 60:5565-5570, 2000

[5]   Abdollahi A, Lipson KE, Han X, *et al.* SU5416 and SU6668 attenuate the angiogenic effects of radiation-induced tumor cell growth factor production and amplify the direct anti-endothelial action if radiation *in vivo*. Cancer Res 63:3755-3763, 2003

[6]   Zips D, Krause M, Hessel F, *et al.* Experimental study on different combination schedules of VEGF-receptor inhibitor PTK787/ZK222584 and fractionated irradiation. Anticances Res 23:3869-3876, 2003

[7]   Geng L, Donnoly E, McMahon G, *et al.* Inhibition of vascular endothelial growth factor receptor signaling leads to reversal of tumor resistance to radiotherapy. Cancer Res 61:2413-2419, 2004

[8]   Mc Donnel CO, Holden G, Sheridan ME, *et al.* Improvement in efficacy of chemoradiotherapy by addition of an antiangiogenic agent in a murine tumor model. J Surg Res 116:19-23, 2004

[9]   Verhoeff JJ, Stalpers LJ, Van Noorden CJ, *et al.* Angiogenesis inhibitor DC101 delays growth of intracerebral glioblastoma but induces morbidity when combined with irradiation. Cancer Lett, 2009

[10]   Tong RT, Boucher Y, Kozin SV, *et al.* Vascular normalization by vascular endothelial growth factor receptor 2 blockade induces a pressure gradient across the vasculature and improves drug penetration in tumors. Cancer Res 64:3731-3736, 2004

[11]   Ma J, Pulfer S, Li S, *et al.* Pharmacodynamic-mediated reduction of temozolomide tumor concentrations by the angiogenesis inhibitor TNP-470. Cancer Res 61:5491-5498, 2001

[12]   Ma J, Li S, Reed K, *et al.* Pharmacodynamic-mediated effects of the angiogenesis inhibitor SU5416 on the tumor disposition of temozolomide in subcutaneous and intracerebral glioma xenograft models. J Pharmacol Exp Ther 305:833-839, 2003

[13]   Senger DR, Galli SJ, Dvorak AM, *et al.* Tumor cells secrete a vascular permeability factor that promotes accumulation of ascites fluid. Science 219:983-985, 1983

[14]   Senger DR, Perruzzi CA, Feder J, *et al.* A highly conserved vascular permeability factor secreted by a variety of human and rodent tumor cell lines. Cancer Res 46:5629-5632, 1986

[15]   Bruce JN, Criscuolo GR, Merrill MJ, *et al.* Vascular permeability induced by protein product of malignant brain tumors: inhibition by dexamethasone. J Neurosurg 67:880-884, 1987

[16]   Batchelor TT, Sorensen AG, di TE, *et al.* AZD2171, a pan-VEGF receptor tyrosine kinase inhibitor, normalizes tumor vasculature and alleviates edema in glioblastoma patients. Cancer Cell 11:83-95, 2007

[17]   Macdonald DR, Cascino TL, Schold SC, *et al.* Response criteria for phase II studies of supratentorial malignant glioma. J Clin Oncol 8:1277-1280, 1990

[18]   Cairncross JG, Macdonald DR, Pexman JHW, *et al.* Steroid-induced CT changes in patients with recurrent glioma. Neurology 38:724-726, 1988

[19]   van den Bent MJ, Vogelbaum MA, Wen PY, *et al.* End point assessment in gliomas: novel treatments limit usefulness of classical Macdonald's Criteria. J Clin Oncol 27:2905-2908, 2009

[20]   Chen W, Delaloye S, Silverman DH, *et al.* Predicting treatment response of malignant gliomas to bevacizumab and irinotecan by imaging proliferation with [18F] fluorothymidine positron emission tomography: a pilot study. J Clin Oncol 25:4714-4721, 2007

[21]   Sorensen AG, Batchelor TT, Zhang WT, *et al.* A "vascular normalization index" as potential mechanistic biomarker to predict survival after a single dose of cediranib in recurrent glioblastoma patients. Cancer Res 69:5296-5300, 2009

[22]   Norden AD, Young GS, Setayesh K, *et al.* Bevacizumab for recurrent malignant gliomas: efficacy, toxicity, and patterns of recurrence. Neurology 70:779-787, 2008

[23]   Narayana A, Kelly P, Golfinos J, *et al.* Antiangiogenic therapy using bevacizumab in recurrent high-grade glioma: impact on local control and patient survival. J Neurosurg 110:173-180, 2009

[24]   Paez-Ribes M, Allen E, Hudock J, *et al.* Antiangiogenic therapy elicits malignant progression of tumors to increased local invasion and distant metastasis. Cancer Cell 15:220-231, 2009

[25]   Ebos JM, Lee CR, Cruz-Munoz W, *et al.* Accelerated metastasis after short-term treatment with a potent inhibitor of tumor angiogenesis. Cancer Cell 15:232-239, 2009

[26]   Loges S, Mazzone M, Hohensinner P, *et al.* Silencing or fueling metastasis with VEGF inhibitors: antiangiogenesis revisited. Cancer Cell 15:167-170, 2009

[27]   Raymond E, Fabbro M, Boige V, *et al.* Multicentre phase II study abd pharmacokinetic analysis of irinotecan in chemotherapy-naïve patients with glioblastoma. Ann Oncol 14:603-614, 2003

[28]   Tol J, Koopman M, Rodenburg CJ, *et al.* A randomised phase III study on capecitabine, oxaliplatin and bevacizumab with or without cetuximab in first-line advanced colorectal cancer, the CAIRO2 study of the Dutch Colorectal Cancer Group (DCCG). An interim analysis of toxicity. Ann Oncol 19:734-738, 2008

CHAPTER 23

Bevacizumab (Avastin®) and Malignant Glioma: Is there a Role? A European Perspective

Michael Weller*

University Hospital Zurich, Switzerland

Abstract: Bevacizumab (Avastin®) is an antibody to the vascular endothelial derived growth factor (VEGF) that has been approved for the treatment of several human cancers, including in May 2009 in the US, recurrent glioblastoma. Approval for recurrent glioblastoma was based on an increased response rate defined by neuroradiology and on favourable outcome measures regarding surrogate parameters of quality of life and overall survival, compared with historical controls. The approval of bevacizumab despite the lack of an appropriate controlled registration trial has provoked a heated discussion on the minimal requirements for approval of an agent in an orphan-like indication with urgent medical need, such as recurrent glioblastoma. A registration trial for bevacizumab in newly diagnosed glioblastoma is planned.

INTRODUCTION

The introduction of bevacizumab (Avastin®), an antibody to the vascular endothelial growth factor (VEGF), into the repertoire of the medical management of malignant gliomas has markedly influenced the field of glioma treatment. Bevacizumab was approved for the treatment of recurrent glioblastoma in the US in May 2009 and a decision regarding the approval of bevacizumab alone or in combination with irinotecan in Europe is awaited for the end of the year. Along with bevacizumab, several other candidate competitor antiangiogenic agents including the VEGF receptor antagonist, cediranib, as well as cilengitide and enzastaurin seek or have sought approval for recurrent or newly diagnosed glioblastoma.

STRENGTHS OF BEVACIZUMAB

The most prominent change in neuro-oncology brought about by the introduction of bevacizumab was the high response rate based on T1-weighted magnetic resonance imaging (MRI) with gadolinium enhancement. After decades of aiming at stopping tumor growth and inducing "stable disease" as defined by Macdonald and colleagues [1], neuro-oncologists were suddenly confronted with objective response rates at frequencies of 30-60% [2-4] Table **1**. The progression-free survival (PFS) rate at 6 months, defined again by neuroimaging, our current gold standard of assessing novel treatments for recurrent glioblastoma, may be in the range of 30-50% with bevacizumab-containing regimens, which may be superior to the figure of around 30% which is achieved with dose-intense regimens of temozolomide in patients pre-exposed to temozolomide [5-6]. Moreover, bevacizumab is overall well tolerated in this patient population which is otherwise prone to side effects from tumor-specific therapies, and many patients are able to reduce or even discontinue steroids at least transiently when treated with bevacizumab.

Table 1: Efficacy of Bevacizumab in Recurrent Glioblastoma

		CR+PR (%)	Median PFS	PFS at 6 months (%)
Vredenburgh *et al.* [2] (n=32)	Bevacizumab plus irinotecan	61	23	38
Kreisl *et al.* [4] (n=48)	Bevacizumab	35	16	31
Cloughesy *et al.* [3] (n=85)	Bevacizumab	20		35
Cloughesy *et al.* [3] (n=82)	Bevacizumab plus irinotecan	33		50

*Address correspondence to Michael Weller: University Hospital Zurich, Switzerland; Email: michael.weller@unituebingen.de

CONTROVERSIES SURROUNDING BEVACIZUMAB

VEGF was initially also referred to as vascular permeability factor (VPF) and it is well recognized that VEGF is a major mediator of blood brain barrier disturbance in glioblastoma patients. Accordingly, it is not too surprising that an antibody blocking VEGF bioavailability will score favourably on a scoring system [1] that focuses almost entirely on T1-weighted gadolinium-enhanced imaging. We are therefore still uncertain in how the high response rate seen with bevacizumab translates into a gain in survival and whether not new imaging endpoints are required to more adequately judge the efficacy of antiangiogenic agents such as bevacizumab or cediranib [7]. Moreover, it was interesting to note that the overall response rate judged to be 41% by the investigators was restated to be 28% by Genentech`s review and to be 26% by the independent FDA review, suggesting biases or simply that our current criteria are difficult to apply.

Further, as predicted by preclinical observations [8-9], continuous exposure to antiangiogenic therapies may provoke the development of a more invasive tumor phenotype, leading specifically in glioblastoma to an altered pattern of recurrence reminiscent of gliomatosis cerebri [10]. How common this risk is at present can only be determined in prospective studies with standardized neuroimaging and preferably a bevacizumab-free control population.

WEAKNESSES OF BEVACIZUMAB

The efficacy of bevacizumab alone in recurrent glioblastoma is limited. The PFS rate of 29% at 6 months [4] leaves a lot of room for improvement most likely to be achieved by identifying a suitable combination partner for bevacizumab. The initial reports of the unexpected impressive effects of the combination of bevacizumab and irinotecan suggested a strong synergistic potential of two agents which appeared to have limited activity when administered alone. Yet, the results from the randomized trial of bevacizumab alone versus bevacizumab plus irinotecan [3] confirmed that irinotecan is contributing little to the effect of the novel combination. Switching patients who progressed under bevacizumab to the combination of bevacizumab and irinotecan did not induce objective responses and was overall not effective either [4]. The last two ASCO meetings each had a series of abstracts reporting on the combination of bevacizumab and various cytotoxic agents, but the nature of these small phase II-like series did not permit firm conclusions on which agent to choose for an appropriately powered phase III trial.

In terms of safety and tolerability, although clinically relevant intratumoral hemorrhage seems to be rare in bevacizumab-treated patients, other relevant complications such as craniotomy site dehiscence and the risk of surgical procedures during bevacizumab therapy may become new problems in the favourable subgroup of recurrent glioblastoma patients who are offered multiple lines of treatment for recurrent disease [11].

CONCLUSIONS

Bevacizumab provides symptomatic clinical benefit for many patients with recurrent glioblastoma and helps to reduce dose of - or even to discontinue - steroids. This is likely to represent a meaningful clinical benefit translating into improved quality of life. Yet, the efficacy of bevacizumab alone regarding tumor control at 6 months is modest and a suitable partner for combination therapy awaits identification. No indisputable impact on PFS or overall survival has been demonstrated so far. Safety and efficacy in the frontline setting are currently being explored.

REFERENCES

[1] Macdonald DR, Cascino TL, Schold SC, *et al.* Response criteria for phase II studies of supratentorial malignant glioma. J Clin Oncol 1990;8:1277-1280.

[2] Vredenburgh JJ, Desjardins A, Herndon 2nd JE, *et al.* Phase II trial of bevacizumab and irinotecan in recurrent malignant glioma. Clin Cancer Res 2007;13:1253-1259.

[3] Cloughesy TF, Prados MD, Wen PY, *et al.* A phase II, randomized, non-comparative clinical trial of the effect of bevacizumab (BV) alone or in combination with irinotecan (CPT) on 6-month progression free survival (PFS6) in recurrent, treatment-refractory glioblastoma (GBM). J Clin Oncol 2008;26:2010b(May 20 suppl).

[4] Kreisl TN, Kim L, Moore K, *et al.* Phase II trial of single-agent bevacizumab followed by bevacizumab plus irinotecan at tumor progression in recurrent glioblastoma. J Clin Oncol 2009;27:740-745.

[5]   Perry JR, Rizek P, Cashman R, *et al.* Temozolomide rechallenge in recurrent malignant glioma by using a continuous temozolomide schedule. The "Rescue" approach. Cancer 2008;113:2152-2157.

[6]   Wick A, Pascher C, Wick W, *et al.* Rechallenge with temozolomide in patients with recurrent gliomas. J Neurol in press

[7]   Batchelor TT, Sorensen AG, di Tomaso E, *et al.* AZD2171, a pan-VEGF receptor tyrosine kinase inhibitor, normalizes tumor vasculature and alleviates edema in glioblastomas patients. Cancer Cell 2007;11:83-95.

[8]   Kunkel P, Ulbricht U, Bohlen P, *et al.* Inhibition of glioma angiogenesis and growth *in vivo* by systemic treatment with a monoclonal antibody against vascular endothelial growth factor receptor-2. Cancer Res 2001;61:6624–6628.

[9]   Paez-Ribes M, Allen E, Hudock J, *et al.* Antiangiogenic therapy elicits malignant progression of tumors to increased local invasion and distant metastasis. Cancer Cell 2009;15:220-231.

[10]   Norden AD, Young GS, Setayesh K, *et al.* Bevacizumab for recurrent malignant gliomas. Efficacy, toxicity, and patterns of recurrence. Neurology 2008;70:779–787.

[11]   Chamberlain MC. Bevacizumab plus irinotecan in recurrent glioblastoma. J Clin Oncol 2008;26:1012-1013.

CHAPTER 24

The European Perspective Regarding Avastin and Malignant Gliomas

Wolfgang Wick*, Michael Platten and Antje Wick

University of Heidelberg, Heidelberg, Germany

Abstract: Although, therapies directed to the vasculature of malignant gliomas are equally attractive in Europe and the United States of America (US), limited access to both trials and lack of approval by the European Medicines Agency (EMEA) prevented a *de facto* introduction into the current standard of care as seen in the US, where the compound is registered for recurrent glioblastoma since 05/2009. To date, the STEERING trial using the protein kinase C beta (PKC-β) inhibitor enzastaurin, the REGAL trial applying the vascular endothelial receptor inhibitor (VEGFR) cediranib, the PTK787/ZK trial and the upcoming dasatinib trial comprise the only structured European experience with such molecularly targeted drugs. Several national initiatives using bevacizumab (Avastin®) are now in place to fill the obvious gap. Despite the clear medical need for novel therapies for recurrent malignant glioma, neurooncology in Europe advocates randomized rather than uncontrolled trials to obtain additional data clarifying the role for bevacizumab in malignant gliomas.

INTRODUCTION

In contrast to newly diagnosed glioblastoma, where clinical practice in most European countries as well as national guidelines will adhere to a common standard of care comprising postsurgical radiochemotherapy with temozolomide [1], the situation is less clear in recurrent glioblastoma and anaplastic gliomas. At recurrence further resection, reirradiation and another course of alkylating therapies plus enrolment into studies is the current practice [2]. Since 2007, an increasing number of patients has also received bevacizumab, mostly as third- or fourth-line treatment. After approval by the FDA, bavcizumab is more frequently used at earlier stages, despite its off-label status in Europe. In addition to the scientific challenges that have occurred during the approval process, considerable national differences with respect to access based on the registration status, lack of trials trials (Tables **1** and **2**), pricing, and reimbursement regulations have been particularly problematic for European investigators.

Table 1: Trials with European participation with antiangiogenic therapies in malignant gliomas

Regimen (reference)	Trial [yes/no]	Patients [n]	Response [%]	PFS [months, (95% CI)]	Toxicity	OS [months, (95% CI)]
Recurrent glioblastoma						
Enzastaurin versus lomustine (16)	yes, phase III	174/92	2.9/4.3 (CR + PR)	1.51 (1.45-2.1)/1.64 (1.48-2.79)	minor for enzastaurin	6.6 (5.22-7.75)/7.13 (6.01-8.8)
Cediranib versus cediranib plus lomustine versus lomustine	yes, phase III	Accrual finished 09/2009				
Sunitinib	yes, phase II	Trial stopped 07/2009				
Newly diagnosed glioblastoma						
Radiochemotherapy with temozolomide and cilengitide (26)	yes, phase I/II	46	/	34/52 (65.4% [95% CI, 50.9-78.0%])	3/52 (5.7%): constitutional symptoms, elevated liver function tests, deep venous thrombosis and pulmonary embolism	/
Radiochemotherapy with temozolomide and PTK-787 (27)	yes, phase I	18	/	/	liver enzyme elevation, arterial hypertension, fatigue	/

*****Address correspondence to Wolfgang Wick:** Department of Neurooncology, University Hospital of Heidelberg, Im Neuenheimer Feld 400, D-69120 Heidelberg, Germany; Tel: +49 6221 56 7075, Fax: +49 6221 56 7554, Email: wolfgang.wick@med.uni-heidelberg.de

Table 2: European experience with bevacizumab in malignant gliomas

Histology / regimen (reference)	Trial [yes/no]	Patients [n]	Response [%, CR, PR]	PFS [months, (95% CI)]	Toxicity	OS [months]
Recurrent O / bev + iri (28)	no	25	20/52	4.6 (3.9-nd)	20% treatment discontinuation 24% i.tu. hemorrhage 4% sympt. bleeding	not reached
Recurrent HGG / bev + iri (29)	no	52	25% CR+PR (30% grade IV, 15% grade III glioma)	5	8% treatment discontinuation (cerebral haemorrhage, cardiac arrhythmia, intestinal perforation and diarrhoea	6.8

Abbreviations: Bevacizumab (bev), complete reponse (CR, 14), confidence interval (CI), high-grade glioma (HGG), irinotecan (iri), oligodendroglial tumors (O), partial response (PR, 14)

The standard of care for all patients with anaplastic gliomas is to use postoperative radio- or chemotherapy alone, although European neurooncologists increasingly apply regimens developed for the treatment of patients with glioblastoma [3-5]. This discrepancy between evidence from randomized trials and daily practice may in part be due to the diagnostic uncertainties associated both with typing and grading of gliomas as well as the still grim prognosis of patients with anaplastic gliomas.

Phase II trials and larger published series of treatment with bevacizumab mostly in combination with irinotecan have been reported from the large US sites [5-10]. The high response rates (30-60%) reported are unusual and had never been seen in malignant glioma trials before. The reported progression-free survival (PFS) and overall survival (OS) rates were not particular impressive (6-month PFS 30-50%; median OS: 8-10 months), but still remarkable with antibody-based regimens. Comparisons to historical data remain a field of controversy and should probably avoided if possible.

Currently bevacizumab is certainly welcome as a potential new weapon for the treatment of malignant gliomas. The accepted mode of action of anti-vascular endothelial growth factor (VEGF)/VEGF receptor (VEGFR) compounds includes normalization of the vasculature by inhibiting pathological proliferation of endothelial cells leading to immature vessels [11]. This results in an often marked effect on the peritumoral edema as well as in a reduction of contrast enhancement. Apart from more extensive data on toxicity and considerations on the best treatment dose and regimen in brain tumors, three main questions that need to be addressed in clinical trials emerge:

I.   The positive effect on the tumor vasculature opens opportunities for combinations with other agents that benefit from the normalization of blood-flow. Therefore, it is generally believed that a combination of a classical cytostatic drug and a targeted agent or a cocktail of targeted agents would be necessary to optimize the activity of targeted compounds. It has been shown that VEGF-targeting agents in combination with cytotoxic agents can be safely administered to malignant glioma patients. However, the combinations of daily temozolomide or irinotecan or other compounds and bevacizumab show only marginal additional activity against glioblastoma progressive after radiochemotherapy over bevacizumab alone [5,6,7,12].

II. Preclinical data suggest that in addition to the combinations of treatment and their timing the sequence of treatments is influencing the efficacy of the treatments [11]. Therefore it might not be equivalent to use bevacizumab at first or second recurrence or, as done in many European centers outside trials, in the terminal stage of the disease. Further, from the randomized trial [5] it can be deducted that while PFS and OS are favourable, the time between progression and death is very short. Whether this is due to the notion that a tumor progressing under bevacizumab is not likely to be controlled by another treatment regimen [7] or wrong sequencing is unclear.

III. Preclinical studies suggest that anti-angiogenic VEGF-targeting compounds may enhance the invasiveness of tumor cells [13, 14]. Uncontrolled trials with bevacizumab [8,9] also suggest an increase in invasive tumor at recurrence both in the context of an objective response or a progression according to the Macdonald criteria [15]. This increased invasiveness is commonly termed "gliomatosis-like phenotype" and best depicted on fluid attenuated inversion recovery (FLAIR) magnetic resonance imaging (MRI) sequences so far [9].

Only a thorough understanding of the biological activity and solid data from controlled trials will help define the role of bevacizumab in malignant glioma therapy with respect to timing, dose, duration and combination with other agents.

GENERAL CONSIDERATIONS ON BEVACIZUMAB IN EUROPE

In contrast to the US the question whether bevacizumab is the new standard of care and should be favored as a salvage treatment over cytotoxic chemotherapy for recurrent disease is still a matter of debate. This is mainly due to the off-label status of the drug and the subsequent use at later, palliative stages in most European countries. In other European countries bevacizumab has not been available at all for brain tumor patients since the costs are not reimbursed by the health care system. Further, many patients in Europe regard treatment with bevacizumab as the last chance because the data indicate that once failure to treatment with bevacizumab is diagnosed by conventional radiographic methods [15], most patients experience rapid deterioration and die shortly afterwards [5]. It is generally believed that patients willing to participate in clinical trials exploring novel treatment options should do so prior to starting bevacizumab, which is also reflected by the inclusion criteria of the respective trial protocols.

New methods and radiographic criteria for detecting disease progression are needed. Cost-effectiveness of bevacizumab in gliomas deserves further investigation. The role of irinotecan in this combination remains unclear. At this time, bevacizumab should only be used in newly diagnosed malignant gliomas in the setting of a clinical trial.

COMBINATION PARTNERS

Given the minimal efficacy of lomustine after standard primary treatment in glioblastoma [16] it will be difficult to argue that nitrosoureas are the most promising agents at recurrence. Maybe in contrast to many US sites, European centers frequently use temozolomide, mostly within more intensified regimens, although patients had been pretreated with conventional temozolomide before [17-19]. Nevertheless, in Europe lomustine is still a reasonable combination partner or counterpart both in current practice and in control arms of clinical trials.

The situation is different in anaplastic gliomas, where nitrosoureas still play an important role in the first and second-line treatment [4]. Similar to recurrent glioblastoma, a phase II trial in recurrent anaplastic gliomas demonstrated encouraging activity of irinotecan combined with bevacizumab with partial responses (15) in 61% and a PFS at 6 months of 55% [20]. Given this interesting data it is difficult to understand that a randomized trial – per se minimizing selection biases - is missing and that the role of irinotecan obviously needs to be redefined in anaplastic glioma after limited activity was demonstrated in glioblastoma [5]. Currently the European Organization for Research and Treatment of Cancer (EORTC) is developing a trial proposal in recurrent low-grade and anaplastic gliomas.

PSEUDORESPONSE

Pseudoresponse or -regression is a clinically relevant reduction of T1-contrast enhancing tumor, which is considered to be a consequence of reduced blood-brain-barrier permeability and vascular normalization and not as reduction of viable tumor mass [21]. Bevacizumab and VEGFR inhibitors, such as the tyrosine kinase inhibitor cediranib, are producing marked decrease in contrast enhancement within 24-48 h after initiation of therapy [5,22]. Pseudoresponses are partly due to normalization of abnormally permeable tumor vessels and not necessarily to a true antitumor effect. As a result, radiological responses in studies with antiangiogenic agents have to be interpreted with caution. There is a disappointing disparity between the high response rates in recurrent glioblastoma and the modest, potential survival benefit. It has to be shown, whether this at least partly is explained by the limited effect on the tumor mass itself [21]. In Europe, the duration of a response or stability or even better the OS are considered to be more accurate indicators of the therapeutic activity of a compound.

European sites are also aware of the frequent discrepancy between T1-contrast responses and T2/FLAIR progression occurring at the same time. Particularly the risk of promoting invasiveness [9] that is at least preclinically observed with antiangiogenic therapies as well as several clinical observations [8, 13] warrant a careful consideration, when to use bevacizumab and call for clinical study data.

TOXICITY

As with any therapy, both the knowledge of accurate use, limitations and potential unwanted effects are pivotal for the broad success of its implementation. Amongst others, the encountered positive effects have to be balanced with new or increased toxicities. Combining chemotherapy with anti-VEGF approaches may be expected to increase fatigue, myelotoxicity and the risk for trombo-embolic events both in the venous and the arterial system. Although the total numbers of bevacizumab treated patients are > ½ million in the general oncology population, only a few hundred specific treatments in primary brain tumors have been reported thus far. Therefore, rare but relevant unwanted effects (toxicities) for Neurooncology may have been missed til date. In fact, craniotomy site wound dehiscence has been reported to be more than an unique cumbersome adverse effect following antiangiogenic treatment in brain tumor patients, and problems with local wound healing, at least in within weeks from surgery, which was followed by bevacizumab treatment have been observed [23].

Amongst others, the incidences of arterial hypertension need to be recorded carefully and structured recommendations for their treatment needs to be provided. Interestingly, different from other indications [24], in glioblastoma, the clinical efficacy of bevacizumab is not predictable by the increase in arterial blood pressure [25].

In summary, European Neurooncologists advocate more scientific experience in managing recurrent malignant glioma patients with an important drug. At the moment, several proposals to the company Roche/Genentech are discussed to assess the impact of bevacizumab in recurrent low-grade and anaplastic gliomas and additionally to determine the best place, first or second recurrence, for bevacizumab in gliobastoma. It is regarded extremely important, that future approval processes take the European perspective before filing the documents and the experts in the particular disease scientifically assess that compounds, and that is Neurooncologists with respect to bevacizumab in malignant gliomas.

CONFLICT OF INTEREST

W. Wick has been consultant to and has received honoraria from Roche, the company marketing bevacizumab in Europe.

REFERENCES

[1]   Stupp R, Mason WP, van den Bent MJ, *et al.* Radiotherapy plus concomitant and adjuvant temozolomide for glioblastoma. N Engl J Med 2005 Mar 10;352(10):987-96.

[2]   Van den Bent MJ, Carpentier AF, Brandes AA, *et al.* Adjuvant procarbazine, lomustine, and vincristine improves progression-free survival but not overall survival in newly diagnosed anaplastic oligodendrogliomas and oligoastrocytomas: a randomized European Organisation for Research and Treatment of Cancer phase III trial. J Clin Oncol 2006 Jun 10;24(18):2715-22.

[3]   Cairncross G, Berkey B, Shaw E, *et al.* Phase III trial of chemotherapy plus radiotherapy compared with radiotherapy alone for pure and mixed anaplastic oligodendroglioma: Intergroup Radiation Therapy Oncology Group Trial 9402. J Clin Oncol 2006 Jun 20;24(18):2707-14.

[4]   Wick W, Hartmann C, Engel C, *et al.* for the Neurooncology Working Group (NOA) of the German Cancer Society. NOA-04 Randomized Phase III Trial of Sequential Radiochemotherapy of Anaplastic Glioma With PCV or Temozolomide. J Clin Oncol 2009 in press

[5]   Friedman HS, Prados MD, Wen PY, *et al.* Bevacizumab Alone and in Combination With Irinotecan in Recurrent Glioblastoma. J Clin Oncol 2009 Aug 31. [Epub ahead of print]

[6]   Nghiemphu PL, Liu W, Lee Y, *et al.* Bevacizumab and chemotherapy for recurrent glioblastoma: a single-institution experience. Neurology 2009 Apr 7;72(14):1217-22.

[7]   Kreisl TN, Kim L, Moore K, *et al.* Phase II trial of single-agent bevacizumab followed by bevacizumab plus irinotecan at tumor progression in recurrent glioblastoma. J Clin Oncol 2009 Feb 10;27(5):740-5.

[8]   Zuniga RM, Torcuator R, Jain R, *et al.* Efficacy, safety and patterns of response and recurrence in patients with recurrent high-grade gliomas treated with bevacizumab plus irinotecan. J Neurooncol 2009 Feb;91(3):329-36.

[9]   Norden AD, Young GS, Setayesh K, *et al.* Bevacizumab for recurrent malignant gliomas: efficacy, toxicity, and patterns of recurrence. Neurology 2008 Mar 4;70(10):779-87.

[10]   Vredenburgh JJ, Desjardins A, Herndon JE 2nd, *et al.* Bevacizumab plus irinotecan in recurrent glioblastoma multiforme. J Clin Oncol 2007 Oct 20;25(30):4722-9.

[11]   Shaked Y, Henke E, Roodhart JM, *et al.* Rapid chemotherapy-induced acute endothelial progenitor cell mobilization: implications for antiangiogenic drugs as chemosensitizing agents. Cancer Cell 2008;14:263-73

[12]   Maron R, Vredenburgh JJ, Desjardins A, *et al.* Bevacizumab and daily temozolomide for recurrent glioblastoma multiforme (GBM). J Clin Oncol 2008; 26:S15, abstr 2074

[13]   Kunkel P, Ulbricht U, Bohlen P, *et al.* Inhibition of glioma angiogenesis and growth *in vivo* by systemic treatment with a monoclonal antibody against vascular endothelial growth factor receptor-2. Cancer Res 2001 Sep 15;61(18):6624-8

[14]   Lucio-Eterovic AK, Piao Y, de Groot JF. Mediators of glioblastoma resistance and invasion during antivascular endothelial growth factor therapy. Clin Cancer Res 2009 Jul 15;15(14):4589-99

[15]   Macdonald DR, Cascino TL, Schold SC Jr, Cairncross JG. Response criteria for phase II studies of supratentorial malignant glioma. J Clin Oncol 1990 Jul;8(7):1277–80

[16]   Wick W, Puduvalli VK, Chamberlain M, *et al.* Enzastaurin versus lomustine in the treatment of recurrent intracranial glioblastoma: A phase III study. J Clin Oncol in press

[17]   Brandes AA, Tosoni A, Cavallo G, *et al.* Temozolomide 3 weeks on and 1 week off as first-line therapy for recurrent glioblastoma: phase II study from gruppo italiano cooperativo din euro-oncologia (GICNO). Br J Cancer 2006 Nov 6;95(9):1155-60

[18]   Wick A, Felsberg J, Steinbach JP, *et al.* Efficacy and tolerability of Temozolomide in an one week on/one week off regimen in patients with recurrent glioma. J Clin Oncol 2007 Aug 1;25(22):3357-61.

[19]   Wick A, Pascher C, Wick W, *et al.* Rechallenge With Temozolomide in Patients with Recurrent Gliomas. J Neurol 2009 May;256(5):734-41 Epub 2009 Feb 25

[20]   Desjardins A, Reardon DA, Herndon JE 2nd, *et al.* Bevacizumab plus irinotecan in recurrent WHO grade 3 malignant gliomas. Clin Cancer Res 2008 Nov 1;14(21):7068-73.

[21]   Kamoun WS, Ley CD, Farrar CT, *et al.* Edema control by cediranib, a vascular endothelial growth factor receptor-targeted kinase inhibitor, prolongs survival despite persistent brain tumor growth in mice. J Clin Oncol. 2009 May 20;27(15):2542-52. Epub 2009 Mar 30.

[22]   Batchelor TT, Sorensen AG, di Tomaso E, *et al.* AZD2171, a pan-VEGF receptor tyrosine kinase inhibitor, normalizes tumor vasculature and alleviates edema in glioblastoma patients. Cancer Cell 2007 Jan;11(1):83-95.

[23]   Lai, A., Filka, E., McGibbon, B., W. *et al.* Phase II pilot study of bevacizumab in combination with temozolomide and radiotherapy for up-front treatment of patients with newly diagnosed glioblastoma multiforme: Interimanalysis of safety and tolerability. Int J Radiat Oncol Biol Phys 2008;71:1372-80

[24]   Mir O, Ropert S, Alexandre J, Goldwasser F. Hypertension as a surrogate marker for the activity of anti-VEGF agents. Ann Oncol 2009 May; 20(5):967-970

[25]   Wick A, Schäfer N, Dörner N, *et al.* Arterial hypertension and bevacizumab treatment in glioblastoma: no correlation with clinical outcome. J Neurooncol 2009 Aug 29 [Epub ahead of print]

[26]   Stupp R, Goldbrunner R, Neyns B, *et al.* Phase I/IIa trial of cilengitide (EMD121974) and temozolomide with concomitant radiotherapy, followed by temozolomide and cilengitide maintenance therapy in patients (pts) with newly diagnosed glioblastoma (GBM). J Clin Oncol 2007 Vol 25, No. 18S (June 20 Supplement), 2007: 2000

[27]   Brandes AA, Stupp R, Hau P, *et al.* EORTC Study 26041–22041: Phase I/II study on concomitant and adjuvant temozolomide (TMZ) and radiotherapy (RT) with or without PTK787/ZK222584 (PTK/ZK) in newly diagnosed glioblastoma—Results of a phase I trial. J Clin Oncol Vol 25, No 18S (June 20 Supplement), 2007: 2026

[28]   Taillibert S, Vincent LA, Granger B, *et al.* Bevacizumab and irinotecan for recurrent oligodendroglial tumors. Neurology 2009 May 5;72(18):1601-6

[29]   Poulsen HS, Grunnet K, Sorensen M, *et al.* Bevacizumab plus irinotecan in the treatment patients with progressive recurrent malignant brain tumours. Acta Oncol. 2009;48(1):52-8.

CHAPTER 25

Sunitinib for the Treatment of Central Nervous System Glioma

Neyns Bart*

Clinical Professor Medical Oncology, UZ Brussel, Laarbeeklaan 101, 1090 Brussel, Belgium

Abstract: Sunitinib malate (sunitinib) is an orally absorbed small molecule inhibitor of multiple cellular kinases including the family of "Vascular Endothelial Growth Factor Receptors" (VEGFRs), "Platelet Derived Growth Factor Receptors" (PDGFR–alfa and –beta), c-Kit, FLT1, FLK1/KDR, the FLT3 and RET kinases. Treatment with sunitinib offers a proven survival benefit and is registered for the treatment of patients with advanced renal cell carcinoma and GIST (two respectively HIF/VEGF and PDGFR or KIT dependent cancers) but sunitinib has also demonstrated meaningful anti-tumor activity against a subset of other common cancers (including breast, colon and non-small cell lung cancer). Increased receptor tyrosine kinase signaling involving the VEGF/VEGFR ligand/receptors but also KIT and PDGFR receptor signaling causes profound neo-angiogenesis and may contribute to cellular proliferation and survival of high-grade gliomas (HGG) of the central nervous system (CNS). Furthermore, the KIT, PDGFRa and VEGFR2 genes are frequently amplified and over-expressed in HGG and therefore represent an attractive molecular target for inhibition by sunitinib. Notwithstanding its attractive drug profile, sunitinib has so far not been widely investigated for the treatment of central nervous system glioma. Only recently, the first results from an exploratory clinical trial of sunitinib for recurrent HGG have become available. These early results (obtained with a continuous 37,5 mg/day regimen) indicate that sunitinib has a measurable but transient inhibitory effect on the pathological increase in cerebral blood volume and -flow within recurrent gliomas but that this effect is transient in time and associated with limited clinical benefit. In addition considerable "off target" toxicity (mainly skin and hematological toxicity) were observed that may interfere with further development of sunitinib in this indication. Ongoing phase II studies on sunitinib should further delineate the potential role of this drug in the treatment of CNS glioma at diagnosis and recurrence. Potentially, individual molecular profiling of gliomas to predict their dependence on specified kinase signaling will aid to determine the utility of sunitinib treatment over alternative more specific VEGF(R) targeted agents.

INTRODUCTION

Gliomas are the most frequent primary brain tumors and represent approximately 2% of all malignant diseases. Their annual incidence is about 11.47 new cases per 100.000 persons per year [1]. According to the WHO criteria gliomas are divided into low-grade (grade I and II) and high-grade gliomas (grade III or anaplastic glioma and grade IV or glioblastoma multiforme, GBM) [2]. Based on the histopathological characteristics further distinction is made among grade II and III gliomas between astrocytoma, oligodendroglioma and mixed oligo-astrocytoma.

All gliomas of grade II-IV are lethal cancers for which the cure rate remains extremely low. Despite aggressive surgery, radiotherapy and temozolomide chemotherapy, median time to recurrence for the most common type of glioma, the glioblastoma, is 6.9 months and median overall survival 14.6 months [3]. The prognosis of patients with grade II-III glioma is much more heterogeneous but following initial treatment, the tumor recurs after a median of 2-3 years and is fatal within less than 5 years from diagnosis in most patients. There exists an unmet need for more effective treatment for patients with high-grade glioma.

Sunitinib malate (SU011248) is a small molecule kinase inhibitor with the molecular formula $C_{22}H_{27}FN_4O_2$. Malate is well absorbed following oral administration and may be administered irrespective to meals. There is extensive plasma protein binding of sunitinib (approximately 95% in humans).

Sunitinib is metabolized primarily by the cytochrome P450 enzyme, CYP3A4, to produce the active N-desethyl metabolite, SU012662. The terminal elimination half-life of sunitinib and SU012662 are approximately 40 hours and 80 hours, respectively. Plasma drug concentrations plateau during the first 2 weeks of dosing. Accumulation across multiple cycles of treatment has not been observed.

*Address correspondence to Neyns Bart: Medical Oncology, UZ Brussel, Laarbeeklaan 101, 1090 Brussel, Belgium; Tel.: +3224776415: Fax: +322476012; E-mail: Bart.Neyns@uzbrussel.be

Sunitinib is a small molecule inhibitor of a defined number of cellular kinases, many of which are cell surface receptor tyrosine kinases (RTK). These RTK are transmembrane proteins that transduce extracellular signals to the internal signal transduction pathways within the cell. Typically such RTK contain an extracellular ligand-binding domain, a transmembranar domain and an intracellular catalytic domain; The binding of ligands induces dimerization of the RTK resulting in autophosphorylation of the catalytic domains and activation of tyrosine kinase activity. This further stimulates multiple downstream signal transduction pathways that control cellular proliferation, survival, migration and differentiation. The predominant RTK demonstrated to be inhibited by sunitinib are VEGF, PDGF, bFGF, KIT, FLT3, CSF-1, and RET. The inhibitory capacity (IC50 (μM)) of sunitinib on the VEGFR2, PDGFR-a and –b, and KIT are respectively: 0.004‡ (2.09 ng/mL), 0.069‡ (36.0 ng/mL), 0.039‡ (20.4 ng/mL),and 0.001-0.01 (0.52-5.2 ng/mL).

Sunitinib has been evaluated in several phase 1, 2 and 3 studies for different cancers. The primary dose limiting toxicity in the phase 1 studies was fatigue/asthenia, which generally occurred around 10 to 15 days after start of therapy, and was reversible over a 3 to 7 day period following discontinuation of sunitinib treatment. Additional frequent adverse events associated with sunitinib treatment have been gastrointestinal (nausea, vomiting, diarrhea), and hematologic (neutropenia, thrombocytopenia). Generally, adverse event severity has correlated with higher drug exposure, lower patient performance status or exposure to previous chemotherapy in comparison to chemotherapy-naïve patients. Cardiac toxicity (significant decreases in cardiac ejection fraction) was observed in <3% of solid tumor patients, either with or without a prior history of cardiovascular disease or anthracycline exposure. The maximum tolerated dose of sunitinib has been defined as 50 mg/day on a 4 out of 6 weeks schedule or 37,5 mg/day on a continuous daily regimen.

Antitumor activity of sunitinib has been demonstrated in patients with various solid tumors in phase 1 studies (confirmed partial responses have been achieved with the following solid tumors: GIST, renal cell carcinoma, neuroendocrine tumor, sarcoma, thyroid carcinoma, non-small-cell lung carcinoma, and malignant melanoma). The properties and clinical activity of Sunitinib has been the subject of recent review [4].

In a preclinical animal model of glioblastoma, sunitinib was reported to potently inhibited angiogenesis that was stimulated by implantation of U87MG and GL15 glioblastoma cells into organotypic brain slices at concentrations as low as 10 nM (a concentration that would be sufficient to inhibit VEGFR2 signaling but not PDGFR and KIT signaling in human subjects). At higher doses (10 microM), sunitinib induced direct anti-proliferative and pro-apoptotic effects on GL15 cells and decreased invasion of these cells implanted into brain slices. These concentrations would however not be achieved with conventional dosing regimens of sunitinib in humans. In addition, anti-invasive activity was not observed *in vivo* at the highest dose level utilized (80 mg/kg per day) but experiments in athymic mice bearing intracerebral U87MG GBM demonstrated that this dose level improved median survival by exhibiting a potent antiangiogenic activity in this animal model. These data support the potential utility of sunitinib in the treatment of GBM as an antiangiogenic and possibly cystostatic agent.

We investigated the activity of sunitinib as a single agent in patients with recurrent high-grade glioma and prospectively assessed the anti-angiogenic activity by means of dynamic contrast-enhanced MR imaging (DCE-MRI) of the brain and the metabolic response by fluorinated fenyl-methyl-alanine-PET (FMP-PET) (Neyns et al; poster presentation at the ASCO 2009 annual meeting).

METHODS

Patients with recurrent high-grade glioma (> 18 years and a PS of > 60%) were recruited to this study according to a 2-stage phase II design (Simon two stage Minimax design [alfa 0.1 and beta 0.1]). Macdonald tumor response criteria were used as the primary endpoint for efficacy and accrual of 18 response-assessable patients was planned for the first stage of the study (this population would also be considered as a phase IB study population for the objective of evaluating the antiangiogenic effect of sunitinib) [5]. If no responses were observed among the first 18 patients, no additional patients would be accrued, and it would be concluded that the true best overall tumor response rate is unlikely to be ≥ 5%.

Patients initiated sunitinib treatment at a daily dose of 37.5 mg. This continuous daily regimen was preferred over the more frequently investigated 4 out of 6 weeks regimen in order to prevent the diminishing of biologic effects during the drug-free intervals that could have clinical relevance in patients with recurrent CNS glioma (e.g. intracranial hypertension due to tumor edema).

T1- with and without Gadolinium and T2-weighted MRI images of the brain were obtained after 4 and 8 wks of sunitinib and every 8 weeks thereafter. The antiangiogenic effect of sunitinib was assessed by calculating the cerebral blood volume (CBV) and cerebral blood flow (CBF) from dynamic susceptibility (DSC) based perfusion MRI and calculation of the lesion-to-normal-white matter CBV (CBV_{LTN}) and CBF (CBF_{LTN}) ratios. Uptake of fluorinated fenyl-methyl-alanine (FMP, a fluorinated amino acid PET-tracer) within the CNS was assessed by positron emission tomography (PET) at baseline and re-assessed in responding patients. Treatment could be continued until progression, unacceptable toxicity or patient refusal and one dose reductions was allowed (to a single daily dose of 25 mg) in case of severe hematological toxicity (i.e. an absolute neutrophil count of less than 1500/mm³ and/or a thrombocyte count of less than 100.000/mm³) or grade 3 or 4 non-hematological toxicity (which needed to recover to grade 1 or baseline within a maximum treatment interruption of 2 weeks before treatment was resumed).

RESULTS

Twenty-one consecutive patients were enrolled (with a median age of 43 years (range 34 to 71 years); 15 male and 6 female; a baseline Karnofky performance status of 90-80 in 11 patients, KPS of 70-60 in 10 patients). All patients had progressive disease (PD) following surgery, radiation therapy (RT) and temozolomide chemotherapy. A total of 142 treatment weeks (range 2-84 weeks) were administered and evaluated; 81% of the administrations were at the 37,5 mg-, 19% at the 25 mg dose level. The most frequently encountered treatment related adverse events (AEs) were: skin toxicity (CTCAE v3.1 grade 2 in 1 patient; grade 3 in 1 patient), fatigue (grade 2 in 4 patients), hypertension (grade 2 in 3 patients), diarrhea (grade 2 in 2 patients), mucositis (grade 3 in 1 patient), afebrile- (grade 2 in 3 patients) and febrile neutropenia (grade 3 in 1- and grade 4 [listeria monocytogenes sepsis] in 1 patient), thrombocytopenia (grade 2 in 4- and grade – in one and grade 4 in 1 patient(s)), and lymphocytopenia (grade 2 in 2- and grade 3 in 4 patients) (Fig. **1**).

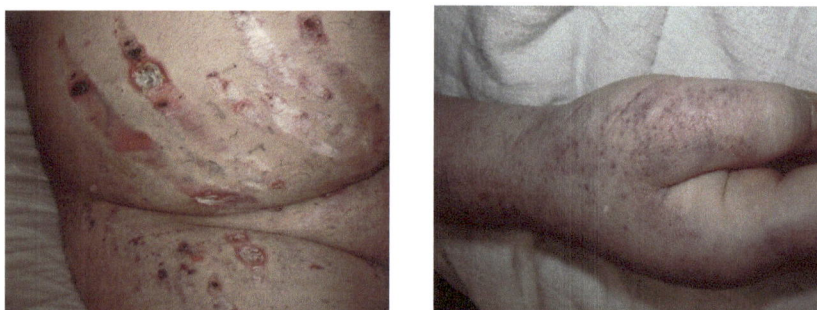

Figure 1: Skin toxicity during treatment with sunitinib. (A) Ulceration of abdominal wall skin striae that preexisted in a patient treated concomitantly with high doses of corticoids (2x 32 mg per day). (B) Petichial rash at the hand (in the absence of thrombocytopenia or coagulopathy).

A stabilization or slight decrease in CBV_{LTN} and CBF_{LTN} was observed in 6 out of 14 evaluable patients (25%) after 4 weeks of sunitinib treatment. This effect however was transient and could not be confirmed after 8 week in any of the patients. Reduced gadolinium-enhancement at evaluation by T1-MRI was also observed (Fig. **2**). No patient obtained an objective tumor response according to Macdonald criteria. Five out of 19 (26%) evaluable patients had a stable disease (SD) on T1+/-Gd MRI-imaging of the brain after 8 weeks of treatment but all had progressive disease (PD) before 16 weeks. One patient (1,7%) experienced a marked clinical improvement with a less intense FMP-avidity of his glioma on PET (suggesting a decreased tumor metabolism) (Fig. **3**). When treatment was withheld at progression in this patient, an accelerated neurological deterioration was observed within a few day after stopping treatment. After resuming treatment with sunitinib in this patient, his conditioning improved rapidly and he continued treatment for reasons of symptomatic palliation for a total of 33 weeks. After a median follow-up of 11 months, the median time to progression (TTP) and overall survival (OS) for the total study population are 1,6 and 3,8 months respectively. None of the patients was free from progression at 6 months (0% 6-mths PFS).

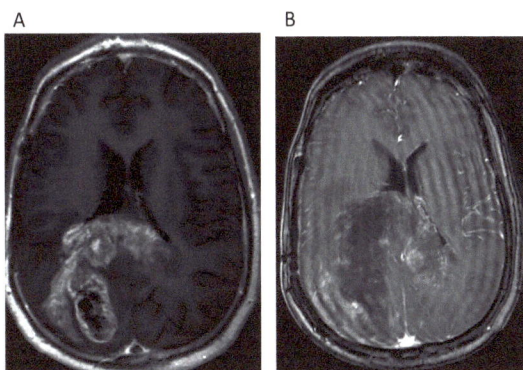

Figure 2: MRI images (T1 with gadolinium) showing marked reduction of gadolinium enhancement following 4 weeks of sunitinib treatment (B) as compared to baseline (A). Tumor dimensions however increased.

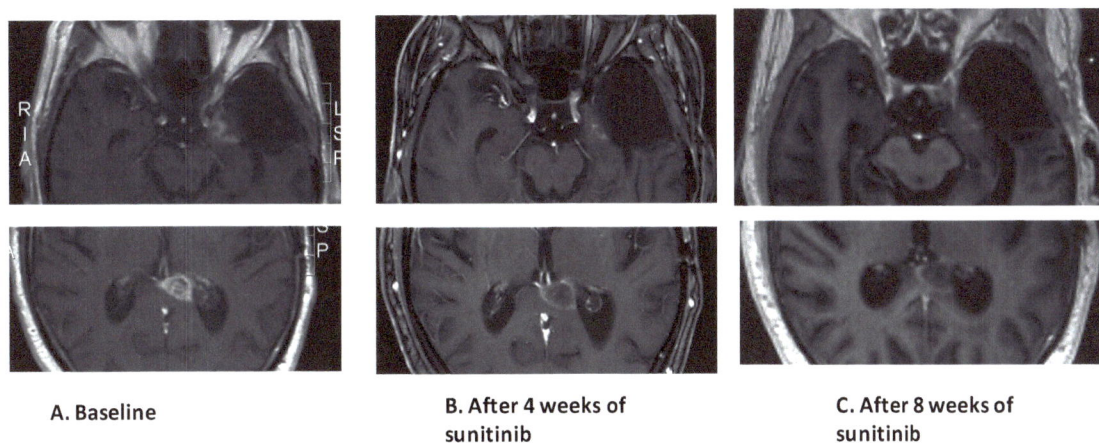

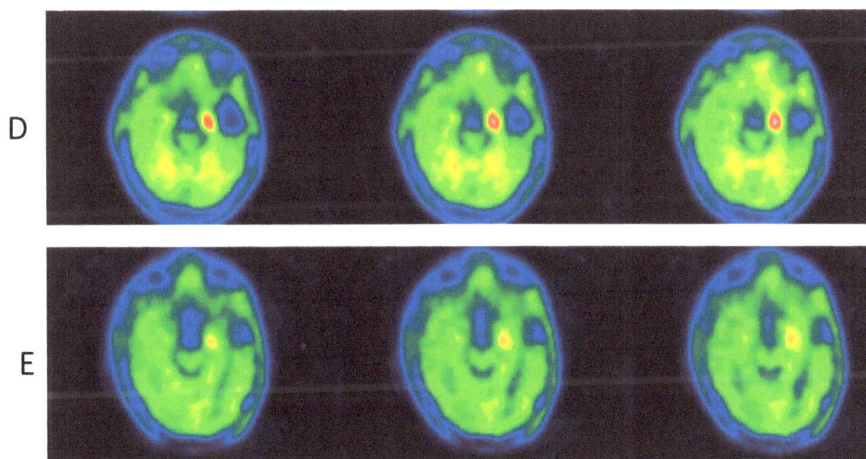

Figure 3: MRI images (T1 with gadolinium) during Sunitinib therapy in a 60 year old male patient with recurrent glioblastoma following surgery (left temporal lobectomy) and recurrence at the medial side of the resection cavity and at a new distant site median of the left posterior horn of the lateral ventricle. A gradual decrease in gadolinium enhancement is observed following 4 (A) and 8 weeks (B) of sunitinib treatment. The crossectional diameters of the paraventricular lesion however remain unchanged. On metabolic imaging (FMP-PET) a marked reduction of enhancement is observed at the recurrence at the border of the resection cavity after 8 weeks of sunitinib therapy (E) as compared to baseline (D).

Gene amplification of the VEGFR2, PDGFRa and KIT genes has been observed in glioblastomas and to a lesser extends in anaplastic gliomas [6-7]. An exploratory characterization was performed to determine the gene copy number for VEGFR2, PDGFRa and Kit genes. An informative test result by *chromogenic in situ hybridization*

(CISH) was obtained on all except 2 patients. Co-amplification (> 6 gene copies per cell) for all three genes was found in the tumor cells from 2 patients (isolated gene amplification for the three genes tested were not detected in any tumor). Both patients with amplified tumors however did not respond to treatment with sunitinib.

Of potential interest is the off-study observation on three patients with a secondary glioblastoma (all had an age of less than 40 year at recruitment) who achieved an objective partial response (according to Macdonald criteria and confirmed after at least 4 weeks in 2 patients) when administered CCNU (at a dose of 80 mg/m^2) at the time of progression under sunitinib mono-therapy. TTP of these patients was 2, 8 and +80 months respectively). In the one patient with the longest TTP, CCNU was initially administered immediately after stopping study treatment with sunitinib and thereafter on day 15 of a 4 week administration of sunitinib (repeated every 6 to 8 weeks).

Our single center study on sunitinib has meanwhile been amended and we have initiated recruitment of a second cohort of patients with recurrent secondary glioblastomas (patients should have had an initial diagnosis of low-grade or anaplastic glioma and have recurrent disease following prior surgery, radiation therapy and alkylating chemotherapy). Sunitinib is initiated at a daily dose of 25 mg and CCNU is administered at a dose of 80 mg/m^2 on day 15 of a 6 week treatment cycle).

Additional phase I/II trials on sunitinib in patients with CNS glioma have been initiated worldwide among which are 2 protocols for patients with recurrent disease sponsored by the NCI [NCT00499473, NCT00713388], a trial conducted within the EU [NCT00535379], and a phase I study that will administer sunitinib concomitantly with RT [NCT00437372] .

CONCLUSIONS

Sunitinib is a multi-targeted cellular kinase inhibitor that has demonstrated both anti-angiogenic as well as cytotoxic effects in different types of cancers. Early clinical results suggest that sunitinib may have considerable toxicity in patients with recurrent glioma who had prior exposure to radiation therapy and alkylating chemotherapy. Especially hematological adverse events might be more frequent and more important as compared with the adverse events related to treatment with the VEGF-targeted monoclonal antibody bevacizumab and possibly also as compared to some other small molecule VEGFR-targeted kinase inhibitors that are currently under development for the treatment of recurrent glioma (some with more restricted targeting to the VEGFR). Inhibition of FLT3 (fms-related tyrosine kinase, Flk2, stk-2), a kinase that is expressed on immature hematopoietic progenitors, as well as some mature myeloid and lymphoid cells and that regulates the survival and proliferation of hematopoietic progenitor cells is likely to be responsible for the hematological toxicity of sunitinib [8]. In addition, Kit is also expressed on c-KIT is produced by the KIT gene, which is expressed on hematopoietic progenitor cells. Patients with prior exposure to alylating agents such as temozolomide and/or the nitrosurea (e.g. BCNU [carmustine] and CCNU [lomustine]) may be more susceptible to this toxicity

Whether the study of sunitinib for the treatment of CNS gliomas is indicated beyond the ongoing early phase I/II trials is likely to depend on the fact whether the more broad spectrum of kinase inhibition offered by sunitinib is advantageous as compared to alternative, more restricted VEGF(R) targeted agents. Such agents are currently available and some are under study for the treatment of CNS gliomas (such as the monoclonal antibody bevacizumab, the VEGF targeted agent aflibercept or the small molecule VEGFR-TKI cediranib; or potentially also axitinib (AG-013736, an alternative small molecule TKI developed by Pfizer that exhibits a VEGFR2 inhibitory activity at a more than 10-fold lower concentration as compared to sunitinib) [9]. Given the potential role of KIT and PDGFR in the biology of some gliomas, sunitinib might be particularly advantageous in these subsets of patients. Sunitinib may also have the potential for synergy in combination with alkylating agents (at least in gliomas that are sensitive to these agents). Such combinations might not only be of interest because of the known potential enhancement of VEGF-inhibition with cytotoxic agents but also because of the inhibition of additional growth an survival promoting signal transduction pathways by sunitinib. Individual molecular-genetic profiling of gliomas, e.g. in terms of expression and amplification of VEGFR2, KIT and PDGFRa as potential targets for sunitinib, e.g. Epidermal Growth Factor Receptor amplification/mutation or MET amplification as potential factors for resistance, and e.g. the methylation status of the MGMT gene promoter as predictor for sensitivity to alkylatig cytotoxic agents is likely to be useful to identify the subpopulation of glioma patients that could benefit from sunitinib.

AUTHOR DISCLOSURE INFORMATION

B. Neyns received research funding and financial compensation for public speaking from Schering-Plough and Pfizer.

REFERENCES

[1] DeAngelis L.M. Brain tumors. N Engl J Med 2001; 344(2): 114-23.

[2] Louis D.N. The 2007 WHO classification of tumours of the central nervous system. Acta Neuropathol 2007; 114(2): 97-109.

[3] Stupp R. Radiotherapy plus concomitant and adjuvant temozolomide for glioblastoma. N Engl J Med 2005; 352(10): 987-96.

[4] Chow L.Q., S.G. Eckhardt. Sunitinib: from rational design to clinical efficacy. J Clin Oncol 2007; 25(7): 884-96.

[5] Macdonald D.R. Response criteria for phase II studies of supratentorial malignant glioma. J Clin Oncol 1990; 8(7): 1277-80.

[6] Joensuu H. Amplification of genes encoding KIT, PDGFRalpha and VEGFR2 receptor tyrosine kinases is frequent in glioblastoma multiforme. J Pathol 2005; 207(2): 224-31.

[7] Puputti M. Amplification of KIT, PDGFRA, VEGFR2, and EGFR in gliomas. Mol Cancer Res 2006; 4(12): 927-34.

[8] Chow L.Q.M., S.G. Eckhardt. Sunitinib: From Rational Design to Clinical Efficacy. J Clin Oncol 2007; 25(7): 884-896.

[9] Batchelor T.T. AZD2171, a pan-VEGF receptor tyrosine kinase inhibitor, normalizes tumor vasculature and alleviates edema in glioblastoma patients. Cancer Cell 2007; 11(1): 83-95.

CHAPTER 26

Cilengitide: A Novel Integrin Antagonist, in Malignant Glioma

L. Burt Nabors*

Neuro oncology Program, University of Alabama at Birmingham, 510 20th Street South, FOT 1020, Birmingham, AL 35294

Abstract: Cilengitide is a novel cyclic peptide that demonstrates anti-integrin activity. In laboratory studies, cilengitide binds with high affinity to the intergrins $\alpha v \beta 3$ and $\alpha v \beta 5$. It blocks proliferation of cells expressing this class of integrins and results in antiangiogenic and antitumor activity in animal models. Cilengitide has found a niche for clinical development in the population of patients affected by malignant glioma. The clinical evaluation has thus far found an overall high safety profile with limited toxicity and improved clinical outcomes in both recurrent and newly diagnosed glioma patients. This review intends to provide an overview of the preclinical development, summary of clinical trials to date, and update on ongoing and active therapeutic studies.

INTRODUCTION

Cilengitide is a novel antagonist of the integrins, $\alpha v \beta 3$ and $\alpha v \beta 5$ that has found a unique role in clinical trial development for glioblastoma multiforme (GBM). GBM is the most common of the malignant gliomas for which therapy brings a median overall survival of around 15 months [1]. Unfortunately, this survival is often associated with a substantial decline in neurological function resulting in a loss in quality of life and increasing stress on caregivers. Malignant gliomas are characterized by cellular behaviors promoting intense angiogenesis with tumor infiltration and invasion of the normal brain. It is these phenotypes that contribute significantly to the morbidity and mortality suffered by patients. An improved understanding of the underlying molecular events which result in these behaviors should advance and improve our ability to more effective treat this disease.

Integrins are a class of cell surface molecules implicated in the survival and migration of cells [2,3]. The class compromises a group of 24 transmembrane receptors composed of paired alpha and beta domains. The domain pairing influences interactions with extracellular matrix ligands and impact cellular functions [4]. The cerebral microenvironment of astrocytic tumors is characterized by high levels of vitronectin [5]. The arginine-glycine-aspartic acid (RGD) peptide sequence in vitronectin is recognized by the integrins, $\alpha v \beta 3$ and $\alpha v \beta 5$. Engagement of the integrin with the appropriate ligand promotes cell survival and migration. In the context of central nervous system tumors, there is expression of the integrins $\alpha v \beta 3$ and $\alpha v \beta 5$ by both the proliferating tumor-associated vessels but also the glioma cells themselves [6,7]. Preclinical studies relevant to glioma have demonstrated universal expression of the integrins $\alpha v \beta 3$ and $\alpha v \beta 5$ by established glioma cells [8]. In addition, the treatment of rodent models of human glioma with anti-integrin agents either alone or in combination with radiation therapy results in a marked improvement in animal survival [8,9]. Interestingly, a preferential sensitivity of tumor xenografts placed in the brain versus subcutaneously exist for cyclic-RGD containing compounds. MacDonald et al demonstrated tumor response only within the context of the brain microenvironment and an absence of response to flank placed tumors [10]. Thus the preclinical evaluation of integrin and ligand expression in cerebral tumors as well as the behavior in tumor models supports the clinical exploration of integrin antagonist in glioma.

Cilengitide (EMD 121974, Merck KGaA, Darmstadt, Germany) is a cyclic pentapeptide (Arg-Gly-Asp-DPhe-(NMeVal)). The RGD peptide sequence binds with high affinity to the integrins $\alpha v \beta 3$ and $\alpha v \beta 5$. *In vitro* binding studies and cell-based assays indicate a binding affinity in the nanomolar range and integrin antagonism in the low micromolar range [11]. Based on the presence of the cilengitide target and encouraging studies in cell and animal models, human clinical trials were undertaken to define the safety and activity in malignant glioma.

*Address correspondence to L. Burt Nabors: Neuro oncology Program, University of Alabama at Birmingham, 510 20th Street South, FOT 1020, Birmingham, AL 35294; Tel: 205-934-1813, Email: bnabors@uab.edu

CLINICAL TRIALS

Phase I

The initial clinical trial in glioma was a phase I completed by the New Approached to Brain Tumor Therapy (NABTT) National Cancer Institute consortium under an agreement between the manufacture of cilengitide (EMD 121974), Merck KGaA (Darmstadt, Germany) and the Cancer Therapy and Evaluation Program (CTEP) (Fig. **1**). At the time this trial was initiated, cilengitide had completed early phase studies in systemic solid cancers where it was well-tolerated but did not illicit a suggestion of biological activity [12]. The NABTT trial was designed as a dose escalation study open to patients with recurrent malignant glioma. The investigational agent was started at a dose of 120 mg/m^2 and escalated to 2400 mg/m^2 without the delineation of a maximum tolerated dose (MTD). Only a single grade 3 hematological toxicity was described. The remainder of the grade 3 or 4 adverse events include thrombosis, myalgia, arthralgia, or abnormal serum chemistries. No patient in this study had a tumor-associated hemorrhage. Intensive pharmacokinetics were performed that demonstrated a relatively short half-life (t $_{1/2}$) of 2.5 hours, renal clearance, and no real impact by hepatic enzyme-inducing anticonvulsant drugs. Of the total 51 patients enrolled, there were two complete responses, three patients with partial responses, and four with stable disease. In addition, perfusion MRI was longitudinally completed on enrolled subjects and a pharmacodynamic model developed to model changes in the perfusion parameters (rCBF and rCBV) with pharmacokinetic parameters (Cmax and AUC). This suggested a relationship between higher doses of cilengitide and perfusion decreases [13]. This trial concluded that cilengitide was tolerated in this patient population, flat dosing of the drug was feasible, and higher doses of the compound were more likely to promote perfusion changes.

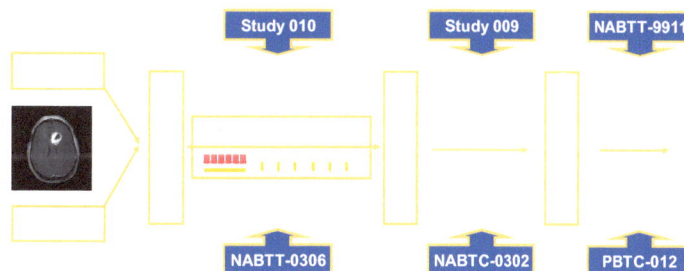

Figure 1: The schematic illustrates the clinical development of cilengitide in malignant glioma.

A companion phase I trial of cilengitide as monotherapy in patients with recurrent or refractory brain tumors also occurred in the pediatric population. This study followed a similar design and treatment schedule as the NABTT trial. In the pediatric study, cilengitide was escalated from 120 mg/m^2 to 2400 mg/m^2 without dose limiting toxicities and again an MTD was not defined. However, 3 of 13 patients treated at the 2400 mg/m^2 dose level experienced grade 3 or 4 intratumoral hemorrhage possibly related to study drug. It was commented that by current toxicity criteria, two of the hemorrhages were asymptomatic and would be classified as grade 1. Biological activity was again suggested as three patients completed one-year of treatment with one GBM patient having a complete response [14] (Fig. **2**).

Phase II

A total of three phase II trials were undertaken with cilengitide in both the recurrent and newly diagnosed settings. In both situations, the trials became more focused enrolling glioblastoma multiforme (GBM) exclusively. The initial effort was led by David Reardon and focused on recurrent disease GBM with a randomized phase II design of two different flat doses of cilengitide in an effort to better define the optimal dose. This trial assigned patients to either receive 500 mg or 2000 mg by twice a week intravenous infusion. A total of 81 patients were randomized. The two arms were well matched for age, gender, functional status, and previous surgery. Overall, this trial provided additional data that cilengitide is well tolerated in the GBM population. There was a trend toward increased activity with the higher dose of cilengitide, 2000 mg than 500 mg. For progression-free survival, at 6 months the 2000 mg cohort was 15% and the 500 mg was 10%. Median overall survival also favored the 2000 mg dose at 10 months versus 7 months for the 500 mg dose [15]. This trial continued to support the tolerability of cilengitide in the malignant glioma population and the randomized design demonstrated that higher doses of the drug (2000 mg) appeared to have more biological activity.

Pretreatment   **Post cycle 24**

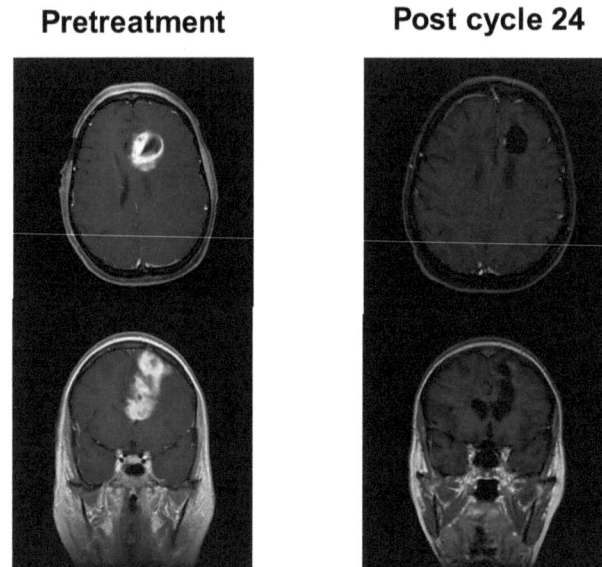

Figure 2: A post-contrast MRI in both the axial (top) and coronal (bottom) planes demonstrating the resolution of enhancement following administration of cilengitide.

The next step in cilengitides development saw the compound move to the newly diagnosed setting and utilize a combination approach with standard of care radiation therapy and temozolomide. A phase II trial combining the low dose of cilengitide (500 mg) with chemoradiation for newly diagnosed GBM was completed using progression free survival (PFS) as a primary endpoint [16]. In this trial, 52 GBM patients received cilengitide by a twice a week IV infusion concurrent with temozolomide and radiation therapy followed by 6 months of temozolomide and cilengitide. Overall, the 6 month PFS was 69% with a PFS of 8 months which compared favorably to the EORTC phase III trial of temozolomide and radiation therapy of 6.9 months. A retrospective subgroup analysis based on patient methyl-guanine methyltransferase (MGMT) status found a PFS in patients with methylated MGMT promoter of 13.4 months suggesting an enhanced benefit in this population. Concurrent to this trial, a U.S. trial sponsored by CTEP enrolled 112 patients in a safety-run in followed by a randomized phase II trial for newly diagnosed GBM. The randomized phase II component utilized the low dose of 500 mg and the high dose of 2000 mg for the cohorts. The safety-run used three predefined doses of 500, 1000, and 2000 mg of cilengitide. A total of 18 patients were enrolled to evaluate the tolerability and safety of cilengitide when given with radiation and chemotherapy. There were no DLTs related to cilengitide. The randomized phase II component enrolled 94 patients. The trial is closed to accrual and patients continue to be followed for survival.

Phase III

Cilengitide has completed a fairly rigorous and comprehensive clinical study in malignant glioma in both the recurrent and newly diagnosed settings. Trials evaluated safety as well as evidence to support biological activity both in adults and children and when given as monotherapy as well as in combination with standard malignant glioma radiation and chemotherapy. Based on an acceptable safety profile and clear evidence for an advantage with the higher flat dose (2000 mg), cilengitide was entered a world-wide, randomized phase III trial in late 2008. This trial is designed as a prospective molecular characterization of eligibility with only patients demonstrating methylation of the MGMT promoter eligible. Patients are randomized to either a standard treatment arm of radiation therapy with concurrent temozolomide or to an arm of cilengitide at 2000 mg twice a week with radiation therapy and concurrent temozolomide.

SUMMARY

The development of cilengitide in central nervous system malignancies offers unique insights into glioma biology and therapy development. Despite the lack of a clinical signal in systemic solid cancer clinical trials, a clear indication of biological activity arose in early phase glioma trials. This activity became more focused and clear with larger studies and with the inclusion of combination therapy utilizing standard of care modalities for glioma. The identification of the exact mechanism in which integrin antagonism exerts a clinical benefit is not as clear. Two possible mechanisms exist. The first, as an anti-angiogenic compound for which cilengitide was originally conceived, exist but may not be the primary mechanism in glioma. The expression of integrins by glioma cells themselves and a role in tumor invasion, the clinical and pathological hallmark of this disease, supports a role as an anti-proliferative and anti-invasion mechanism as well. Given the clear clinical benefit of anti-angiogenic compounds targeted toward vascular endothelial growth factor (VEGF) inhibition, the future clinical development of cilengitide in combination with these compounds suggest an opportunity to promote synergistic effects toward multiple tumor behaviors that lead to tremendous morbidity and mortality for patients.

REFERENCES

[1]   Stupp R, Mason WP, van den Bent MJ, *et al.* Radiotherapy plus concomitant and adjuvant temozolomide for glioblastoma. N Engl J Med. 2005 Mar 10;352(10):987-96.

[2]   Varner JA, Cheresh DA. Integrins and cancer. Curr Opin Cell Biol. 1996 Oct;8(5):724-30.

[3]   Stromblad S, Cheresh DA. Integrins, angiogenesis and vascular cell survival. Chem Biol. 1996 Nov;3(11):881-5.

[4]   Barczyk M, Carracedo S, Gullberg D. Integrins. Cell Tissue Res. 2009 Aug 20.

[5]   Gladson CL, Wilcox JN, Sanders L, *et al.* Cerebral microenvironment influences expression of the vitronectin gene in astrocytic tumors. J Cell Sci. 1995 Mar;108 (Pt 3):947-56.

[6]   Schnell O, Krebs B, Wagner E, *et al.* Expression of integrin alphavbeta3 in gliomas correlates with tumor grade and is not restricted to tumor vasculature. Brain Pathol. 2008 Jul;18(3):378-86.

[7]   Bello L, Francolini M, Marthyn P, *et al.* Alpha(v)beta3 and alpha(v)beta5 integrin expression in glioma periphery. Neurosurgery. 2001 Aug;49(2):380-9; discussion 90.

[8]   Chatterjee S, Matsumura A, Schradermeier J, *et al.* Human malignant glioma therapy using anti-alpha(v)beta3 integrin agents. J Neurooncol. 2000;46(2):135-44.

[9]   Mikkelsen T, Brodie C, Finniss S, *et al.* Radiation sensitization of glioblastoma by cilengitide has unanticipated schedule-dependency. Int J Cancer. 2009 Jun 1;124(11):2719-27.

[10]   MacDonald TJ, Taga T, Shimada H, *et al.* Preferential susceptibility of brain tumors to the antiangiogenic effects of an alpha(v) integrin antagonist. Neurosurgery. 2001 Jan;48(1):151-7.

[11]   Germer M, Kanse SM, Kirkegaard T, *et al.* Kinetic analysis of integrin-dependent cell adhesion on vitronectin--the inhibitory potential of plasminogen activator inhibitor-1 and RGD peptides. Eur J Biochem. 1998 May 1;253(3):669-74.

[12]   Eskens FA, Dumez H, Hoekstra R, *et al.* Phase I and pharmacokinetic study of continuous twice weekly intravenous administration of Cilengitide (EMD 121974), a novel inhibitor of the integrins alphavbeta3 and alphavbeta5 in patients with advanced solid tumours. Eur J Cancer. 2003 May;39(7):917-26.

[13]   Nabors LB, Mikkelsen T, Rosenfeld SS, *et al.* Phase I and correlative biology study of cilengitide in patients with recurrent malignant glioma. J Clin Oncol. 2007 May 1;25(13):1651-7.

[14]   MacDonald TJ, Stewart CF, Kocak M, *et al.* Phase I clinical trial of cilengitide in children with refractory brain tumors: Pediatric Brain Tumor Consortium Study PBTC-012. J Clin Oncol. 2008 Feb 20;26(6):919-24.

[15]   Vredenburgh JJ, Desjardins A, Herndon JE, 2nd, *et al.* Phase II trial of bevacizumab and irinotecan in recurrent malignant glioma. Clin Cancer Res. 2007 Feb 15;13(4):1253-9.

[16]   Stupp R, Goldbrunner R, Neyns B, *et al.* Phase I/IIa trial of cilengitide (EMD121974) and temozolomide with concomitant radiotherapy, followed by temozolomide and cilengitide maintenance therapy in patients with newly diagnosed glioblastoma (GBM). J Clin Oncol. 2007;25

CHAPTER 27

Development of Sorafenib in Malignant Gliomas: Rationale and Early Clinical Experience

Rachel Grossman[1],* and Jaishri Blakeley[2]

Department of Neurosurgery[1] and Neurology[2] and Johns Hopkins School of Medicine, Baltimore, MD

Abstract: Sorafenib is a multi-targeted receptor tyrosine kinase inhibitor (TKI), with activity against vascular endothelial growth factor receptor-1 (VEGFR-1), VEGFR-2, VEGFR-3, Raf-1, B-Raf, C-Raf, and platelet-derived growth factor receptor (PDGFR) -α and -β. Currently, sorafenib has regulatory approval for use in metastatic renal cell carcinoma and hepatocellular carcinoma. An attractive activity profile, pre-clinical evidence of antitumor activity in human malignant glioma models and a promising safety profile have led to recent phase I/II clinical trials for patients with malignant gliomas. Here we review the current data, and future directions for the development of sorafenib for malignant glioma.

INTRODUCTION

Glioblastoma Multiforme (GBM) is the most common primary brain tumor in adults and accounts for more than 50% of all gliomas. It is also the most deadly of the gliomas and despite advances in neurosurgical techniques, radiation therapy and chemotherapy, the median survival remains roughly 12-14 months [1]. The current standard of care includes maximal tolerated tumor resection, intensity modulated radiation therapy (RT) and temozolomide (TMZ). Recognizing the critical need for new approaches to improve the outcome for patients with malignant gliomas, dozens of antineoplastic agents have been tested in clinical trials for patients with malignant gliomas. A major area of interest is in small molecules that are expected to be better able to cross the blood brain barrier (BBB) to reach brain cancer cells and have a more favorable side effect profile than traditional cytotoxic therapies. Small molecule inhibitors have been developed to target a variety of pathways thought to be critical to the development, progression and migration of brain cancers [2,3,4].

Angiogenesis, and the many pathways that contribute to regulation of angiogenesis, are important in the development of all solid tumors. However, it is particularly important in malignant gliomas as these tumors are known to be among the most vascular of all solid tumors. Angiogenesis not only plays an important role in driving tumor growth and development, but also in the signs and symptoms experienced by patients due to peritumoral edema [5]. Recently bevacizumab, a monoclonal antibody against vascular endothelial growth factor (VEGF), became the first anti-angiogenesis drug approved for use in patients with recurrent GBM via accelerated approval by the Food and Drug Administration (FDA). This was in large part based on its ability to reduce tumor related edema and therefore improve patient function. However, bevacizumab is a large monoclonal antibody that may not have an access to tumor cells and it targets only VEGF. This single site inhibition may allow tumors to forge alternative angiogenic pathways and therefore become resistant to VEGF inhibition [6]. Hence, it is of great importance to identify agents that may complement bevacizumab potentially allowing for both improvement in patient function and longer term tumor control in malignant gliomas.

Development of Sorafenib for Solid Tumors

Sorafenib (Nexavar; Bayer HealthCare Pharmaceuticals, West Haven, CT, and Onyx Pharmaceuticals, Emeryville, CA) is a multi-targeted receptor TKI that inhibits tumor-cell proliferation and tumor angiogenesis by targeting:

- The serine-threonine kinases Raf-1, B-Raf, and C-Raf

- The receptor tyrosine kinases of VEGFR-1, VEGFR-2, VEGFR-3, and platelet-derived growth factor receptors (PDGFR)-α and -β. [7]

*Address correspondence to Rachel Grossman:** The Johns Hopkins Oncology Center, 600 North Wolfe Street, Baltimore, MD, 21287, US; Tel: 410-955-8837 Email: grossman@jhmi.edu

Thomas C. Chen (Ed)

Hence, it targets many of the proteins central to angiogenic pathways. It is possible that by inhibiting these multiple pro-angiogenic targets, an agent can avoid "angiogenic escape" that may more readily occur with single target inhibition [6,8]. It is an attractive agent in that it is oral, has been widely tested and therefore has well described pharmacokinetics and predictable and manageable side effects. Moreover, it has been used safely in combination with other TKIs and cytotoxic therapies in systemic solid tumors [9,10]. Thus far, sorafenib has been approved by the FDA and the European Commission for the treatment of advanced renal cell carcinoma and advanced hepatocellular carcinoma.

Renal Cell Carcinoma (RCC)

In 2005, sorafenib was the first drug to be approved for the treatment of advanced RCC by the US FDA since 1992 [11]. Following encouraging results of a phase I study [12], the efficacy of sorafenib in the treatment of RCC was suggested by a phase II randomized study of 65 patients [13]. Median progression-free survival (PFS) was significantly longer among the sorafenib-treated patients in comparison with those receiving placebo (24 vs. 6 weeks, P =0.0087). A subsequent phase III study investigated 903 patients with RCC refractory to standard therapies randomized to receive sorafenib or placebo [14]. There was significantly better PFS for patients receiving sorafenib in comparison with those receiving placebo (5.5 months vs. 2.8 months; P < 0.0001). Although there was a trend in benefit for overall survival (OS), this did not reach statistical significance [14].

Hepatocellular Carcinoma (HCC)

Sorafenib is the only approved drug that has shown improvement in OS in patients with advanced HCC to date [7]. An international, phase III, placebo-controlled Sorafenib HCC Assessment Randomized Protocol (SHARP) trial was conducted and demonstrated a longer OS and time-to-tumor progression (TTP) for sorafenib treated patients compared to placebo [15]. The median OS was 10.7 months in the sorafenib group and 7.9 months in the placebo group (hazard ratio 0.69; 95% CI 0.55-0.87, P< 0.001). Sorafenib also extended the median TTP (5.5 months sorafenib versus 2.8 months placebo) (P < 0.001) [15].

Breast Carcinoma

A multinational, open-label phase II study investigated sorafenib 400mg BID continuous dosing in patients with metastatic breast cancer progressive after standard chemotherapy. No complete responses were observed in the 54 patients treated, however, 2% and 37% of the patients had partial response and stable disease, respectively. In 22% of the patients, disease stabilization was maintained for $\geq$16 weeks. The most common drug-related grade 3 adverse events were rash (6%), hand-foot skin reaction (4%), and fatigue (4%) [16]

Non Small Cell Lung Carcinoma (NSCLC)

Currently, there are several trials with sorafenib in non-small cell lung cancer (NSCLC). Results of a multicenter, phase II trial were recently reported for 54 patients with relapsed or refractory NSCLC [17]. Stable disease (SD) was achieved in 30 of the 51 evaluable patients (59%) and maintained for a median of 5.5 months. Median PFS was 2.7 months, and median OS was 6.7 months. As in other solid tumor trials, grades 3-4 treatment-related toxicities included hand-foot skin reaction (10%), hypertension (4%), fatigue (2%), and diarrhea (2%). Nine patients died within a 30-day period after discontinuing sorafenib, and one patient experienced pulmonary hemorrhage thought to be drug related [17].

Thyroid Carcinoma

A patient with thyroid cancer in a phase II trial for advanced solid tumors showed tumor shrinkage [18]. This prompted two phase II trials in patients with metastatic thyroid carcinoma. The first study involved 30 patients with metastatic thyroid carcinoma [19]. After minimum 16 weeks of 400mg sorafenib BID, 23% of the patients had partial response, and 53% had stable disease. The median PFS was 79 weeks. The second study, included 41 patients with metastatic papillary thyroid carcinoma (PTC) [20]. Median PFS was 15 months and 15% of patients had a partial response; 56% had stable disease for more than 6 months. Grade 3 toxicities again included hand-foot skin reaction, musculoskeletal pain, and fatigue. Although sorafenib has not yet been approved for the treatment of thyroid carcinomas, based on these results sorafenib is often prescribed for select patients with advanced thyroid carcinoma [21].

RATIONAL FOR DEVELOPING SORAFENIB IN GLIOMA

As mentioned, sorafenib targets multiple pathways shown to be important in the proliferation and migration of malignant gliomas. It has a low molecular weight of 464.8 g/mol suggesting it is amenable to transport across the BBB. By way of comparison, the molecular weight of Gd-DTPA commonly used as a contrast agent for magnetic resonance imaging (MRI) of brain tumors is 590g/mol. There is further pre-clinical evidence that it has the potential to reach effective concentrations in brain as it may not be subject to the ATP-binding cassette (ABC) transporters that often exclude chemotherapies from brain [22]. In analysis of the effect of ABC transporters on sorafenib pharmacokinetics, Hu et. al. showed that although it subject to some of the transporters, it still achieves brain concentrations in the range of 300 ng/mL [22]. This is substantially lower than plasma concentrations (roughy 3% of plasma), however, it may be sufficient for clinical activity and indeed reponses in brain metastases from solid tumors have been reported with single agent sorafenib [22, 23, 24].

PRE-CLINICAL EVIDENCE FOR SORAFENIB IN GLIOMAS

Preclinical investigation of sorafenib in glioma models showed sorafenib results in decreased cell proliferation, G1 phase growth arrest, and impaired migration via prevention of VEGFR and PDGFR phosphorylation [25, 26]. Jane *et al.*studied U87 and T98G cell lines *in vitro* and found that sorafenib inhibited the phosphorylation of several receptors of tyrosine kinases including VEGFR-2, mouse VEGFR-3, mouse PDGFR-β, Flt-3, c-KIT, and fibroblast growth factor receptor-1 (FGFR-1) at low micromolar concentrations. Furthermore, they reported that sorafenib was capable of inhibiting cellular proliferation in a dose-dependent manner in several human malignant glioma models. Sorafenib also induced mitochondrially mediated apoptotic cell death and limited the migration of U87 and T98G cells [25]. Additional studies have shown that sorafenib in combination with bortezomib (a proteosome inhibitor) act synergistically to cause apoptosis in U251 and D37 glioma cell lines [26].

CLINICAL EXPERIENCE IN GLIOMA

The safety and toxicity of sorafenib has been investigated in several phase I studies [27, 28, 29] in patients with solid tumors (n = 173). Doses ranged from 50 mg to 800 mg once or twice daily. The maximal tolerated dose (MTD) was 400 mg given continuously twice daily. The most common dose limiting toxicities were diarrhea, fatigue, and rash. Additional toxicities noted were hand-foot neuropathy and hypertension. Based on the toxicity data, 400mg twice-daily dose was the recommended dose for efficacy trials in systemic solid tumors.

However, systemic solid tumor trials may yield different dose recommendations than phase I studies in patients with gliomas based on the specific features of glioma management and pathophysiology (i.e. need for anti-epileptics, underlying nervous system disease). In addition, it is recognized that combination therapy will likely be required for meaningful efficacy in gliomas and phase I trials are required to determine the toxicity and tolerability of multi-agent combinations. This is particularly true when assessing combinations of TKIs that may have overlapping toxicities. Hence, several phase I/II trials have been initiated in patients with malignant gliomas (Table 1). The clinical experience of sorafenib in glioma are not yet published in manuscripts. Hence, the clinical data presented is based on presentations from recent scientific meetings.

Table 1: Ongoing Clinical Studies of Sorafenib in Glioma

Design	Location and Clinicaltrials.gov Identifier	Study Start Date	Estimated Study Completion Date	Primary outcome Measure
Recurrent GBM: Phase I				
A Phase I Trial of sorafenib for Patients With Recurrent or Progressive Malignant Glioma	National Cancer Institute (NCI) NCT00093613	November 2004	Unspecified	• Maximum tolerated dose of sorafenib (+/- EIACDs). •Determine dose-related toxic effects of sorafenib. •Compare pharmacokinetics of sorafenib +/- EIACDs. •Determine overall survival
Phase I/II Studies of	NCI	April 2006	February 2010	•Sequential enrollment design

Sorafenib in Combination With Erlotinib, Tipifarnib or Temsirolimus in Patients With Recurrent GBM or Gliosarcoma	NCT00335764			•Maximum tolerated dose (Phase I) •Progression-free survival (PFS) at 6 months (Phase II)
A Phase I/II Trial of Sorafenib and Temsirolimus in Combination With Recurrent GBM. Phase II Trial of Bevacizumab in Combination With Sorafenib in Recurrent GBM.	NCI NCT00329719	March 2006	March 2010	•Progression-free survival at 6 months
Recurrent GBM: Phase II				
Phase II Study of Sorafenib Plus Protracted Temozolomide in Recurrent Glioblastoma Multiforme	Duke University Bayer Schering-Plough NCT00597493	September 2007	September 2011	•6 month progression free survival
A Phase II Trial of Erlotinib (OSI-774) and Sorafenib for Patients With Progression or Recurrent Glioblastoma Multiforme	NCI NCT00445588	January 2007	August 2009	•Overall survival
Phase II Trial of Bevacizumab in Combination With Sorafenib in Recurrent Glioblastoma Multiforme	NCI NCT00621686	September 2008	February 2009	•6-month progression-free survival •Safety, toxicity, and adverse events
Newly Diagnosed GBM: Phase I				
A Phase I/II Study of Sorafenib With Radiation and Temozolomide in Newly Diagnosed Glioblastoma or Gliosarcoma	M.D. Anderson Cancer Center Bayer NCT00734526	August 2008	August 2011	•To find the highest tolerable dose of sorafenib that can be given in combination with temozolomide.
Phase I Dose Finding Study of Sorafenib in Combination With Radiation Therapy and Temozolomide as a First Line Treatment of Patients With High Grade Glioma	University Hospital, Geneva,Bayer NCT00884416	March 2009	March 2011	•To evaluate safety and tolerability of sorafenib in combination with radiation and temozolomide chemotherapy in patients with newly diagnosed high grade glioma [Time Frame: 35 weeks
Newly Diagnosed GBM: Phase II				
A Phase II Trial of Concurrent Radiation Therapy and Temozolomide Followed by Temozolomide Plus Sorafenib in the First-Line Treatment of Patients With Glioblastoma Multiforme	Sarah Cannon Research Institute SCRI Oncology Research Consortium Bayer NCT00544817	April 2007	April 2009	•Feasibility, toxicity, efficacy, and be progression-free survival.

Recurrent Malignant Glioma

There are several phase I trials of sorafenib in malignant gliomas. The first study investigated sorafenib as a monotherapy (NABTT# 0401; NCT00093613). In a multi-institutional, dose escalation study maximum tolerated dose (MTD) of sorafenib in patients with recurrent malignant glioma was assessed. Thirty five patients, stratified based on the use of enzyme inducing anticonvulsants (EIAC) or not (non-EIAC) were investigated. The DLTs were: hand-foot-syndrome, pruritis, hypophosphatemia and joint pain. The MTD for the EIAC arm was 600 mg BID. The MTD for the non-EIAC arm was 800 mg BID [30].

Another phase I study (NABTC# 05-02; NCT00335764) is evaluating the tolerability of sorafenib in combination with either erlotinib, tipifarnib or temsirolimus [31]. Erlotinib is an inhibitor of the epidermal-like growth factor (EGFR). The EGFR pathway is thought to promote signal cascades leading to cell proliferation, angiogenesis and inhibition of apoptosis. Temsirolimus (CCI-779) is an inhibitor of the mammalian target of rapamycin (mTOR) [32], and tipifarnib is farnesyl protein transferase inhibitor [33]. In patients with recurrent GBM erlotinib was started on day 1 followed by sorafenib on day 2. The MTD was defined as 400 mg of sorafenib twice a day with 100 mg of erlotinib once a day. The sorafenib pharmacokinetics (PK) were not affected by the co-administration of erlotinib. However, sorafenib affected the erlotinib PK resulting in decreased erlotinib concentrations. The major grade 3 or 4 toxicities were transaminitis, hypertension, hypophosphatemia, and increased lipase [31]. Although this combination was relatively well tolerated, the MTD was lower than seen in prior studies. The phase II portion of this study has completed enrollment, but is not yet reported.

Sorafenib and erlotinib has also been tested in a phase II trial in patients with progressive or recurrent GBM through the NABTT consortium (NABTT #0502; NCT00445588). The primary endpoint of that trial is OS, however, additional correlative endpoints such as tumor and blood sampling for immunohistochemistry and geneomic analyses of markers of the targeted pathways (EGFR, ras-raf-ERK, P13K-Akt-mTOR) are included to allow assessment of the relationship between biomarkers and clinical outcome. This study is completed and undergoing analysis with results expected in early 2010.

In another arm of the NABTC#05-02 trial (NCT 000335764), sorafenib was combined with temsirolimus. In 13 patients, the MTD was determined to be 400mg BID of sorafenib and 25 mg of temsirolimus weekly. Much like the sorafenib and erlotinib combination, the major toxicities were transaminitis, hypophosphatemia, fatigue, diarrhea, and hyperlipidemia. Unlike the erlotinib combination, there was no significant interaction between sorafenib and temsirolimus PKs. The phase II portion of this study assessed the 6 month PFS for patients with recurrent GBM at the MTD doses and found that of 19 patients, none remained progression free at 6 months. Hence, the study was stopped due to lack of efficacy [34].

Another phase I trial of sorafenib given with temsiroliums led by the North Central Cancer Treatment Group (NCCTG) resulted in a MTD of 200mg BID for sorafenib and 25mg/weekly for temsirolimus. At this dose 1/6 patients had a DLT (grade 3 thrombocytopenia). Again, the combination therapy resulted in a nearly 10-fold dose reduction in temsirolimus than what had been seen in prior single agent phase I studies in GBM [35]. Despite this, the NCCTG phase II trial (NCT00329719) met their interim analysis criteria for efficacy and tolerability to continue enrollment. In addition to assessing sorafenib 200mg BID and temsirolimus 25mg/week in standard recurrent GBM, this trial will incorporate two novel arms: a surgical arm to assess delivery and activity of sorafenib and temsirolimus in brain tissue as well as an arm assessing the activity of this combination for progressive disease after an anti-VEGF based therapy [36].

The third arm of NABTC#05-02 will assess sorafenib with tipifarnib. Tipifarnib is an oral farnesyltransferase inhibitor thought to sensitize glioma cells to alkylating therapies and influence several glioma promoting pathways. It has been tested as monotherapy in patients with malignant glioma and now will be combined with sorafenib to determine the optimal dose of each agent given in combination [37]. This arm remains under phase I investigation and is currently enrolling.

Finally, sorafenib is being assessed in glioma with either protracted temozolomdie or bevacizumab in the recurrent disease setting. Sorafenib at 400mg po BID is combined with daily temozlomide at 50mg/m2 in a phase II study for patients with recurrent GBM. The primary endpoint is 6 month PFS. The study has enrolled, but no results are yet available (NCT00597493). The NCCTG is assessing bevacizumab every two weeks with daily sorafenib in 14 day cycles. Thus far, 33 of the planned 53 patients have been accrued. The primary endpoints is 6 month PFS and tolerability. This study will also assess the feasibility of using DCE-MRI as a predictor of response to this treatment regimen as well as determine the relationship between the tumor biomarkers and circulating biomarkers of vascular response and clinical outcome (NCT00621686).

Newly Diagnosed Malignant Glioma

There are three ongoing studies assessing sorafenib in combination with upfront therapies for newly diagnosed malignant gliomas. The first is a phase I study to determine the MTD of sorafenib given in combination with temozolomide and radiation therapy. This is a single site study in Geneva, Switzerland (NCT00884416). A second single site phase I study at MD Anderson Cancer Center will assess the MTD of sorafenib given with concurrent radiation and temozololide and then dose intense temozolomide (75mg/m2 daily for 21/28 days) or standard adjuvant (150-200mg/m2 for 5/28 days) for cycle 1 followed by low dose temozolimde (75mg/m2 for 5/28 days) dosing for the remaining cycles (NCT00734526). The SCRI Oncology Research Consortium is investigating sorafenib added to temozolomide in the adjuvant setting of a multicenter phase II study (NCT00544817). Four weeks after completion of standard radiation therapy and concomitant temozolomide, patients with GBM receive temozolomide (150mg/m2 po days 1-5, repeated every 21 days for 6 cycles) plus sorafenib (400mg po bid daily for 24 weeks). To date, 45 patients have been enrolled and 39 completed radiation and comcomitant temozolomide therapy. Six patients were excluded from adjuvant sorafenib and temozolomide due to toxicity from standard therapy. Of the 39 patients who began treatment with temozolomide and sorafenib, 3 have completed all planned treatment, 8 remain on treatment, and 28 stopped treatment early. The preliminary results show that 2% had complete response, 11% had partial response, 49% had stable disease, and 31% had progressive disease. Grade 3/4 toxicities were uncommon, however, 16% of the patients required dose reduction of sorafenib [38].

POTENTIAL BENEFITS AND LIMITATIONS OF SORAFENIB IN GLIOMA

Sorafenib is a promising agent for malignant gliomas as it is a small molecule with a molecular weight that likely allows some access to brain tissue. It has a long half-life (25-48 hours) and high oral bioavailability [12]. It is well tolerated with limited toxicities as a monotherapy, although it has been associated with significant non-traditional toxicities when used in combination. Importantly, it inhibits multiple receptor and intracellular tyrosine kinases important for glioma development and proliferation and exhibits antiangiogenic activity [39]. Finally, unlike other tyrosine inhibitors, sorafenib does not appear to rely on active transport for cell entry and does not appear to be a high-affinity substrate for the common ABC efflux transporters [22].

However, there are several limitations including the drug related side effects [11]. The most common toxic effects are diarrhea (55%), fatigue (39%), hypertension (35%), neuropathy (22%), rash (26%), hand-foot skin reaction (23%), and stomatitis (7%). Rash in particular is very common and 91% of the 85 patients with RCC analyzed as part of a prospective study had at least 1 cutaneous reaction; 60% of the patients experienced hand-foot skin reaction [40]. Sorafenib has also been associated with significant and sustained increase in blood pressure. Regular blood pressure monitoring and strategies to address elevated blood pressure are advised [41]. Pouessel *et al.*[42] reported four patients with brain metastases from RCC who were treated with sunitinib or sorafenib that died from intra-cranial hemorrhage (ICH). However, in a phase III, randomized, double-blind, placebo-controlled trial of sorafenib that included 903 patients with RCC, no ICH was reported [14]. There are also reports of increased intracranial peritumoral edema and seizures in the setting of combination sunitinib and sorafenib therapy in patients with solid tumor brain metastases [43]. However, multiple phase I trails with other TKI combination therapies have not reported this in gliomas.

An important consideration in developing sorafenib will be establishing adequate criteria for measuring its clinical activity in brain cancer. Reliable biomarkers have not yet been identified, however, several of the studies discussed above are working to develop these for sorafenib in glioma. In solid tumor trials, sorafenib did not meet the criteria for anti-tumor activity as assessed by response using traditional radiological evaluations such as RECIST (response evaluation criteria in solid tumors). This may be due to a cytostatic more than cytotoxic mechanism of sorafenib or due to inability of traditional imaging techniques to adequately capture the clinical effect [14]. This may also be true when McDonald criteria is applied in the assessment of malignant gliomas [44]. Hence, various imaging approaches that assess the biologic effect of this antiangiogenesis therapy are in development.

Several studies have been published recently regarding the use of DCE-MRI as a marker of response to sorafenib in solid tumors. Flaherty *et al.*[45] found that DCE-MRI was a predictor to PFS after sorafenib treatment in a pilot study of patients with RCC. However, in a prospective, randomized trial, Hahn *et al.*[46] found that the DCE-MRI results before and after sorafenib treatment were too variable to reliably predict PFS in patients with metastatic RCC. Still, DCE-MRI is increasingly better understood in the setting of glioma therapy and is being used to assess treatment response to angiogenesis therapies in several trials. It will be one of the endpoints in the combination phase II trial of bevacizumab and sorafenib trial discussed above (NCT00621686).

Another potential limitation of sorafenib may be limited access to cancer cells and portions of the tumor microenvironment. A critical factor in the treatment of brain cancers is access of the drug to the tumor. As mentioned above, early investigations of sorafenib showed the brain penetration to be relatively low at 3% of plasma [22]. This is lower than other TKIs, but ongoing trials are directly measuring the delivery of sorafenib to various regions of brain tumors and its activity at targets of interest in brain cancer [22, 39]. Moreover, a portion of sorafenib's effect may be in areas (i.e., endothelium) that do not require high brain concentrations.

A final theoretical limitation of sorafenib for glioma, is that several studies of sorafenib in malignant melanoma have been dissapointing when sorafenib has been used as a monotherapy or in combination with cytotoxic therapies [47, 48]. This may be relevant as GBM and melanoma have many overlapping pathological and clinical features [49, 50]. However, a yet to be defined optimal combination with sorafenib may yield an effective and tolerable approach for both of these traditionally chemo-resistant cancers.

CONCLUSIONS

Sorafenib, a multikinase inhibitor of targets important to glioma pathobiology including VEGFR-1, VEGFR-2, VEGFR-3, Raf-1, B-Raf, C-Raf, and PDGFR -α and –β, is well into development for GBM. It is poised to deliver promising results in combination with complementary agents. However, the optimal dose for efficacy in combination is not yet clear. In phase I studies, sorafenib was well tolerated as a monotherapy, however, in combination with other agents dose reduction is often required. In ongoing phase II studies, there have been some early disappointing results when combined with temsirolimus or upfront with radiation and temozolomide [34, 38]. The required concentration of sorafenib to achieve efficacy against gliomas in patients is not yet known and there may be synergy with complementary agents that allow lower concentrations. Hence, results from the ongoing phase I trials with biologic endpoints such as tissue concentration and local activity in brain tumors are eagerly awaited (NCT00445588, NCT00329719).

Many of the sorafenib combination trials will be maturing in early 2010 and the role of sorafenib in the management of glioma will be better defined. The properties of sorafenib suggest that it will be an important agent to consider in developing an effective multi-agent strategy for glioma. However, the optimal timing, dosing and sequencing of sorafenib with other agents is not yet clear. In summary, sorafenib holds great promise for the treatment of malignant glioma. In the near future, data from current clinical trials will improve our knowledge regarding its role in treating malignant gliomas.

REFERENCES

[1]   Stupp R, Mason WP, van den Bent MJ, *et al.* European Organisation for Research and Treatment of Cancer Brain Tumor and Radiotherapy Groups; National Cancer Institute of Canada Clinical Trials Group. Radiotherapy plus concomitant and adjuvant temozolomide for glioblastoma. N Engl J Med. 2005 Mar 10;352(10):987-96.

[2]   Koul D, Shen R, Bergh S, *et al.* Inhibition of Akt survival pathway by a small-molecule inhibitor in human glioblastoma.. Mol Cancer Ther. 2006 Mar;5(3):637-44.

[3]   Norden AD, Drappatz J, Wen PY.Novel anti-angiogenic therapies for malignant gliomas. Lancet Neurol. 2008 Dec;7(12):1152-60.

[4]   Huang TT, Sarkaria SM, Cloughesy TF, *et al.* Targeted therapy for malignant glioma patients: lessons learned and the road ahead. Neurotherapeutics. 2009 Jul;6(3):500-12.

[5]   Gerstner ER, Duda DG, di Tomaso E, *et al.* VEGF inhibitors in the treatment of cerebral edema in patients with brain cancer..Nat Rev Clin Oncol. 2009 Apr;6(4):229-36.

[6]   Lucio-Eterovic AK, Piao Y, de Groot JF. Mediators of glioblastoma resistance and invasion during antivascular endothelial growth factor therapy. Clin Cancer Res. 2009 Jul 15;15(14):4589-99.

[7]   Zhu AX, Duda DG, Sahani DV, *et al.* Development of sunitinib in hepatocellular carcinoma: rationale, early clinical experience, and correlative studies Cancer J. 2009 Jul-Aug;15(4):263-8.

[8]   Jain RK, Duda DG, Willett CG, *et al.* Biomarkers of response and resistance to antiangiogenic therapy. Nat Rev Clin Oncol. 2009 Jun;6(6):327-38.

[9]   Choueiri TK, Plantade A, Elson P, *et al.* Efficacy of sunitinib and sorafenib in metastatic papillary and chromophobe renal cell carcinoma. J Clin Oncol. 2008 Jan 1;26(1):127-31.

[10] Hauschild A, Agarwala SS, Trefzer U, *et al.* Results of a phase III, randomized, placebo-controlled study of sorafenib in combination with carboplatin and paclitaxel as second-line treatment in patients with unresectable stage III or stage IV melanoma. J Clin Oncol. 2009 Jun 10;27(17):2823-30.

[11] Hahn O, Stadler W. Sorafenib. Curr Opin Oncol. 2006 Nov;18(6):615-21.

[12] Strumberg D, Richly H, Hilger RA, *et al.* Phase I clinical and pharmacokinetic study of the novel RAF kinase and vascular endothelial growth factor receptor inhibitor BAY 439006 in patients with advanced refractory solid tumors. J Clin Oncol 2005;23:965–72

[13] Ratain MJ, Eisen T, Stadler WM, *et al.* Phase II placebo-controlled randomized discontinuation trial of sorafenib in patients with metastatic renal cell carcinoma. J Clin Oncol 2006;24:2505–12.

[14] Escudier B, Eisen T, Stadler WM, *et al.* TARGET Study Group. Sorafenib in advanced clear-cell renal-cell carcinoma. N Engl J Med. 2007 Jan 11;356(2):125-34.

[15] Llovet JM, Ricci S, Mazzaferro V, *et al.* SHARP Investigators Study Group. Sorafenib in advanced hepatocellular carcinoma. N Engl J Med. 2008 Jul 24;359(4):378-90.

[16] Bianchi G, Loibl S, Zamagni C, *et al.* Phase II multicenter, uncontrolled trial of sorafenib in patients with metastatic breast cancer. Anticancer Drugs. 2009 Aug;20(7):616-24.

[17] Blumenschein GR Jr, Gatzemeier U, Fossella F, *et al.*Phase II, multicenter, uncontrolled trial of single-agent sorafenib in patients with relapsed or refractory, advanced non-small-cell lung cancer..J Clin Oncol. 2009 Sep 10;27(26):4274-80.

[18] Pacey SC, Ratain MJ, O'Dwyer PO, *et al.* Phase II antitumor activity of BAY 43-9006, a novel Raf kinase and VEGFR inhibitor, in patients with sarcoma enrolled in a randomized discontinuation study. Eur J Cancer 2:114, 2004 (abstr)

[19] Gupta-Abramson V, Troxel AB, Nellore A, *et al.* Phase II trial of sorafenib in advanced thyroid cancer. J Clin Oncol. 2008. 26:4714–4719.

[20] Kloos R, Ringel M, Knopp M, *et al.* Significant clinical and biologic activity of RAF/VEGF-R kinase inhibitor BAY 43-9006 in patients with metastatic papillary thyroid carcinoma (PTC): updated results of a phase II study. J Clin Oncol. 2006. 24:5534.

[21] Sherman SI 2008 NCCN practice guidelines for thyroid cancer, version 2008.

[22] Hu S, Chen Z, Franke R, *et al.* Interaction of the multikinase inhibitors sorafenib and sunitinib with solute carriers and ATP-binding cassette transporters. Clin Cancer Res. 2009 Oct 1;15(19):6062-9.

[23] Valcamonico F, Ferrari V, Amoroso V, *et al.* Long-lasting successful cerebral response with sorafenib in advanced renal cell carcinoma. J Neurooncol 2009;91:47–50.

[24] 24. Ranze O, Hofmann E, Distelrath A, Hoeffkes HG. Renal cell cancer presented with leptomeningeal carcinomatosis effectively treated with sorafenib.Onkologie. 2007 Sep;30(8-9):450-1.

[25] Jane EP, Premkumar DR, Pollack IF. Coadministration of sorafenib with rottlerin potently inhibits cell proliferation and migration in human malignant glioma cells. Jane J Pharmacol Exp Ther. 2006 Dec;319(3):1070-80.

[26] Yu C, Friday BB, Lai JP, *et al.* Cytotoxic synergy between the multikinase inhibitor sorafenib and the proteasome inhibitor bortezomib in vitro: induction of apoptosis through Akt and c-Jun NH2-terminal kinase pathways..Mol Cancer Ther. 2006 Sep;5(9):2378-87.

[27] Awada A, Hendlisz A, Gil T, *et al.* Phase I safety and pharma¬cokinetics of BAY 43-9006 administered for 21 days on/7 days off in patients with advanced, refractory solid tumours. Br J Cancer 2005;92:1855–61.

[28] Moore M, Hirte HW, Siu L, *et al.* Phase I study to determine the safety and pharmacokinetics of the novel Raf kinase and vegfr inhibitor BAY 43-9006, administered for 28 days on/7 days off in patients with advanced, refractory solid tumors. Ann Oncol 2005;16:1688–94.

[29] Strumberg D, Richly H, Hilger RA, *et al.* Phase I clinical and pharmacokinetic study of the novel Raf kinase and vascular endothelial growth factor receptor inhibitor BAY 43-9006 in patients with advanced refractory solid tumors. J Clin Oncol 2005;23:965–72.

[30] 30.Nabors LB, Rosenfeld M, Chamberlain M, *et al.* A phase I trial of sorafenib (BAY 43-9006) for patients with recurrent or progressive malignant glioma (NABTT 0401). Journal of Clinical Oncology, 2007 ASCO Annual Meeting Proceedings Part I. Vol 25, No. 18S (June 20 Supplement), 2007: 2058

[31] Prados M, Gilbert M, Kuhn J, *et al.* Phase I/II study of sorefenib and erlotinib for patients with recurrent glioblastoma (GBM) (NABTC 05-02). 2009 ASCO Annual Meeting

[32] Hu X, Pandolfi PP, Li Y, *et al.*mTOR promotes survival and astrocytic characteristics induced by Pten/AKT signaling in glioblastoma. Neoplasia. 2005 Apr;7(4):356-68.

[33] Delmas C, Heliez C, Cohen-Jonathan E, *et al.* Farnesyltransferase inhibitor, R115777, reverses the resistance of human glioma cell lines to ionizing radiation. Int J Cancer. 2002 Jul 1;100(1):43-8.

[34] Wen PY, Cloughesy T, Kuhn J, *et al.* Phase I/II study of sorafenib and temsirolimus for patients with recurrent glioblastoma (GBM) (NABTC 05-02). 2009 ASCO Annual Meeting.

[35]   Galanis E, Buckner JC, Maurer MJ, *et al.* North Central Cancer Treatment Group. Phase II trial of temsirolimus (CCI-779) in recurrent glioblastoma multiforme: a North Central Cancer Treatment Group Study. J Clin Oncol. 2005 Aug 10;23(23):5294-304.

[36]   Schiff D, Sarkaria J, Decker P, *et al.* Phase I study of temsirolimus (CCI-779) and sorafenib in recurrent gliombastoma : North Central Cancer Treatment Group (NCCTG) N0572, Abstracts for the Twelfth Annual Meeting of the Society for Neuro-Oncology (SNO), Neuro-Oncology, October 2007

[37]   Cloughesy TF, Wen PY, Robins HI, *et al.* Phase II trial of tipifarnib in patients with recurrent malignant glioma either receiving or not receiving enzyme-inducing antiepileptic drugs: a North American Brain Tumor Consortium Study. J Clin Oncol. 2006 Aug 1;24(22):3651-6.

[38]   Lamar E, Spigel DR, Burris HA, *et al.* Phase II trial of radiation therapy/temozolomide followed by temozolomide/sorafenib in the first-line treatment of glioblastoma multiforme (GBM). 2009 ASCO Annual Meeting.

[39]   WilhelmS, Carter C, Lynch M, *et al.* Discovery and development of sorafenib: a multikinase inhibitor for treating cancer. Nat Rev Drug Discov 2006;5:835–44.

[40]   Autier J, Escudier B, Wechsler J, *et al.* Prospective study of the cutaneous adverse effects of sorafenib, a novel multikinase inhibitor. Arch Dermatol. 2008 Jul;144(7):886-92.

[41]   Veronese ML, Mosenkis A, Flaherty KT, *et al.*Mechanisms of hypertension associated with BAY 43-9006. J Clin Oncol. 2006 Mar 20;24(9):1363-9.

[42]   Pouessel D, Culine S. High frequency of intracerebral hemorrhage in metastatic renal carcinoma patients with brain metastases treated with tyrosine kinase inhibitors targeting the vascular endothelial growth factor receptor..Eur Urol. 2008 Feb;53(2):376-81.

[43]   Hill KL Jr, Lipson AC, Sheehan JM. Brain magnetic resonance imaging changes after sorafenib and sunitinib chemotherapy in patients with advanced renal cell and breast carcinoma. J Neurosurg. 2009 Sep;111(3):497-503.

[44]   Norden AD, Drappatz J, Wen PY. Antiangiogenic therapies for high-grade glioma..Nat Rev Neurol. 2009 Oct 13.

[45]   Flaherty KT, Rosen MA, Heitjan DF, *et al.* Pilot study of DCE-MRI to predict progression-free survival with sorafenib therapy in renal cell carcinoma. Cancer Biol Ther. 2008 Apr;7(4):496-501.

[46]   Hahn OM, Yang C, Medved M, *et al.* Dynamic contrast-enhanced magnetic resonance imaging pharmacodynamic biomarker study of sorafenib in metastatic renal carcinoma. J Clin Oncol. 2008 Oct 1;26(28):4572-8.

[47]   Eisen T, Ahmad T, Flaherty KT, *et al.* Sorafenib in advanced melanoma: a Phase II randomised discontinuation trial analysis. Br J Cancer. 2006 Sep 4;95(5):581-6.

[48]   Hauschild A, Agarwala SS, Trefzer U, *et al.* Results of a phase III, randomized, placebo-controlled study of sorafenib in combination with carboplatin and paclitaxel as second-line treatment in patients with unresectable stage III or stage IV melanoma. J Clin Oncol. 2009 Jun 10;27(17):2823-30.

[49]   Solomon DA, Kim JS, Cronin JC, *et al.* Mutational inactivation of PTPRD in glioblastoma multiforme and malignant melanoma. Cancer Res. 2008 Dec 15;68(24):10300-6.

[50]   Bleeker FE, Lamba S, Rodolfo M, *et al.* Mutational profiling of cancer candidate genes in glioblastoma, melanoma and pancreatic carcinoma reveals a snapshot of their genomic landscapes. Hum Mutat. 2009 Feb;30(2):E451-9.

CHAPTER 28

Aflibercept (VEGF-Trap) in High-Grade Gliomas

Jan Drappatz[1,2,3], Andrew D. Norden[1,2,3] and Patrick Y. Wen[1,2,3,*]

[1]*Department of Neurology, Division of Cancer Neurology, Brigham and Women's Hospital;* [2]*Center for Neuro-Oncology, Dana Farber Cancer Institute and* [3]*Harvard Medical School*

Abstract: Vascular endothelial growth factor (VEGF) is the key protein in the regulation of pathological angiogenesis, a hallmark of glioblastomas. Inhibition of VEGF has become a major strategy in glioma therapy. Most clinical trial data generated to date have been with bevacizumab, a humanized monoclonal antibody against VEGF. Aflibercept (VEGF Trap; Regeneron, Inc.), is an engineered soluble receptor made from extracellular domains of VEGFR1 and VEGFR2 which binds to all isoforms of VEGF and to placental growth factor (PlGF). The avidity with which aflibercept binds to VEGF-A and VEGF-B is significantly higher than that for bevacizumab. The toxicities observed include hypertension and proteinuria and are similar to those with other therapies targeting the VEGF pathway. A phase II trial in patients with relapsed high-grade glioma demonstrated encouraging activity. Ongoing trials are evaluating aflibercept in combination with temozolomide and radiation in newly-diagnosed glioblastoma.

CURRENT TREATMENT OF PATIENTS WITH HIGH-GRADE GLIOMAS

Standard therapy for patients with newly-diagnosed glioblastomas involves radiation therapy (RT) (60 Gy in 1.8- to 2-Gy fractions), together with concomitant and adjuvant temozolomide [1,2]. However, most patients develop recurrent disease within one year of diagnosis. Bevacizumab, a humanized monoclonal antibody directed against VEGF, showed encouraging activity in phase II trials with 6-month progression free survival (PFS6) rates of 30-50 % [3-9]. As a result, bevacizumab recently received accelerated approval by the Food and Drug Administration for the treatment of recurrent glioblastoma. Nonetheless, not all patients benefit, and only about one third have prolonged disease control. Drugs targeting the VEGF receptor (VEGFR) such as cediranib (VEGFR), sunitinib (VEGFR, PDGFR, and c-kit), sorafenib (VEGFR, PDGFR, and c-kit), XL 184 (VEGFR and c-met), CT-322(VEGFR), and vandetanib (VEGFR and EGFR) are all being studied in high-grade glioma patients [10].

DEVELOPMENT OF AFLIBERCEPT (VEGF TRAP)

Early studies indicated that one of the most effective ways to inhibit the VEGF signaling pathway is to prevent VEGF from binding to its endogenous receptors by administering soluble decoy receptors. In particular, a soluble decoy receptor created by fusing the first three immunoglobulin- like (Ig) domains of VEGFR1 to the constant region (Fc portion) of human IgG1 resulted in a homodimer that acted as a very high affinity inhibitor with 5–20 picomolar binding affinity for VEGF [11].

Despite its high affinity, the VEGFR1-Fc was not a feasible clinical candidate because of its poor pharmacokinetic profile when administered subcutaneously. These characteristics were related to the high positive charge of the protein, resulting in deposition of the agent at the injection site due to adhesion to the extracellular matrix. To circumvent this, the Trap technology platform was used [12]. This involved fusing minimal binding units from different receptor components to generate chimeric fusion proteins that act as high-affinity soluble inhibitors. The result was a chimeric fusion protein containing a modified domain 2 of VEGFR1 and the third Ig domain of VEGFR2 fused to the Fc region of human IgG, resulting in a fully human protein, aflibercept (VEGF Trap) [13] (Fig. **1**). These changes increased bioavailability after subcutaneous administration, with an increase in C_{max} and area under the curve of aflibercept. Aflibercept had an affinity for VEGF of ~1 pmol/L, significantly improved from the 5 pmol/L binding affinity seen with the Trap molecule made solely from VEGFR1 domains [13]. Aflibercept binds to VEGF-A and VEGF-B with significantly higher affinity than bevacizumab, as well as binding placental growth factor (PlGF) [14,15].

*****Address correspondence to Y. Wen:** Center for Neuro-Oncology, Dana Farber Cancer Institute, 44 Binney Street, SW-430D, Boston, MA 02115; Tel: 617-632-2166; Fax: 617-632-4773; Email: Patrick_Wen@dfci.harvard.edu

Thomas C. Chen (Ed)

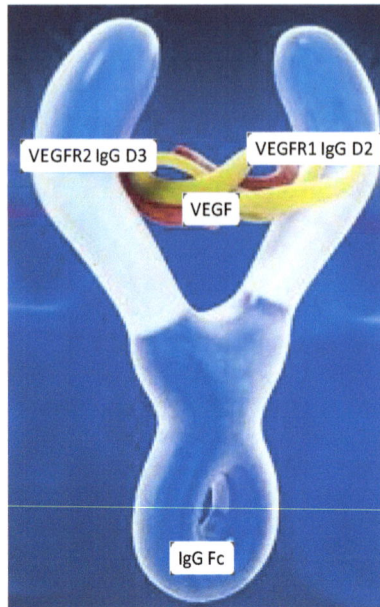

Figure 1: VEGF Trap (Aflibercept) is a chimeric fusion protein containing a modified domain 2 of VEGFR1 and the third Ig domain of VEGFR2 fused to the Fc region of human IgG, resulting in a fully human protein, VEGF Trap.

PRECLINICAL STUDIES OF AFLIBERCEPT

Holash et al examined the therapeutic efficacy of aflibercept in several tumor xenograft models (mouse B16F10.9 melanoma, human A673 rhabdomyosarcoma, and rat C6 glioma) [13]. When given subcutaneously twice weekly, aflibercept led to significant decrease in tumor size for the xenografts tested compared with control animals. Immunohistochemical staining showed a dramatic, dose-dependent reduction in tumor vasculature. To achieve similar growth inhibition of B16F10.9 cells with the anti-VEGFR2 antibody DC101, serum levels 60 times those of aflibercept were required. Studies of aflibercept in neuroblastoma xenografts also showed significant inhibition of tumor growth and decrease in vessel density [16].

Aflibercept significantly prolonged survival in a U-87 orthotopic glioma model [17]. Examination of the brains of animals following prolonged treatment of aflibercept revealed the presence of "secondary structures" or "satellitosis" consisting of aggregations of glioma cells in the perivascular regions, as well as the presence of glioma cells along the Virchow-Robin spaces. This suggested that U-87 MG-derived xenografts acquired an invasive phenotype in response to anti-VEGF therapy. These results are in agreement with a similar pattern of growth observed in intracranial G55 xenografts in animals treated with an antibody against mouse VEGFR-2, DC101 [18]. Clinically, a similar pattern of invasive growth has been observed in a subset of patients treated with bevacizumab [19,20].

Other preclinical studies have examined the combination of aflibercept with radiation and chemotherapy and showed additive or synergistic activity. In a U87 subcutaneous glioma xenograft model, the combination of radiation therapy with aflibercept had additive activity [21]. Hu *et al.* examined the efficacy of aflibercept in combination with paclitaxel in an ovarian cancer xenograft model [22]. They showed >50% decrease in tumor burden with either aflibercept or paclitaxel alone, but the combination resulted in a 98% reduction in tumor volume.

CLINICAL STUDIES OF AFLIBERCEPT

The first phase I trial of aflibercept explored subcutaneous administration [23]. Toxicity data were consistent with inhibition of the VEGF pathway including proteinuria, hypertension, venous thromboembolic disease, and leukopenia. Heavily pretreated patients with a variety of tumor types were enrolled. At the two highest dose levels reported (800 µg/kg weekly or twice weekly), 8 of 10 patients had stable disease for more than 10 weeks. Intravenous aflibercept, given on an every-2-week schedule, showed similar results [24]. Again, toxicities suggestive of VEGF inhibition were seen, such as grade 3/4 proteinuria, hypertension, fatigue, and hoarse voice. The maximum tolerated dose had not been reached at 5 mg/kg every 2 weeks.

Pharmacokinetic data from the subcutaneous and intravenous phase I trials of aflibercept indicate that at doses of 800 µg/kg subcutaneously once weekly, or 2 mg/kg intravenously every 2 weeks, concentrations of free aflibercept were in excess of bound aflibercept, suggesting adequate drug delivery to achieve maximal VEGF binding. There was no evidence that anti-aflibercept antibodies were produced.

More recent phase 1b trials suggest that aflibercept can be safely combined with cytotoxic chemotherapies including FOLFOX4 (oxaliplatin, leucovorin, and 5- fluorouracil) [25] and I-LV5FU2 (irinotecan, 5-fluorouracil, and leucovorin) [26]. Early phase 2 results indicate that aflibercept has activity against recurrent ovarian cancer [27] and non-small cell lung cancer (NSCLC)[28]. Phase II trials in several diseases are ongoing, including gliomas, colorectal cancer, multiple myeloma, non-Hodgkin's lymphoma, prostate cancer, endometrial cancer, breast cancer, melanoma, ovarian cancer and NSCLC. A broad phase III development program includes four phase III studies of aflibercept in combination with chemotherapy that are targeted to enroll a total of approximately 4,000 patients. These studies are being conducted in first-line metastatic pancreatic cancer, first-line metastatic hormone-refractory prostate cancer, second-line non-small cell lung cancer, and second-line metastatic colorectal cancer.

CLINICAL TRIALS IN MALIGNANT GLIOMAS

The North American Brain Tumor Consortium (NABTC) recently completed a phase II trial of aflibercept monotherapy (4 mg/kg every 2 weeks) for recurrent temozolomide-resistant high-grade gliomas (NABTC 06-01). Thirty-two patients with recurrent glioblastomas and 16 patients with recurrent anaplastic gliomas were enrolled. Based on investigator assessment, the response rate for the anaplastic glioma cohort was 50%(4 SD, 5 PR, 2 CR of 14 evaluable patients), and the response rate for patients with glioblastomas was 30% (14 SD, 8 PR of 27 evaluable patients), which are similar to those obtained with bevacizumab. There were two grade 4 adverse events, one patient with ischemic stroke and one patient with systemic hemorrhage. Grade 3 adverse events included fatigue, hypertension, hand-foot syndrome, lymphopenia, thrombosis and proteinuria. In total, 12 patients (25%) discontinued therapy due to toxicity, on average less than 2 months into treatment, suggesting that the dose of 4 mg/kg maybe slightly high [29]. Aflibercept resulted in rapid and sustained decreases in free VEGF levels. Although greater than 95% of PlGF remained bound, free PlGF levels significantly increased over time. Treatment significantly modulated multiple cytokine and angiogenic factors with striking increases in macrophage migration inhibitory factor and stem cell growth factor-β [30].

A 3 arm phase I study of aflibercept with radiation therapy and temozolomide in patients with newly-diagnosed high-grade gliomas is being conducted by the American Brain Tumor Consortium (ABTC). In arm 1, aflibercept is administered in combination with radiation therapy and concomitant temozolomide. Because the ongoing RTOG 0525 study has not yet determined the optimal adjuvant temozolomide dosing schedule, post-radiation patients in arms 2 and 3 of this study receive either aflibercept with standard adjuvant dosing (5 days every 28 days) or a dose-intense regimen (21 days every 28 days). A phase II study using this regimen conducted by the ABTC is planned.

CONCLUSIONS

Emerging data suggest that a number of agents with different mechanisms of targeting the VEGF pathway may have activity in high-grade gliomas. The high VEGF-binding affinity of aflibercept and the additional binding of PlGF raise the possibility that aflibercept may have advantages over the current generations of VEGF-directed therapies. Aflibercept has been moderately well-tolerated and has demonstrated encouraging activity in recurrent high-grade gliomas. Aflibercept is now being evaluated in patients with newly-diagnosed high-grade gliomas in conjunction with TMZ and RT. Preclinical data suggests that patients treated with aflibercept are at risk of developing a invasive phenotype which resembles the diffuse pattern of disease recurrence seen with bevacizumab. Future studies directed at identifying biomarkers of response, and understanding mechanisms of resistance will be necessary. Ultimately, the role of aflibercept is likely to be in combination with other therapies.

REFERENCES

[1]   Stupp R, Hegi ME, Mason WP, *et al.* Effects of radiotherapy with concomitant and adjuvant temozolomide versus radiotherapy alone on survival in glioblastoma in a randomised phase III study: 5-year analysis of the EORTC-NCIC trial. Lancet Oncol 2009;10:459-466.

[2]   Stupp R, Mason WP, van den Bent MJ, *et al.* Radiotherapy plus concomitant and adjuvant temozolomide for glioblastoma. N Engl J Med 2005;352:987-996.

[3]   Cloughesy T, Prados, MD, Wen, PY, *et al.* A phase II, randomized, non-comparative clinical trial of the effect of bevacizumab (BV) alone or in combination with irinotecan (CPT) on 6-month progression free survival (PFS6) in recurrent, treatment-refractory glioblastoma (GBM). J Clin Oncol 26 2008;26:Abstract 2010b.

[4]   Kreisl TN, Kim L, Moore K, *et al.* Phase II trial of single-agent bevacizumab followed by bevacizumab plus irinotecan at tumor progression in recurrent glioblastoma. J Clin Oncol 2009;27:740-745.

[5]   Chamberlain MC, Johnston S. Salvage chemotherapy with bevacizumab for recurrent alkylator-refractory anaplastic astrocytoma. J Neurooncol 2009;91:359-367.

[6]   Vredenburgh JJ, Desjardins A, Reardon DA, *et al.* Experience with irinotecan for the treatment of malignant glioma. Neuro Oncol 2009;11:80-91.

[7]   Fischer I, Cunliffe CH, Bollo RJ, *et al.* High-grade glioma before and after treatment with radiation and Avastin: initial observations. Neuro Oncol 2008;10:700-708.

[8]   Vredenburgh JJ, Desjardins A, Herndon JE, 2nd, *et al.* Bevacizumab plus irinotecan in recurrent glioblastoma multiforme. J Clin Oncol 2007;25:4722-4729.

[9]   Vredenburgh JJ, Desjardins A, Herndon JE, 2nd, *et al.* Phase II trial of bevacizumab and irinotecan in recurrent malignant glioma. Clin Cancer Res 2007;13:1253-1259.

[10]   Chi AS, Norden AD, Wen PY. Antiangiogenic Strategies for Treatment of Malignant Gliomas. Neurotherapeutics 2009;6:513-526.

[11]   Kuo CJ, Farnebo F, Yu EY, *et al.* Comparative evaluation of the antitumor activity of antiangiogenic proteins delivered by gene transfer. Proc Natl Acad Sci U S A 2001;98:4605-4610.

[12]   Economides AN, Carpenter LR, Rudge JS, *et al.* Cytokine traps: multi-component, high-affinity blockers of cytokine action. Nat Med 2003;9:47-52.

[13]   Holash J, Davis S, Papadopoulos N, *et al.* VEGF-Trap: a VEGF blocker with potent antitumor effects. Proc Natl Acad Sci U S A 2002;99:11393-11398.

[14]   Ferrara N, Hillan KJ, Gerber HP, *et al.* Discovery and development of bevacizumab, an anti-VEGF antibody for treating cancer. Nat Rev Drug Discov 2004;3:391-400.

[15]   Rudge JS, Holash J, Hylton D, *et al.* Inaugural Article: VEGF Trap complex formation measures production rates of VEGF, providing a biomarker for predicting efficacious angiogenic blockade. Proc Natl Acad Sci U S A 2007;104:18363-18370.

[16]   Huang J, Frischer JS, Serur A, *et al.* Regression of established tumors and metastases by potent vascular endothelial growth factor blockade. Proc Natl Acad Sci U S A 2003;100:7785-7790.

[17]   Gomez-Manzano C, Holash J, Fueyo J, *et al.* VEGF Trap induces antiglioma effect at different stages of disease. Neuro Oncol 2008;10:940-945.

[18]   Rubenstein JL, Kim J, Ozawa T, *et al.* Anti-VEGF antibody treatment of glioblastoma prolongs survival but results in increased vascular cooption. Neoplasia 2000;2:306-314.

[19]   Quant EC, Norden AD, Drappatz J, *et al.* Role of a second chemotherapy in recurrent malignant glioma patients who progress on bevacizumab. Neuro Oncol 2009.

[20]   Norden AD, Young GS, Setayesh K, *et al.* Bevacizumab for recurrent malignant gliomas: efficacy, toxicity, and patterns of recurrence. Neurology 2008;70:779-787.

[21]   Wachsberger PR, Burd R, Cardi C, *et al.* VEGF trap in combination with radiotherapy improves tumor control in u87 glioblastoma. Int J Radiat Oncol Biol Phys 2007;67:1526-1537.

[22]   Hu L, Hofmann J, Holash J, *et al.* Vascular endothelial growth factor trap combined with paclitaxel strikingly inhibits tumor and ascites, prolonging survival in a human ovarian cancer model. Clin Cancer Res 2005;11:6966-6971.

[23]   Dupont J, Schwartz, L., Koutcher, J., Spriggs, J,. Phase I and pharmacokinetic study of VEGF Trap administered subcutaneously (sc) to patients (pts) with advanced solid malignancies. J Clin Oncol 2004;22:3009.

[24]   Dupont J, Rothenberg, ML, Spriggs, DR, *et al.*. Safety and pharmacokinetics of intravenous VEGF Trap in a phase I clinical trial of patients with advanced solid tumors. J Clin Oncol 2005;23:3029.

[25]   25.Mulay M, Limentani, SA, Carroll, M, Furfine, ES, Cohen, DP, Rosen, LS. Safety and pharmacokinetics of intravenous VEGF Trap plus FOLFOX4 in a combination phase I clinical trial of patients with advanced solid tumors. J Clin Oncol 2006;24.

[26]   Rixe O, Verslype, C, Méric, JB, *et al.* Safety and pharmacokinetics of intravenous VEGF Trap plus irinotecan,5-fluorouracil, and leucovorin (I-LV5FU2) in a combination phase I clinical trial ofpatients with advanced solid tumors. J Clin Oncol 2006;24:13161.

[27]   Moroney JW, Sood AK, Coleman RL. Aflibercept in epithelial ovarian carcinoma. Future Oncol 2009;5:591-600.

[28]   Riely GJ, Miller VA. Vascular endothelial growth factor trap in non small cell lung cancer. Clin Cancer Res 2007;13:s4623-4627.

[29]   De Groot J, Wen, PY, Lamborn, K, Chang, S, Cloughesy, TF *et al.* Phase II single arm trial of aflibercept in patients with recurrent temozolomide-resistant glioblastoma: NABTC 0601. J Clin Oncol 2008;26:2010.

[30]   Piao Y, Heymach, JV, Bekele, B, Camphausen, K, Wen, PY, Liu, J, Yung, WK, De Groot, J;. Circulating cytokine and angiogenic factors as predictive biomarkers of glioblastoma response to aflibercept (VEGF Trap). J Clin Oncol. 2009;27:2029.

CHAPTER 29

Cediranib in Glioblastoma

Elizabeth R. Gerstner, Jörg H. Dietrich, Daphne Wang and Tracy T. Batchelor[*]

Stephen E. and Catherine Pappas Center for Neuro-Oncology, Massachusetts General Hospital, Harvard Medical School, 55 Fruit Street, Yawkey 9E, Boston, MA 02114

Abstract: Targeting tumor-derived angiogenesis has emerged as a promising new treatment strategy in patients with glioblastoma. Cediranib (Recentin™) is a potent oral inhibitor of vascular endothelial growth factor (VEGF) receptors and has demonstrated improved progression-free survival in an uncontrolled phase II study of patients with recurrent glioblastoma. The drug is taken orally, once daily, and has a manageable side effect profile. In addition, it has potent anti-edema and steroid-sparing effects that might improve the quality of life of glioblastoma patients. Several clinical trials are ongoing testing cediranib in patients with gliomas.

INTRODUCTION

Despite advances in diagnostic imaging, surgical techniques, radiation therapy, and the development of new cytotoxic drugs, glioblastoma remains one of the most challenging solid tumors to treat. The survival rate for patients with glioblastoma has improved only modestly in recent decades. Median overall survival for glioblastoma patients treated with current standard radiation and temozolomide chemotherapy remains between 12-15 months from the time of diagnosis [1]. However, an improved understanding of glioma-related angiogenesis has identified a number of promising new therapeutic targets.

Tumor growth beyond approximately 1 mm is critically dependent on the formation of new blood vessels. The complex process of tumor angiogenesis involves activation of endothelial and perivascular cells, tissue remodeling, and dynamic interactions of pro-angiogenic and anti-angiogenic factors. While angiogenesis plays a pivotal role during development, in adults this process occurs mainly at times of wound healing and during cyclical changes in the female reproductive tract. Thus, targeting angiogenesis is very appealing in adult glioma patients where potential off-target side effects may be minimal.

One of the most potent pro-angiogenic mediators is vascular endothelial growth factor (VEGF). Inhibition of VEGF signaling either through neutralizing antibodies against VEGF or VEGF receptor tyrosine kinase inhibitors (TKIs) has produced encouraging results in the treatment of cancer patients. Among a number of novel targeted therapeutics evaluated in preclinical studies and recent clinical trials, the oral pan-VEGF receptor TKI cediranib has emerged as a promising agent with potent anti-angiogenic properties. This review will summarize available pre-clinical and clinical data regarding cediranib in patients with glioblastomas.

TARGETING THE VEGF PATHWAY

VEGF signaling influences numerous processes related to tumor angiogenesis, including activation of endothelial cell precursors, endothelial cell migration and proliferation, modification of protease and integrin expression, capillary tube formation, and vascular permeability [2,3]. A variety of agents that target VEGF signaling are currently under development for gliomas. Bevacizumab, a humanized monoclonal antibody against VEGF-A, was recently approved by the FDA for the treatment of recurrent glioblastoma [4]. In clinical trials in patients with recurrent malignant gliomas, bevacizumab in combination with irinotecan (CPT-11), a cytotoxic topoisomerase I inhibitor, resulted in encouraging objective radiographic responses and improved progression-free survival compared to historical controls [5-7]. However, it remains unclear whether these results will translate into an extension of survival.

---

*Address correspondence to Tracy T. Batchelor: Stephen E. and Catherine Pappas Center for Neuro-Oncology, Yawkey 9E, Massachusetts General Hospital Cancer Center, 55 Fruit Street, Boston, MA 02114; Email: TBatchelor@partners.org

Thomas C. Chen (Ed)

In contrast to bevacizumab, which acts solely by VEGF sequestration, several small-molecule compounds have been developed that function as competitive inhibitors of VEGF receptors and other receptor tyrosine kinases important in angiogenesis such as the platelet-derived growth factor (PDGF) family [8]. Considering the redundancy and complexity of angiogenic signaling, inhibition of a single growth factor pathway is not likely to result in complete inhibition of angiogenesis so multi-targeted kinase inhibitors of several angiogenic growth factor pathways may yield greater clinical efficacy. One member of this group of multi-targeted TKIs in development is cediranib. Cediranib is a potent small molecule receptor TKI with cross activity against PDGFR and c-kit that is currently being tested in the glioblastoma patient population in phase I, II and III clinical trials.

EARLY PHASE STUDIES OF CEDIRANIB

Cediranib (AZD2171; Recentin®) was co-developed by AstraZeneca (London, UK), the National Cancer Institute of the United States and the National Cancer Institute of Canada. It is an indole-ether quinazoline with a molecular weight of 450.51 and potent ATP-competitive inhibition of VEGF signaling by binding to the intracellular domain of all three VEGF receptor tyrosine kinases but mainly VEGFR-2 [9]. In addition, cediranib inhibits tyrosine kinase activity for PDGFR-α, PDGFR-β, c-Kit, and other tyrosine and serine/threonine kinases (fibroblast growth factor receptor (FGFR-1) and epidermal growth factor (EGFR)) (Table 1). Dose-dependent inhibition of VEGF-induced angiogenesis and tumor growth with once daily dosing of cediranib was demonstrated in a range of tumor xenograft mouse models, including colon, lung, prostate, breast and ovary [9]. Significant reduction in tumor vessel density and vascular regression was notable within 52 hours of a once daily administration schedule [9]. Subsequent studies in other human tumor xenograft models were consistent with these findings and revealed potent cediranib-associated reduction in tumor microvessel density mediated via VEGFR-2 inhibition [10-14].

Table 1: Pharmacokinetic and pharmacodynamic parameters of cediranib

IC$_{50}$ values	VEGFR	<0.001µM
	c-Kit	<0.002µM
	PDGFR-β	<0.005µM
	FGFR	<0.026µM
	PDGFR-α	<0.036µM
Monotherapy dose	30mg or 45mg	
Plasma half-life	22 hrs [12.5-35.4 hrs]	
Peak plasma concentration after one single dose	<8hrs	

In Phase I testing, peak plasma concentrations of cediranib were reached 1 to 8 hours after a single dose, and the plasma half-life was 22 hours, supporting the use of a once-daily oral dose in humans. The drug was generally well tolerated as monotherapy up to an oral daily dose of 45mg [15,16].

CEDIRANIB IN CLINICAL TRIALS OF GLIOBLASTOMA

In patients with recurrent glioblastoma, encouraging results were reported from a National Cancer Institute (NCI)-sponsored Phase II study. In this study, cediranib was administered as a 45mg single daily dose to 31 patients with recurrent glioblastoma [17]. The regimen was associated with moderate toxicity, requiring temporary drug suspension in 69% of the initial 16 patients. Adverse effects included diarrhea, fatigue and hypertension. Using volumetric analysis of treatment response, decrease in tumor enhancement by more than 50% was notable in 9/16 patients (56%) and by 25-50% in 3/16 patients (19%). The median progression-free survival of the initial cohort was 111 days, comparing favorably to a historical database of a similar patient population treated with standard therapies [18]. Importantly, cediranib resulted in a significant reduction of tumor-associated vasogenic edema as measured by MRI techniques. This effect was paralleled by a potent steroid-sparing effect in most patients- 11 patients taking steroids were able to reduce or discontinue steroids. Most patients who stopped cediranib required re-initiation of steroids likely because of rebound edema.

Correlative cranial MRI studies using gradient echo, spin echo and contrast enhanced sequences demonstrated that decreased contrast enhancement was associated with reduction in blood vessel size, vascular permeability, blood flow and blood volume, supporting the concept of "vascular normalization" of abnormal tumor blood vessels. Relative tumor vessel size was significantly decreased as early as 1 day after initiation of cediranib, was more pronounced in larger microvessels (>10μM), and was maintained for at least 28 days. However, this effect was transient, and blood vessel size reverted towards abnormal values in most patients within 2 months of treatment and after cessation of drug administration. In patients who required temporary "drug holidays," tumor vessels re-normalized after resumption of cediranib. Unlike the transient changes in vessel size, vascular permeability remained decreased for up to 112 days, suggesting that this feature of vascular normalization was more prolonged.

The phenomenon of vascular normalization appears to be one of the critical features of anti-angiogenic therapies. Through selective pruning and maturation of unstable tumor blood vessels, anti-angiogenic agents have been previously shown to promote the formation of more stable and pericyte-coated smaller blood vessels, which may diminish tumor hypoxia and, consequently, improve the efficacy of concurrently administered radiation therapy and cytotoxic chemotherapy [19-22]. The observation that vascular normalization is a transient phenomenon, suggests that a specific treatment window might exist during which chemotherapy and radiation may be most effective. The mechanism responsible for the re-establishment of pathological vascularization is poorly understood, but may offer an explanation for treatment failure due to up-regulation of alternate pro-angiogenic factors [23,24]

Despite the promising responses to cediranib and other anti-angiogenic drugs, patients have variable responses to these agents so one of the most critical challenges has been the identification and validation of molecular or biological markers of treatment response. An important finding in the Phase II study of cediranib was that the change from baseline to day one of treatment in tumor cerebral blood volume, vascular permeability (as measured by the MRI parameter K^{trans}), and circulating collagen IV levels predicted both progression-free survival and overall survival [25]. This composite biomarker, termed the "vascular normalization index", could serve as an early predictor of patient response to cediranib and potentially other anti-angiogenic TKIs. The ability to identify patients on day 1 of treatment who are less likely to respond to this class of drugs will limit exposure of resistant patients to a potentially toxic drug and potentially shift them to more effective therapies.

This study also provided novel insights into the use of surrogate blood markers of treatment response [17]. Disease progression during ongoing treatment with cediranib correlated with increases in bFGF, SDF1-α and viable circulating endothelial cells (CEC). Tumor progression after drug cessation during "drug holidays", in contrast, correlated with an increase in the number of circulating progenitor cells (CPC), suggesting an independent role of CEC and CPC as biomarkers of treatment response in patients treated with cediranib.

These encouraging results with cediranib in patients with recurrent glioblastoma warrant further investigations to validate these initial trial results, and to explore whether cediranib may have a role in conjunction with radiation and temozolomide as first-line treatment. Consequently several other studies of cediranib in patients with glioblastoma are being conducted (Table **2**). A Phase III international trial (REGAL study) randomizing patients with recurrent glioblastoma to cediranib monotherapy, cediranib + lomustine, or lomustine alone will determine whether the drug has efficacy in this patient population.

Table 2: Ongoing clinical trials of cediranib in brain tumors

Agents	Phase	Diagnosis	Sponsor	Primary Endpoint
Cediranib + CCNU	III	Recurrent GBM	AstraZeneca	PFS
Cediranib + TMZ + RT	Ib/II	New GBM	NCI	PFS (phase-II)
Cediranib + Cilengitide	Ib	Recurrent GBM	NCI/ABTC	Survival
Cediranib	Ib/II	Brain Metastases from NSCLC	NCI	Survival

PFS- progression-free survival; ABTC- Adult Brain Tumor Consortium

ASSESSMENT OF TREATMENT RESPONSE AND BIOMARKERS

Current treatment response criteria in patients with malignant gliomas are based on MRI and are dependent on the degree of contrast enhancement [26]. In patients treated with anti-VEGF therapies, this parameter may be misleading, as the reduction in enhancement may simply be related to the decrease in vascular permeability produced by these agents rather than to an anti-tumor cell effect. This phenomenon likely is the explanation why objective radiographic responses in patients treated with anti-VEGF therapies have so far not translated into prolongation of overall survival. Future trials of cediranib should incorporate advanced imaging modalities, such as dynamic contrast-enhanced MRI, perfusion imaging, diffusion-weighted imaging, magnetic resonance spectroscopy, or positron emission tomography studies (PET) as novel biomarkers to appropriately evaluate treatment effect and anti-tumor response.

There have been increasing concerns about the promotion of tumor infiltration, tumor cell migration and metastasis with anti-angiogenic therapies [27-31]. In an orthotopic rodent glioma model, Rubenstein *at al.* demonstrated that anti-VEGF treatment delayed glioblastoma growth but also resulted in increased tumor cell infiltration and cooption of the native host vasculature [28]. Enhanced tumor cell invasion into surrounding brain parenchyma is poorly detected by conventional contrast-enhanced MRI because native brain vasculature is characterized by an intact BBB and tumor surrounding these blood vessels are not visible on conventional contrast-enhanced images. Although changes in T2/FLAIR hyperintensity have been advocated to assess for non-enhancing tumor and are now being incorporated into glioblastoma radiographic response criteria these changes may reflect not only tumor infiltration but also vasogenic cerebral edema and peritumoral gliosis [32-35]. Other MRI-based techniques including diffusion-weighted imaging may prove more useful for the detection of diffuse tumor infiltration [36].

POTENT ANTI-EDEMA EFFECT OF CEDIRANIB

Tumor-associated vasogenic cerebral edema is a direct consequence of the vascular abnormalities seen in patients with malignant gliomas and constitutes a significant cause of morbidity and mortality in this patient population [36]. The degree of vasogenic edema has been considered to be an important factor in treatment failure due to associated hypoxia and inadequate tumor penetration of chemotherapy agents secondary to increased interstitial tumor pressure. Reduction of vasogenic edema also improves patient quality of life and neurological function. Corticosteroids are the most widely used agents to treat vasogenic edema, but their use is associated with serious short-term and long-term complications [37]. The mechanisms leading to increased vascular hyperpermeability and fluid leakage from the intravascular space into the brain parenchyma are, at least in part, dependent on the up-regulation and activation of the VEGF signaling pathway in glioblastoma [36]. Consequently, anti-angiogenic agents acting through VEGF blockade have been demonstrated to reduce vasogenic edema through vascular normalization in both preclinical and clinical studies [17,38].

Cediranib reduces vasogenic edema and has a steroid-sparing effect in the majority of glioblastoma patients who have received the drug [17]. In orthotopic models of glioblastoma treated with cediranib, intravital microscopy and MRI techniques demonstrated significantly decreased vascular permeability with associated reduction in vasogenic edema [39]. The reduction of vasogenic edema by cediranib significantly prolonged animal survival but had no impact on tumor growth. Based on these pre-clinical observations it appears possible that anti-VEGF agents may be able to exert beneficial effects on progression-free and overall survival through edema control alone even in the absence of significant tumor growth inhibition. Based on its manageable toxicity profile, there may be a role for cediranib as an anti-edema agent in steroid-refractory patients rather than as a direct tumor cytotoxic agent.

TOXICITY PROFILE OF CEDIRANIB

Cediranib and other anti-angiogenic agents are generally well tolerated in patients with glioblastomas. Available toxicity data from clinical trials suggest unique patterns of adverse effects associated with this class of anti-cancer agents (Table **3**). The most commonly reported toxicities include hypertension, fatigue, diarrhea, anorexia, and hoarseness [15,40,41]. Most are manageable with appropriate supportive care. Hypertension is perhaps the most notable and patients on cediranib need to be carefully monitored for hypertension as subjects who develop hypertension can be successfully treated with early initiation of conventional anti-hypertensive agents. The possible mechanisms of hypertension are thought to be VEGF blockade of nitric oxide and prostacyclin synthesis, impaired baroreceptor responses, and perturbation of endothelial cell function.

Table 3: Anti-VEGF agent toxicities

Toxicity	Possible Mechanism
Bleeding Impaired wound healing	platelet dysfunction
Thrombotic events	EC apoptosis, platelet activation
Hypertension	blockade of NO and prostacyclins, decreased capillary density, impaired baroreceptor response
Proteinuria	podocyte dysfunction in kidney glomeruli
Rash Hand-foot syndrome	epidermal cell apoptosis, EC dysfunction
GI perforation	mucosal cell apoptosis, EC dysfunction
Hypothyroidism	decreased thyroid vascularity
Fatigue	hypothyroidism

EC- endothelial cell; NO- nitric oxide; GI- gastrointestinal

Due to the physiological role of VEGF in wound healing and new blood vessel formation, most anti-VEGF/VEGFR agents are associated with a mildly increased risk of bleeding and wound dehiscence, which has been a concern in patients with brain tumors. Prior intratumoral hemorrhage has been considered to be a relative contraindication to the use of cediranib or other anti-VEGF therapy. However, the incidence of intratumoral hemorrhage appears to be relatively low in preliminary studies of these agents. Moreover, therapeutic anti-coagulation with low-molecular weight heparin also appears to be relatively safe, when indicated, in patients receiving anti-VEGF therapy who do not have evidence of active bleeding.

Another concern has emerged from recent studies on the cell-biological basis of cancer therapy-associated neurotoxicity. Conventional cytotoxic agents target neural progenitor cells that are critically important in the maintenance of normal brain function and white matter integrity [42]. The physiological function of normal neural stem cells and progenitor cells is dependent on a number of factors, such as VEGF, FGF, EGF and PDGF, also employed by cancer stem cells. As much as there is the hope that anti-angiogenic therapies may also be beneficial in targeting cancer stem cells, disruption of those signaling pathways may ultimately result in considerable adverse effects, such as cognitive dysfunction, in long-term survivors [43]. Long-term, serial neuropsychological studies need to be performed in this population to determine the extent of this risk in patients receiving anti-VEGF therapies.

SUMMARY AND CONCLUSION

Cediranib has shown promising results in patients with recurrent glioblastoma (see Figs. **1** and **2**). The drug is generally well tolerated with a predictable and dose-dependent toxicity profile. Potent anti-edema and steroid-sparing effects have been observed in patients treated with cediranib. A temporary normalization effect on the tumor vasculature following therapy with cediranib suggests a unique opportunity for combination therapy with cytotoxic agents. Clinical trials are ongoing to determine whether cediranib may have a role in combination with radiation and temozolomide in patients with newly diagnosed glioblastoma or in combination with other agents in patients with recurrent glioblastoma. Development and validation of novel biomarkers is needed to monitor tumor response and emergence of tumor resistance so that the use of cediranib can be optimized. Future studies of cediranib and other VEGF-targeting agents will determine whether there is a survival benefit and will further define the long-term toxicity profile in cancer patients.

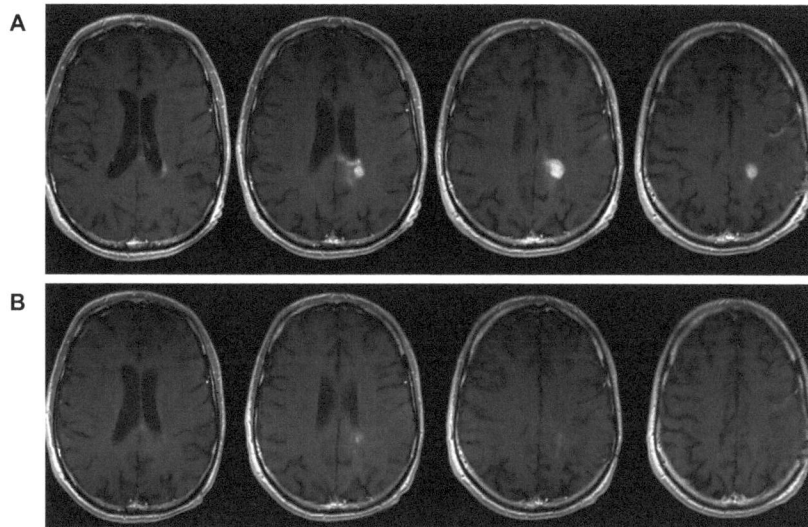

Figure 1: Magnetic resonance imaging (T1 + gadolinium) from a 37 year old patient with L fronto-parietal glioblastoma. **A.** MRI study at baseline prior to initiation of cediranib. **B.** MRI one month after treatment with cediranib, demonstrating a marked decrease in gadolinium enhancement.

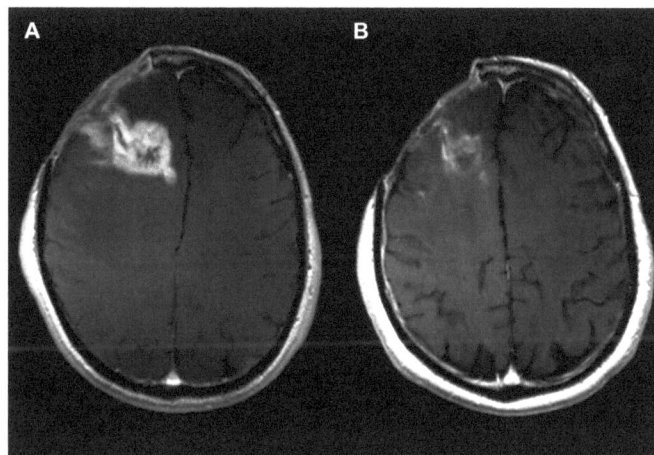

Figure 2: Magnetic resonance imaging (T1 + gadolinium) from a 46 year old patient with right frontal glioblastoma, treated with cediranib. **A.** MRI prior to initiation of cediranib. **B.** MRI one month after initiation of cediranib, showing significant decrease in the amount of vasogenic edema and extent of contrast enhancement.

REFERENCES

[1]   Stupp R, Mason WP, van den Bent MJ, *et al.* Radiotherapy plus concomitant and adjuvant temozolomide for glioblastoma. N Engl J Med 2005, 352(10), 987-996.

[2]   Ferrara N, Gerber HP, LeCouter J. The biology of VEGF and its receptors. Nat Med 2003, 9(6), 669-676.

[3]   Plate KH, Breier G, Weich HA, Risau W. Vascular endothelial growth factor is a potential tumour angiogenesis factor in human gliomas in vivo. Nature 1992, 359(6398), 845-848.

[4]   Hurwitz H, Fehrenbacher L, Novotny W, *et al.* Bevacizumab plus irinotecan, fluorouracil, and leucovorin for metastatic colorectal cancer. N Engl J Med 2004, 350(23), 2335-2342.

[5]   Pope WB, Lai A, Nghiemphu P, *et al.* MRI in patients with high-grade gliomas treated with bevacizumab and chemotherapy. Neurology 2006, 66(8), 1258-1260.

[6]   Vredenburgh JJ, Desjardins A, Herndon JE, 2nd, *et al.* Phase II trial of bevacizumab and irinotecan in recurrent malignant glioma. Clin Cancer Res 2007, 13(4), 1253-1259 (2007).

[7]   Vredenburgh JJ, Desjardins A, Herndon JE, 2nd, *et al.* Bevacizumab plus irinotecan in recurrent glioblastoma multiforme. J Clin Oncol 2007, 25(30), 4722-4729.

[8]   Dietrich J, Norden AD, Wen PY. Emerging antiangiogenic treatments for gliomas - efficacy and safety issues. Curr Opin Neurol 2008, 21(6), 736-744.

[9]   Wedge SR, Kendrew J, Hennequin LF, *et al*. AZD2171: a highly potent, orally bioavailable, vascular endothelial growth factor receptor-2 tyrosine kinase inhibitor for the treatment of cancer. Cancer Res 2005, 65(10), 4389-4400.

[10]   Smith NR, James NH, Oakley I, *et al*. Acute pharmacodynamic and antivascular effects of the vascular endothelial growth factor signaling inhibitor AZD2171 in Calu-6 human lung tumor xenografts. Mol Cancer Ther 2007, 6(8), 2198-2208.

[11]   Gomez-Rivera F, Santillan-Gomez AA, Younes MN, *et al*. The tyrosine kinase inhibitor, AZD2171, inhibits vascular endothelial growth factor receptor signaling and growth of anaplastic thyroid cancer in an orthotopic nude mouse model. Clin Cancer Res 2007, 13(15 Pt 1), 4519-4527.

[12]   Takeda M, Arao T, Yokote H, *et al*. AZD2171 shows potent antitumor activity against gastric cancer over-expressing fibroblast growth factor receptor 2/keratinocyte growth factor receptor. Clin Cancer Res 2007, 13(10), 3051-3057.

[13]   Goodlad RA, Ryan AJ, Wedge SR, *et al*. Inhibiting vascular endothelial growth factor receptor-2 signaling reduces tumor burden in the ApcMin/+ mouse model of early intestinal cancer. Carcinogenesis 2006, 27(10), 2133-2139.

[14]   Miller KD, Miller M, Mehrotra S, *et al*. A physiologic imaging pilot study of breast cancer treated with AZD2171. Clin Cancer Res 2006, 12(1), 281-288 (2006).

[15]   Drevs J, Siegert P, Medinger M, *et al*. Phase I clinical study of AZD2171, an oral vascular endothelial growth factor signaling inhibitor, in patients with advanced solid tumors. J Clin Oncol 2007, 25(21), 3045-3054 (2007).

[16]   Ryan CJ, Stadler WM, Roth B, *et al*. Phase I dose escalation and pharmacokinetic study of AZD2171, an inhibitor of the vascular endothelial growth factor receptor tyrosine kinase, in patients with hormone refractory prostate cancer (HRPC). Invest New Drugs 2007, 25(5), 445-451.

[17]   Batchelor TT, Sorensen AG, di Tomaso E, *et al*. AZD2171, a pan-VEGF receptor tyrosine kinase inhibitor, normalizes tumor vasculature and alleviates edema in glioblastoma patients. Cancer Cell 2007, 11(1), 83-95 (2007).

[18]   Wong ET, Hess KR, Gleason MJ, *et al*. Outcomes and prognostic factors in recurrent glioma patients enrolled onto phase II clinical trials. J Clin Onco 1999, 17(8), 2572-2578.

[19]   Winkler F, Kozin SV, Tong RT, *et al*. Kinetics of vascular normalization by VEGFR2 blockade governs brain tumor response to radiation: role of oxygenation, angiopoietin-1, and matrix metalloproteinases. Cancer Cel 2004, 6(6), 553-563.

[20]   Jain RK. Normalization of tumor vasculature: an emerging concept in antiangiogenic therapy. Science 2005, 307(5706), 58-62.

[21]   Gerber HP, Ferrara N. Pharmacology and pharmacodynamics of bevacizumab as monotherapy or in combination with cytotoxic therapy in preclinical studies. Cancer Res 2005, 65(3), 671-680.

[22]   Jain RK, di Tomaso E, Duda DG, Loeffler JS, Sorensen AG, Batchelor TT. Angiogenesis in brain tumours. Nat Rev Neurosci 2007, 8(8), 610-622.

[23]   Yoshiji H, Harris SR, Thorgeirsson UP. Vascular endothelial growth factor is essential for initial but not continued *in vivo* growth of human breast carcinoma cells. Cancer Res 1997, 57(18), 3924-3928.

[24]   Bergers G, Hanahan D. Modes of resistance to anti-angiogenic therapy. Nat Rev Cancer 2008, 8(8), 592-603.

[25]   Sorensen AG, Batchelor TT, Zhang WT, *et al*. A "vascular normalization index" as potential mechanistic biomarker to predict survival after a single dose of cediranib in recurrent glioblastoma patients. Cancer Res 2009, 69(13), 5296-5300.

[26]   Macdonald DR, Cascino TL, Schold SC, Jr., Cairncross JG. Response criteria for phase II studies of supratentorial malignant glioma. J Clin Oncol 1990, 8(7), 1277-1280.

[27]   Holash J, Maisonpierre PC, Compton D, *et al*. Vessel cooption, regression, and growth in tumors mediated by angiopoietins and VEGF. Science 1999, 284(5422), 1994-1999.

[28]   Rubenstein JL, Kim J, Ozawa T, *et al*. Anti-VEGF antibody treatment of glioblastoma prolongs survival but results in increased vascular cooption. Neoplasia 2000, 2(4), 306-314.

[29]   Loges S, Mazzone M, Hohensinner P, Carmeliet P. Silencing or fueling metastasis with VEGF inhibitors: antiangiogenesis revisited. Cancer Cell 2009, 15(3), 167-170.

[30]   Ebos JM, Lee CR, Cruz-Munoz W, *et al*. Accelerated metastasis after short-term treatment with a potent inhibitor of tumor angiogenesis. Cancer Cell 2009, 15(3), 232-239.

[31]   Paez-Ribes M, Allen E, Hudock J, *et al*. Antiangiogenic therapy elicits malignant progression of tumors to increased local invasion and distant metastasis. Cancer Cell 2009, 15(3), 220-231.

[32]   Lassman AB, Iwamoto FM, Gutin PH, Abrey LE. Patterns of relapse and prognosis after bevacizumab (BEV) failure in recurrent glioblastoma (GBM). J Clin Oncol 2008, 26, 2028 (abstract).

[33]   Zuniga RM, Torcuator R, Doyle T, *et al*. Retrospective analysis of patterns of recurrence seen on MRI in patients with recurrent glioblastoma multiforme treated with bevacizumab plus irinotecan. J Clin Oncol 2008, 26, 13013 (abstract).

[34] Narayana A, Raza S, Golfinos JG, *et al.* Bevacizumab therapy in recurrent high grade glioma: Impact on local control and survival. J Clin Oncol 2008, 26, 13000 (abstract).

[35] Norden AD, Young GS, Setayesh K, *et al.* Bevacizumab for recurrent malignant gliomas: efficacy, toxicity, and patterns of recurrence. Neurology 2008, 70(10), 779-787.

[36] Gerstner ER, Duda DG, di Tomaso E, *et al.* VEGF inhibitors in the treatment of cerebral edema in patients with brain cancer. Nat Rev Clin Oncol 2009, 6(4), 229-236.

[37] Gutin PH. Corticosteroid therapy in patients with cerebral tumors: benefits, mechanisms, problems, practicalities. Semin Oncol 1975, 2(1), 49-56.

[38] Weis SM, Cheresh DA. Pathophysiological consequences of VEGF-induced vascular permeability. Nature 2005, 437(7058), 497-504.

[39] Kamoun WS, Ley CD, Farrar CT, *et al.* Edema control by cediranib, a vascular endothelial growth factor receptor-targeted kinase inhibitor, prolongs survival despite persistent brain tumor growth in mice. J Clin Oncol 2009, 27(15), 2542-2552.

[40] Eskens FA, Verweij J. The clinical toxicity profile of vascular endothelial growth factor (VEGF) and vascular endothelial growth factor receptor (VEGFR) targeting angiogenesis inhibitors; a review. Eur J Cancer 2006, 42(18), 3127-3139.

[41] van Heeckeren WJ, Ortiz J, Cooney MM, Remick SC. Hypertension, proteinuria, and antagonism of vascular endothelial growth factor signaling: clinical toxicity, therapeutic target, or novel biomarker? J Clin Oncol 2007, 25(21), 2993-2995.

[42] Dietrich J, Han R, Yang Y, *et al.* CNS progenitor cells and oligodendrocytes are targets of chemotherapeutic agents *in vitro* and in vivo. J Biol 2006, 5(7), 22.

[43] Dietrich J, Monje M, Wefel J, Meyers C. Clinical patterns and biological correlates of cognitive dysfunction associated with cancer therapy. Oncologist 2008, 13(12), 1285-1295.

CHAPTER 30

Bevacizumab for Malignant Gliomas: Comparative Study with Other Malignancies

Helen Gu[1,*] and Thomas C. Chen[2]

[1]Dept of Medicine, Oncology (USC) and [2]Dept of Neurosurgery and Pathology (USC)

Abstract: Although, the use of temozolomide, as described by Stupp *et al.* has been hailed as one of the landmark breakthroughs for malignant gliomas, this diagnosis still portends one of the worst prognosis in oncology. Bevacizumab (Avastin) was reported to have favorable results and an acceptable toxicity profile in the treatment of glioblastoma multiforme (GBM) patients who progressed on temozolomide. Given the addition of this potent new treatment agent into the glioma arsenal, and the introduction of a new class of treatment medications it represents; it will be useful to review its clinical history and compare and contrast the experience and pitfalls other oncology sub-specialties have had with this agent.

INTRODUCTION

Although the use of temozolomide, as described by Stupp *et al.* has been hailed as one of the landmark breakthroughs for malignant gliomas, an area of continued need is the treatment of temozolomide refractory malignant glioma patients [1]. These patients tend to do quite poorly, and historically used agents such as procarbazine, carboplatin, irinotecan, etoposide, still result in low response rates [2].

In 2007 and 2008, bevacizumab (Avastin) was reported to have favorable results and an acceptable toxicity profile in the treatment of glioblastoma multiforme (GBM) patients who progressed on temozolomide. Vrendenburg *et al.* reported a single center experience at Duke University involving 23 patients with recurrent GBM receiving bevacizumab (10 mg/kg) and irinotecan (CPT-11), a topoisomerase I inhibitor. The response rate was 57% with a 6 months survival rate of 77% [3]. The regimen used was inspired by the colon cancer regimen of bevacizumab and irinotecan that was available at that time. Cloughesy *et al.* subsequently confirmed these findings in a randomized, non-comparative phase II trial [4]. Larger, phase III trials are currently underway utilizing bevacizumab both in recurrent and also upfront clinical settings for GBM.

The preceding chapters have provided perspective on the role of Avastin in the treatment of malignant gliomas. The goal of this chapter is to put everything in perspective by reviewing the role of bevacizumab in treatment of other cancers.

PRE-CLINICAL WORK ON BEVACIZUMAB

The concept that tumor growth is often accompanied by increased vascular proliferation has been known for the greater part of the modern medical century. The ability to explore that potential for clinical gain, however, has eluded much of modern therapeutic development. Even though the idea of a soluble molecule secreted by a neoplasm to obtain neo-vascularization and growth advantage had been around since the 1930's, it was not until the late 1980's when technology and serendipity came together.

In 1989, Ferrara and his laboratory were able to isolate an endothelial cell specific mitogen which they named "vascular endothelial growth factor". Work done in other laboratories showed that this protein was able to induce vascular leakage in the skin. The gene encoding VEGF is organized into eight exons, separated by seven introns. Alternative splicing resulted in the generation of five known iso-forms, ranging from 121 to 206 amino acids. The VEGF ligand that is being most explored clinically is VEGF-A. Its actions are a rate-limiting step in normal and pathological blood vessel growth [5].

*Address correspondence to Helen Gu**: Norris Cancer Center, 1441 Eastlake Ave, Los Angeles CA 90033, Tel: (323) 865-3945, E-mail: helen.gu@gmail.com

Thomas C. Chen (Ed)

Multiple human tumors, including lung, breast, gastrointestinal tract, and renal cell have shown VEGF mRNA expression levels. In particular, GBM and other tumors that have necrosis as a hallmark pathological feature, have high VEGF mRNA levels in the hypoxic tumor cells adjacent to the necrotic zone [6].

Bevacizumab is a monoclonal antibody that binds to VEGF. It was fully humanized in 1997; however, it began development as a mouse anti-human antibody tested against three human tumor cell lines, A673 rhabdomyosarcoma, G55 glioblastoma, and SK-LMS-1 leiomyosarcoma [7]. The robust pre-clinical response (inhibition of VEGF on the order of 70 to 90%) allowed it to be further developed.

EARLY CLINICAL TRIALS

Phase I data examining the safety and pharmacokinetics of bevacizumab determined a half-life of 17 to 21 days and a safety profile appropriate for use in combination with cytotoxic agents [8]. In 1998, five phase II trials investigating the efficacy of bevacizumab use in specific tumor types were launched – castration resistant prostate cancer, metastatic breast cancer, renal cell cancer, metastatic colon cancer, and stage III/IV non-small cell lung cancer. Overall, 333 patients were exposed to a variety of dosage schedules, ranging from 3 mg/kg weekly to 15 mg/kg every 3 weeks. Interestingly, the renal cell data showed an effective treatment dose to be 10mg/kg every 2 weeks; however, that same dose was the inferior regimen when compared to 5mg/kg every 2 weeks in the colorectal cohort [9,10]. The reason behind this is still a matter of debate.

PIVOTAL CLINICAL TRIALS

Colon Cancer

Based on the robust phase II data, two large, prospective, randomized phase III trials were undertaken in colorectal cancer. Hurwitz *et al.* randomized a group of metastatic colon cancer patients who had never received treatment to receive IFL (irinotecan, fluorouracil, leucovorin) with or without bevacizumab at a dose of 5mg/kg every two weeks. A large number of patients (813) were enrolled and randomized with the primary endpoint of the study being survival. The results were strongly in favor of IFL + bevacizumab, with a median survival of 20.3 months in the plus bevacizumab group versus 15.6 months in the chemotherapy alone group (Hazard Ratio 0.66, p value <0.001) [11]. Minimal additional toxicity was reported, primarily in hypertension and proteinuria.

The Eastern Cooperative Oncology Group (ECOG) released the interim analysis of their E3200 trial in which patients who have received prior therapy for their metastatic colorectal cancer were randomized to 3 different arms, FOLFOX 4 (Fluorouracil, leucovorin, oxaliplatin), FOLFOX 4 plus bevacizumab (10mg/kg), or bevacizumab (10 mg/kg) as monotherapy. The monotherapy arm was closed early as it was demonstrated to be inferior to FOLFOX 4. The interim data was presented at ASCO 2005, indicating a statistically significant hazard ratio of 0.7, favoring the FOLFOX4 arm plus bevacizumab [12].

Bevacizumab has also been evaluated in the adjuvant setting for colon cancer. NSABP C-08 reported their 3 years follow-up data at ASCO 2009. This study randomized stage II/III colon cancer patients to receive FOLFOX 4 for six months or FOLFOX 4 plus bevacizumab (5 mg/kg), with an extension of bevacizumab as monotherapy for six additional months. One total year of anti-VEGF therapy was planned on the experimental arm. Nearly three thousand patients have been recruited to date, with the primary end point being disease free survival. The DFS curves favored the bevacizumab arm in the first two years of follow-up; after the third year, the DFS curves demonstrated no overall significant benefit between the three arms [13].

This trial had revived a long-standing debate amongst the medical oncology community regarding the timing and duration of administering this biological agent, especially in face of its prohibitive price tag. Many have pointed to NSABP C08 as proof that bevacizumab does not actually aid in augmenting the tumoricidal capability of the accompanying cytotoxic regimen, but rather produces a cohort of biologically quiescent tumor cells that will reactivate if and when VEGF suppression is withdrawn.

In summary, bevacizumab has received FDA indication for treatment of first and second line metastatic colorectal cancer at a dosage of 5mg/kg when combined with IFL and 10 mg/kg when combined with FOLFOX 4. From a practice standpoint, these guidelines are rather loosely followed, and the GI-oncologists at Norris Cancer Center have used either 5mg or 10mg per kg dosing when combined with FOLFOX or FOLFORI, the two standard chemotherapy stems for metastatic colorectal cancer.

Lung Cancer

The pivotal phase III trial for treatment of non-small cell lung cancer is ECOG 4599. The results of the entire study have yet to be published, it was presented at the plenary session at ASCO 2005.

Eight hundred seventy eight patients with untreated, unresectable non-squamous cell carcinoma with no history of brain metastasis and no history of hemoptysis, were randomized to receive paclitaxel/carboplatin alone or the same regimen with bevacizumab (15mg/kg every 3 weeks). Paclitaxel/carboplatin was given every 3 weeks for six cycles. Bevacizumab for the treatment arm was continued as monotherapy until disease progression or unacceptable toxicity. Squamous cell histology was excluded secondary to phase II data that had shown an unacceptable bleeding risk in this cohort of patients. The primary endpoint was overall survival. The data presented at ASCO 2005 indicated a statistically significant benefit to overall survival with the addition of bevacizumab. Median survival was 12.3 months for the treatment group and 10.3 months for the control group. This was the first trial in metastatic NSCLC that showed a median survival of more than one year, leading the FDA to approve bevacizumab for the treatment of unrespectable non-small lung cancer in front-line setting [14].

While the data contained in E4599 was sufficient enough for the FDA, in practice reimbursement for bevacizumab has been varied. Most private insurers will reimburse for use of bevacizumab in this population. However, several large government payers, citing financial reasons and lack of published data, will not pay for the addition of bevacizumab to standard platinum doublet therapy in the treatment of this patient population.

Breast Cancer

Several large phase III trials utilizing similar treatment regiments to colorectal and non-small cell lung carcinoma have been performed in breast cancer patients. The largest one, and the one that lead to the approval of bevacizumab for front-line metastatic breast cancer patient was ECOG 2100. The treatment schema was relatively simple, with the use of paclitaxel with or without the addition of bevacizumab. Seven hundred twenty two subjects were enrolled on to the trial, with CNS metastasis as exclusion criteria. Significant controversy exists regarding E2100's primary endpoint -- disease free survival. When the data was presented at ASCO 2005, patients had a highly significant DFS (11.3 months versus 5.8 months); overall survival, however, was not statistically significant [15]. The FDA granted approval for bevacizumab for treatment of metastatic breast cancer in 2008; however, in doing so, it went against the recommendation of its panel of independent advisors who voted 5 to 4 against approval, citing the lack of survival data.

Because the survival data advantage in breast cancer was missing, it can be difficult in practice to get insurance authorizations for bevacizumab. Moreover, because of the large number of available agents that may be potentially used for metastatic breast cancer, failure of authorization in the case of bevacizumab often results in the usage of an alternative chemotherapy.

Renal Cell

The rationale behind using anti-VEGF therapy in the treatment of this neoplasm is well established. RCC is a tumor that is traditionally resistant to both chemotherapy and radiotherapy. RCC is closely associated with mutations in the von-Hippel Lindau gene, which in turn lead to an overproduction of VEGF via upregulation of hypoxia-inducing factor (HIF) [16]. The suppression of VEGF appears to be a logical choice in the treatment of this disease.

The two pivotal trials for renal cell carcinoma are CALGB 90206 and BO177705. Over 1300 patients were enrolled between the two trials. They were both designed very similarly; all patients received interferon alpha for treatment. Patients were then randomized to receive or not receive bevacizumab on a 1:1 randomization scheme. The primary endpoint in the CALGB 90206 study was overall survival, the BO177705 study's endpoint was disease free survival at 5 months. At ASCO-GU 2008, CALGB reported positive data for progression free survival and response rate; but overall survival data is still pending. The expected side-effects and toxicities from bevacizumab were once again seen in treated cohort, with hypertension and proteinuria being the most common grade 3, 4 toxicities. There was also a 1-2% bleeding risk that has been reported [17].

Ovarian Cancer

Epithelial ovarian cancer (>95% of diagnosed ovarian cancer) represents a significant clinical burden, being the most lethal of gynecological malignancies. Median survival for patients diagnosed with stage III or IV disease, representing the majority of the patient population, ranges from 3 to 4 years [18]. A poor prognostic indication in this patient population is the development of platinum-resistance, as evidenced by refractory or recurrent disease within 6 months of platinum treatment. A number of cytotoxic therapies have been evaluated in this patient population.

In 2005, the first reported case study using bevacizumab in patient was published describing single-agent activity in a patient who was heavily pre-treated [19]. Since that time, three significant phase III trials were published – GOG 170-D; AVF 2949, sponsored by Genetech; and a Californa Cancer Consortium/NCI trial [20-22]. GOG 170-D examined efficicacy of bevacizumab as a single agent, and found a 17.7% response rate, with two complete responders. Genentech sponsored AVF 2949 also incorporated a single agent approach in recurrent ovarian cancer patients. The trials was terminated early due to an unacceptable 5 GI perforations in the first 44 patients enrolled. The reported response on the industry trial was 16%.

Garcia et. al reported a CCC/NCI phase II trial involving bevacizumab in addition to oral cyclophosphamide. The bevacizumab dose used here was 10mg/kg weekly for 3 weeks, then 10mg/kg in every 2 week fashion until disease progression. This particular trial reported a response rate of 24%, but a clinical benefit rate (SD + PR) of 87%. Median time to progression was 7.2 months and median survival was 16.9 months [22]. There were three treatment-related deaths, GI perforation and pulmonary hypertension (secondary to right atrial thrombus) were established as culprits in two of the cases.

Currently, two large phase III trials involving stage III and IV ovarian cancer patients have completed accrural. Both GOG 218 and ICON7 are expected to report results in the next two years. The primary objectives of both trials are overall survival.

CLINICAL EXPERIENCE WITH BEVACIZUMAB

Bevacizumab entered into clinical practice in 1998 as a compound with a novel mechanism of action. A decade later, we are still trying to optimize the use of this medication in the field of oncology. Bevacizumab currently holds five FDA indications, colon cancer, lung cancer, breast cancer, renal cell carcinoma and GBM. The strength of data supporting each indication is quite different. Two of those indications (colon, lung) are based on studies that show overall survival benefit, one of the tumor types (breast) show no overall survival benefit; and we are still waiting for data regarding survival on the other two (brain and renal).

Bevacizumab also demonstrated its efficacy in combination with a variety of agents, fluoropyridine, platinum, taxane, and immunotherapies (interferon) to name a few. Despite the temptation to use it in any and every combination, results of the recent CAIRO2 study in colorectal cancer, where a combination of chemotherapy and dual receptor blockade with bevacizumab and cetuximab actually appeared to have decreased the survival of patients (non significant p-value). Even more disturbing, this was in the presence of a response rate that favors the combination arm [18].

The current dosage of bevacizumab approved for GBM treatment is 10 mg/kg every two weeks, much like the dosage used in combination treatment for renal cell cancer and breast cancer. NSCLC and colon cancer physicians tend to give 15 mg/kg every 3 weeks and 5 mg/kg every 2 weeks respectively. The FDA's bevacizumab approval for GBM is unique in that it is the only cancer where bevacizumab is approved as a single agent. This approval was given despite the fact when bevacizumab was given as monotherapy in the colorectal cohort (ECOG 3200); that arm closed early as it had a dismal outcome with a median survival of 2.3 months. Whether a cytotoxic agent is actually necessary for full clinical benefit when using bevacizumab is still a matter of debate in the neuro-oncology community.

Bevacizumab use has also opened up a number of unforeseen issues such as pseudo-response and pseudo-progression. There is general consensus that a lack of a satisfactory unifying system to evaluate and standardize response and clinical benefit in this disease will hinder further research. Before measuring benefit, the ruler needs to be defined first. Future research into this field must take into account this deficiency. Large scale phase III studies using bevacizumab is underway and will help further clarify the role of this agent in treatment of patients with malignant gliomas, whether in the upfront or recurrent setting.

Table 1: Summary of large human clinical cancer trials for Avastin

Tumor type	Study	Year	No. in study	Randomized?	Phase?	Regimens tested	Primary Endpoint	Results	P-value	FDA approved	Adverse effects?
Colorectal (Metastatic)	Hurwitz	2004	813	Y	3	A: IFL B: IFL + Bev 5mg/kg (q2wks)	OS	15.6 mo. Vs. 20.3 mo	<0.001	Y	Hypertension 22.4%. 3 bleeds in bev groupå
Colorectal (Metastatic)	ECOG 3200	2005	822	Y	3	A: FOLFOX B: FOLFOX + Bev 10mg/kg (q 2 wks) with Bev continued for 6 additional mo. C: Bev 10mg/kg (q2 wks) CLOSED early	OS PFS RR	12.5 mo. Vs. 10.7 mo.	--	Y	Hypertension Proteinuria GI Perforationß
Colorectal (Adjuvant for stage II/III)	NSABP C-08	2009	2710	Y	3	A: FOLFOX B: FOLFOX + Bev 5mg/kg (q2 wks)	3 years DFS	HR 0.89	0.15	N	Hypertension Proteinuria
NSCLC (Metastatic)	ECOG 4599	2006	878	Y	3	A: Carboplatin/Paclitaxel B: Carboplatin/Paclitaxel + Bev 15mg/kg (q3wks) with Bev continued until progression	OS	12.3 mo vs. 10.3 mo	0.003	Y	Bleeding risk in squamous etiology (excluded in phase III trial) Hypertension Proteinuria
Breast (Metastatic)	ECOG 2100	2007	722	Y	3	A: Paclitaxel B: Paclitaxel + Bev 10mg/kg (q2 wks)	PFS	11.3 mo vs. 5.8 mo	<0.001	Y	Hypertension Proteinuria Cardiovascular Ischemia
Renal (Metastatic)	CALGB 90206	2008	732	Y	3	A: Interferon B: Interferon + Bev 10 mg/kg (q2wks)	OS Secondary: PFS, RR	Pending for OS data PFS: 8.5 mo. Versus 5.2 mo.	<0.0001	Y	Hypertension Fatigue Anorexia Proteinuria
Brain (GBM)	Cloughsey	2008	167	Y	2	A: CPT-11 + Bev 10mg/kg (q2 wks) B: Bev 10mg/kg (q2wks)	6 mo. PFS	9.2 mo. Versus 8.7 mo.	Non sig P-value	Y	Wound healing Intracranial hemorrhage Thrombotic events
Ovarian (Metastatic)	Garcia	2008	70	N	2	A: Metronomic Cyclophosphamide B: Cyclophosphamide + Bev 10mg/kg	6 mo. PFS	56%	--	N	GI perforation Pulmonary Hypertension

REFERENCES

[1]   Stupp R. *et al.* Radiation plus concomitant and adjuvant temozolomide for gliomas. New Engl J Medicine 12: 987-96, 2005.

[2]   Wen PY, Kesari T. Malignant gliomas in adults. New Engl J Med 359: 492-503, 2008.

[3]   Vredenburgh, J *et al.* Bevacizumab plus irinotecan in recurrent glioblastoma multiforme. J. Clin. Oncol. 25, 4722-4729 (2007)

[4]   Cloughesy, T. *et al.* A phase II, randomized, non-comparative clinical trial of the effect of bevacizumab (BV) alone or in combination with irinotecan (CPT) on 6-month progression free survival (PFS6) in recurrent, treatment-refractory glioblastoma (GBM) J. Clin Oncol 26: 2008 (May 20 suppl; abstr 2010b)

[5]   Ferara, N. and Hanzel, W.J. Pituitary follicular cells secrete a novel heparin binding growth factor specific for vascular endothelial cells. Biochem. Biophys. Res. Commun. 161; 851-858 (1989)

[6]   Plate, K.H. *et al.* Vascular endothelia growth factor is a potential tumour angiogenesis factor in human gliomas in vivo. Nature 359, 843-845 (1992).

[7]   Kim, K.J. *et al.* Inhibition of vascular endothelia growth factor-induced angiogenesis suppresses tumor growth in vivo. Nature 362, 841-844 (1993).

[8]   Gordon, M. S. *et al.* Phase I safety and pharmacokinetic study of recombinant human anti-vascular endothelia growth factor in patients with advanced cancer. J. Clin. Oncol. 19, 843-850 (2001)

[9]   Yang, J.C. *et al.* A randomized trial of bevacizumab, an anti-VEGF antibody, for metastatic renal cancer. N. Engl. J. Med. 349, 427 – 434 (2003)

[10]   Kabbinavar, F. *et al.* Phase II, randomized trial comparing bevacizumab plus fluorouracil (FU)/leucovorin (LV) with FU/LV alone in patients with metastatic colorectal cancer. J. Clin. Oncol. 21, 60-65 (2003)

[11]   Hurwitz, H. *et al.* Bevacizumab plus Irinotecan, Fluorouracil, and Leucovorin for Metastatic Colorecal Cancer. N. Engl. J. Med 350; 2335-2342 (2004).

[12]   Giantonio, B. *et al.* High-dose bevacizumab improves survival when combined with FOLFOX 4 in previously treated advanced colorectal cancer: Results from the Eastern Cooperative Oncology Group (ECOG) study E3200. ASCO annual meeting, abstract 2.

[13]   Wolmark N, *et al.* ASCO 2009. Results of NSABP C-08: mFOLFOX6 +/- bevacizumab in stage II/III colon cancer patients. ASCO 2009. Abstract LBA4.

[14]   Sandler, AB. *et al.* Paclitaxel-Carboplatin Alone or with Bevacizumab for Non-Small-Cell Lung Cancer. N. Engl. J. Med. 2006;355:2542-50.

[15]   Miller, K.D. *et al.* Paclitaxel plus Bevacizumab versus Paclitaxel Alone for Metastatic Breast Cancer. N. Engl. J. Med. 2007;357:2666-76.

[16]   Rini, B.I. *et al.* CALGB 90206: A phase III trial of bevacizumab plus interferon-alpha versus interferon-alpha monotherapy in metastatic renal cell carcinoma. ASCO Genitourinary Cancer Symposium, 2008, abstr: 350.

[17]   Tol, J. *et al.* Chemotherapy, Bevacizumab, and Cetuximab in Metastatic Colorectal Cancer. N. Engl. J. Med. 360:563-572 (2009).

[18]   Burger, R. Experience with Bevacizumab in the Management of Epithelial Ovarian Cancer. J. Clin. Oncol. 25, 2902-2908 (2007).

[19]   Monk, B.J., *et al.* Activity of bevacizumab (rhuMAB VEGF) in advanced refractory epithelial ovarian cancer. Gynecol. Oncol. 96: 902-905 (2005).

[20]   Burger, R. *et al.* Phase II Trial of Bevacizumab in Persistent or Recurrent Epithelial Ovarian Cancer or Primary Peritoneal Cancer: A Gynecologic Oncology Group Study. J. Clin. Oncol. 25, 5165-5171 (2007).

[21]   Cannistra S.A., *et al.* Bevacizumab in patients with advanced platinum-resistant ovarian cancer. J. Clin. Oncol. 24: 257s, 2006 (suppl; abstr).

[22]   Garcia, A. *et al.* Phase II Clinical Trial of Bevacizumab and Low-Dose Metronomic Oral Cyclophosphamide in Recurrent Ovarian Cancer: a Trial of the California, Chicago, and Princess Margaret Hospital II Consortia. J. Clin. Oncol. 26, 76-82 (2008).

AUTHOR INDEX

INDEX

A

ADC histogram analysis-65
Aflibercept (Regeneron)-171
Aflibercept and toxicity-173
Anaplastic astrocytoma-127
Angiogenesis-1
Angiogenesis and radiation-20
Astrocytes-120
AVGLIO-30
$\alpha v\beta 3$, $\alpha v\beta 5$–158

B

Bevacizumab (Avastin) 1, 3
Bevacizumab and anaplastic gliomas-111
Bevacizumab and anticoagulation-51,52
Bevacizumab and anti-invasion agents-24
Bevacizumab and arterial hypertension-148
Bevacizumab and breast cancer-186
Bevacizumab and colon cancer-185
Bevacizumab and complications in newly diagnosed GBM-29
Bevacizumab dosing-55,56
Bevacizumab and erlotinib-9,10
Bevacizumab and etoposide -9,10
Bevacizumab and European usage-136,140,142,149
Bevacizumab and failures-25
Bevacizumab and gastrointestinal perforation-47
Bevacizuma b and hypofractionated radiation-19
Bevacizumab and intracranial metastases-111
Bevacizumab and intracranial sacromas-111
Bevacizumab and intratumoral hemorrhage-47
Bevacizumab and irinotecan -8,9,10
Bevacizumab and lung cancer-186
Bevacizumab and monotherapy-12,13
Bevacizumab and newly diagnosed GBM-13,29
Bevacizumab and non-glioma tumors-111
Becvaciumab and optic neuropathy-48
Bevacizumab and ovarian carcinoma-187
Bevacizumab and posterior reversible encephalopathy syndrome (PRES)-47
Bevacizumab and proteinuria-46
Bevacizumab and pseudoprogression-111
Bevacizumab and radiation induced injury treatment-111,117
Bevaciumab and radiation optic neuropathy-111
Bevacizumab and radiotherapy-33-35,37
Bevacizumab and recurrence-14
Bevacizumab and recurrent anaplastic glioma-12,127,128,133,134,144,145
Bevacizumab and renal cell carcinoma-186,187
Bevacizumab and schedule of administration-56
Bevacizumab and stereotactic irradiation-20
Bevacizumab and surgery-100,103,107,108
Bevacizumab and temozolomide-9,10

www.ingramcontent.com/pod-product-compliance
Lightning Source LLC
Chambersburg PA
CBHW041659210326
41598CB00007B/460

9 781608 055197